THE
CHEST
X-RAY

THE CHEST X-RAY

A SURVIVAL GUIDE

Gerald de Lacey, MA, MB, B Chir, FRCR
Consultant Radiologist
Radiology Red Dot Courses, London and www.radiology-courses.com

Simon Morley, MA, BM, BCh, MRCP, FRCR
Consultant Radiologist and Honorary Senior Lecturer
University College Hospitals, London

Laurence Berman, MB, BS, FRCP, FRCR
Lecturer and Honorary Consultant Radiologist
University of Cambridge and Addenbrooke's Hospital, Cambridge

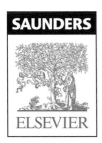

SAUNDERS

ELSEVIER

Philadelphia • Edinburgh • London • New York • Oxford • St Louis • Sydney • Toronto • 2008

SAUNDERS
ELSEVIER

An imprint of Elsevier Limited
© 2008 Elsevier Limited. All rights reserved.

First published 2008

The right of Gerald de Lacey, Simon Morley and Laurence Berman to be identified as authors of this work has been asserted by them in accordance with the Copyright, Designs and Patents Act 1988.

ISBN 978-0-7020-3046-8
  Reprinted 2008 (twice), 2011 (twice), 2012, 2013 (three times), 2014 (twice), 2015 (three times)

British Library Cataloguing in Publication Data
A catalogue record for this book is available from the British Library

Library of Congress Cataloging in Publication Data
A catalog record for this book is available from the Library of Congress

Notice
Medical knowledge is constantly changing. Standard safety precautions must be followed, but as new research and clinical experience broaden our knowledge, changes in treatment and drug therapy may become necessary or appropriate. Readers are advised to check the most current product information provided by the manufacturer of each drug to be administered to verify the recommended dose, the method and duration of administration, and contraindications. It is the responsibility of the practitioner, relying on experience and knowledge of the patient, to determine dosages and the best treatment for each individual patient. Neither the Publisher nor the author assume any liability for any injury and/or damage to persons or property arising from this publication.

The Publisher

Printed in China

Last digit is the print number: 17 16 15 14

Commissioning Editor: **Michael J Houston**
Project Manager: **Cheryl Brant**
Copyeditor/Designer: **Claire Gilman**
Illustrator: **Philip Wilson**

The
publisher's
policy is to use
**paper manufactured
from sustainable forests**

CONTENTS

PREFACE

Despite the continuing development and increasing sophistication of computed tomography (CT) and magnetic resonance imaging (MRI), the chest x-ray (CXR) is still the most frequently requested radiology investigation in a general hospital. Swiftly, inexpensively, and with a high degree of accuracy the CXR enables the physician to detect or rule out numerous disorders, diseases and abnormalities. It will also help to exclude several serious therapeutic complications. A normal CXR will time and again provide valuable clinical reassurance. The CXR remains the most appropriate examination in many circumstances—it is a bedrock imaging test.

Yet there is an important caveat. Accurate CXR interpretation requires a sound understanding of basic principles. The increasing reliance on CT and MRI has caused these essential competencies to become neglected. They are in danger of being lost altogether. The aim of this book is to assist in reversing this trend, by providing a convenient and informative white coat pocket guide to complement the numerous excellent bench reference volumes.

The structure of this book derives from the Radiology Red Dot teaching course "The CXR: A Survival Course" (www.radiology-courses.com), and from the regular questions and concerns of its participants. **Part A** concentrates on the core knowledge—describing normal and abnormal thoracic anatomy, CXR appearances occuring with several common conditions, and also CXR findings in the intensive care and neonatal intensive care units. **Part B** focuses on specific clinical problems—including those CXR appearances about which our students most frequently seek guidance.

The English author C.C. Colton identified three difficulties in authorship: to write anything worth publishing, to find honest people to publish it, and to get sensible people to read it. In attending to these we added our own fourth requirement…to find an outstanding medical illustrator. Explanatory drawings were always crucial to achieving our main goal—to describe and explain how assessment of the CXR depends upon an informed and organised analytical approach. Happily, we found that exceptional illustrator, Philip Wilson.

Finally, a couple of quick notes about our use of language. We use the word "physician" to include all medical doctors (rather than just those covered by the parochial British usage of the word). Our choice of pronoun (*he* or *she*) occurs randomly and arbitrarily throughout the book.

Whether you are a senior doctor, a doctor in training, or a medical student learning the fundamental and important aspects of our craft, we hope that you will have as much enjoyment reading and using this book as we had creating it.

Gerald de Lacey,
Simon Morley,
Laurence Berman,
July 2007

ACKNOWLEDGEMENTS

We owe debts of gratitude to so many individuals. Our priority was to utilise a large number of exquisitely precise drawings within an overall structure and design layout that would assist in explaining the basic concepts that underpin accurate analysis of the plain CXR. To achieve this we needed to assemble a team that included a skilled medical illustrator and a first class designer/editor. These were our principle objectives before we set about making the first keystrokes. We had worked with Claire Gilman previously and her design skills, imagination, and superb professionalism have proved to be more than invaluable—they have been priceless. We sought and found a wonderfully skilful medical artist, Philip Wilson, who created 250 figurative and realistic artworks of the very highest quality. Michael Houston and Cheryl Brant of Elsevier completed the team and with predictable expertise guided the project through to completion.

We could not have completed this Survival Guide without the help of Pam Golden who typed numerous drafts and revisions. Others who helped us included Floss (Tracey Wilson) who carried out supplementary typing. Dr Denis Remedios, Dr Emily Tam and Jeremy Weldon of Northwick Park Hospital, Julian Evans and Dr Nick Screaton of the University of Cambridge, and Dr Tracey Kilborn of Red Cross Children's Hospital, Cape Town, South Africa, assisted us with material for illustration. Professor Colin Morley (Professor of Neonatal Medicine, Royal Womens' and Royal Childrens' Hospitals, Melbourne, Victoria, Australia) provided practical and constructive advice when reviewing important parts of the manuscript.

It would be very wrong to write a book on the plain CXR without acknowledging the influence of numerous internationally renowned masters and past masters. We have appropriated and utilised their original observations and explanations time and time again. There are too many of these experts for us to list. Nevertheless, two maestros must be mentioned. Firstly, Professor Peter Armstrong, recently of St Bartholomew's Hospital, London, and previously radiologist at the University of Virginia Medical School. Peter is the principal faculty member on our advanced plain CXR course held in London. Every year we learn something new from his clear and logical analyses. He will surely forgive us for adapting several of his descriptions in order to explain and illustrate various anatomical concepts—particularly around the hilum of the lung. Another renowned expert, Dr Benjamin Felson, through his writings and enduring teachings had long ago stimulated our interest in the diagnostic subtleties underpinning CXR analysis. Dr Felson, once a radiologist at the University of Cincinnati College of Medicine, was the acknowledged pioneer in developing the scientific approach to CXR assessment. His enduring legacy remains an academic and clinical treasure chest. Dr Felson's numerous and exquisitely perceptive observations retain a relevance and a freshness which remain fully appropriate to 21st century medicine and modern day medical imaging. We owe all these individuals a very great debt. Thank you.

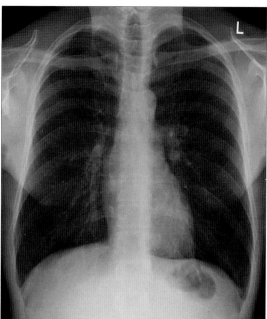

A normal CXR

Below are representations indicating the positions of the three lobes of the right lung and the two lobes of the left lung. The dotted lines represent the lung fissures which separate the lobes.

RUL = right upper lobe
ML = middle lobe
RLL = right lower lobe
LUL = left upper lobe
LLL = left lower lobe

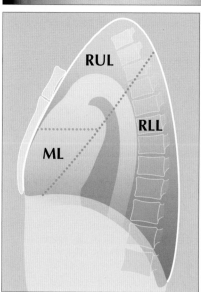

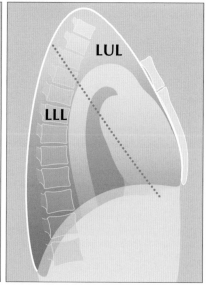

Part A
Core Knowledge

1 CHEST RADIOLOGY: THE BASIC BASICS

You will need a basic understanding of some of the technical factors affecting chest radiography, if only to recognise when a particular appearance arises not from pathology but from suboptimal technique. This chapter concentrates on the frontal CXR. We discuss the lateral CXR in Chapter 2.

THE RADIOGRAPHIC IMAGE

Table 1.1 Attenuation of the x-ray beam.

Tissue absorption		Effect on the radiograph (see Fig. 1.1)
Least	Air or gas	Black image
↓	Fat	Dark grey image
	Soft tissue	Grey image
Most	Bone or calcium	White image

THE FRONTAL CXR

This standard CXR is obtained at a fixed distance between the x-ray tube and the cassette of 180 cm (6 ft). The patient faces the cassette and the x-ray beam passes through in the posterior to anterior direction, i.e. PA (Fig. 1.2).

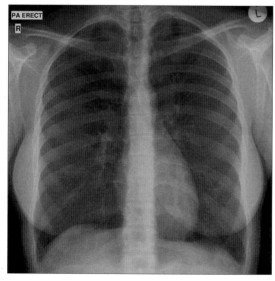

Figure 1.1 *Normal PA CXR. Standard radiographic technique allows comparison of the heart size on any previous or subsequent PA CXR.*

The PA CXR is preferred because the radiographic technique is standard. This allows accurate and valid comparison between repeated PA CXRs.

If the patient is unable to stand erect then he faces the x-ray tube and an antero–posterior (AP) chest radiograph is obtained. AP CXRs are acquired:

▪ At the bedside or with a seriously ill or frail patient in the emergency department. The patient may be lying supine (Fig. 1.3) or sitting up.

▪ In the radiology department when the patient is either too frail or too unsteady to stand erect. The radiographer (technologist) sits the patient on a chair with his back to the cassette (Fig. 1.4).

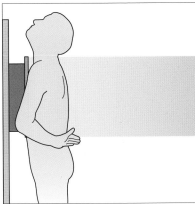

Figure 1.2 *Patient positioning for a standard PA CXR. The 180 cm (6 ft) x-ray tube to cassette distance results in a beam that is minimally divergent. In effect, the x-rays are parallel when they impact on the thorax.*

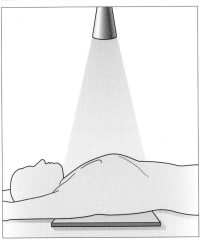

Figure 1.3 *Bedside (i.e. portable) radiograph, patient supine. AP CXR. The distance from the x-ray source to the cassette is much less than 180 cm (6 ft).*

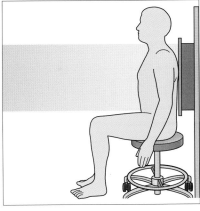

Figure 1.4 *Frail patient. Departmental radiograph, patient sitting up. AP CXR.*

THE BEDSIDE (PORTABLE) AP CXR HAS DISADVANTAGES

The AP CXR should always be interpreted with caution (Fig. 1.5). The following factors may cause misleading appearances:

▪ The mediastinum is magnified (Figs 1.6 and 1.7).

▪ When lying supine a patient is often unable to take a full inspiration. Also, he may be rotated because of difficulty in cooperating. Therefore some AP CXRs are of inferior quality in comparison with a departmental PA radiograph.

Be careful of making a major diagnosis (e.g. hilar mass) too readily. But don't be too gloomy. Many AP radiographs, even if not meeting the quality expected of a PA CXR, will usually confirm whether or not the lungs are clear.

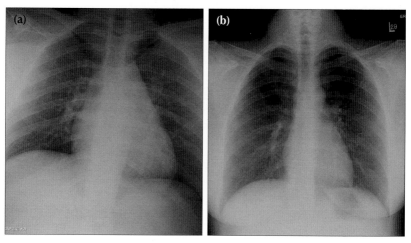

Figure 1.5   *Age 24. (a) AP CXR. Is the heart enlarged? It looks big but it is difficult to be sure because the radiographic technique produces magnification of the cardiac shadow. (b) PA CXR one day later. The CXR is entirely within normal limits.*

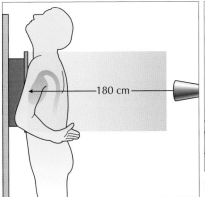

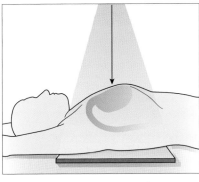

Figure 1.7 *On a bedside (portable) AP CXR the heart is situated well away from the cassette. The x-ray beam diverges at the margins of the heart causing magnification. A second cause for magnification is the shorter distance from the x-ray tube to the cassette. This is invariably less than 180 cm and produces a divergent x-ray beam.*

Figure 1.6 *On a PA CXR the heart is situated anteriorly in relation to the cassette. The 180 cm distance means that there is minimal divergence of the x-ray beam. Cardiac magnification is limited.*

MAGNIFICATION ON AN AP CXR: DOES IT MATTER?

Magnification occurs because of two factors:

1. A shortened distance between the x-ray tube and the cassette compared with the standard 180 cm PA CXR distance. This results in a diverging x-ray beam at the margins of the heart (Fig. 1.7).

2. The heart and mediastinum are situated further from the cassette than is the case with a PA CXR (Figs 1.6 and 1.7).

The drawbacks of magnification are:

■ A false impression of cardiac, mediastinal and/or aortic enlargement.

■ Precise comparison of the mediastinal appearance with an earlier or subsequent PA radiograph is a risky business.

THE COIN GROWS BIGGER	
Demonstration:	A coin is taped to the front of a chest (phantom) and another coin is taped to the back. An AP CXR is obtained.
CXR result:	The coin on the back of the phantom (close to the cassette) appears of near normal size. The coin on the front of the phantom (further away from the cassette) appears much larger.

DEPTH OF INSPIRATION: DOES IT MATTER?

Rule of thumb: If the anterior aspects of at least six ribs do not lie above the left dome of the diaphragm, then suspect a shallow inspiration (see Chapter 16, p. 237).

Shallow inspiration is common in the elderly, those in pain, unconscious patients, and with bedside radiography. Two problems occur when an inspiration is shallow:

1. The transverse cardiac diameter (see p. 148) may appear spuriously enlarged. The diaphragm is attached to the under-surface of the heart and this muscle pulls the heart downwards on a full inspiration. This downward pull is less when an inspiration is shallow. Consequently the side-to-side diameter of the heart will appear larger.

2. The failure to distend the lungs fully can cause crowding of vessels at the lung bases. The resulting appearance may simulate basal lung infection or areas of subsegmental collapse.

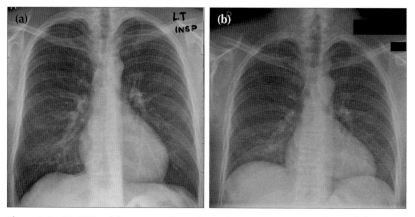

Figure 1.8   *PA CXRs of the same patient taken minutes apart: (a) was obtained during a good inspiration, and (b) was obtained during a poor inspiration. In (b) the heart appears enlarged…but this is bogus. A shallow inspiration can cause spurious cardiomegaly and also crowding of vessels at the lung bases. The latter appearance can mimic infection.*

PATIENT ROTATION: DOES IT MATTER?

Rule of thumb: The patient is not rotated if a vertical line drawn through the centre of the vertebral bodies (T1–T5) is equidistant from the medial end of each clavicle. Rotation is present when one of the clavicles is further away from this vertical line (Fig. 1.9).

A rotated CXR will cause various structures to be projected towards the right or left side. Potential problems:

■ Rotation to the right on a PA CXR…the manubrium and/or superior vena cava and/or vessels arising from the arch of the aorta may become unusually prominent on the right. This can simulate a mediastinal mass.

■ Rotation to the left on an AP CXR…the aortic arch may appear enlarged. Rotation is a common cause for one lung appearing blacker than the opposite side (see p. 257).

Rotation is often a problem in drowsy or ill adults, and in little children who wriggle around and do not like being held still.

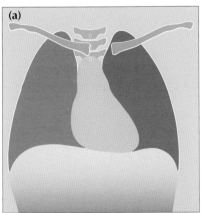

(a)

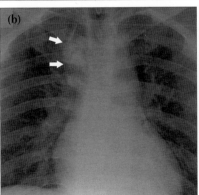

(b)

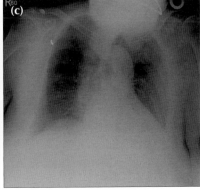

(c)

Figure 1.9   *Patient rotation. (a) Rotation to the left. (b) Male. Age 43. AP CXR. Rotation to the right projects the manubrium and aortic arch vessels (arrows) over the right upper zone, mimicking a mass. (c) Female. Age 87. Rotation to the left makes the aortic arch appear unduly prominent.*

OVEREXPOSURE / UNDEREXPOSURE — BE CAREFUL

With analogue chest radiography a poor exposure (film too dark or film too pale) can lead to errors in diagnosis because some areas or structures cannot be seen. With digital imaging the ability to alter (i.e. window) the image electronically will often help to overcome these problems.

SCAPULA POSITION — BE CAREFUL

The frontal CXR should have the scapulae rotated off the thorax and projected well away from the lungs (Fig. 1.10). This is not always easy to achieve in elderly, frail or sick people. Misleading shadows (e.g. a spurious pneumothorax) can be produced when part of a scapula overlies a lung.

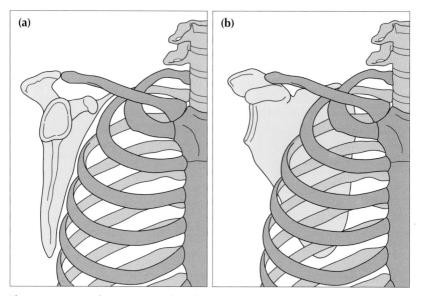

Figure 1.10 *Scapula position on a frontal projection: (a) good; (b) poor.*

OCCASIONAL PITFALL—BEDSIDE RADIOGRAPHS AND BEAM ANGULATION ARTEFACT

Rule of thumb: On PA and AP CXRs both domes of the diaphragm should be well-defined. If either dome is obliterated—in part or in whole—then disease in the adjacent lower lobe is highly likely (pp. 46–47). This rule is an application of the silhouette sign (Chapter 4, pp. 42–51).

With bedside radiographs this rule of thumb still applies, but with a caveat. On occasion the x-ray beam may not be perpendicular to the patient's chest, but may be angled upwards. Angulation can cause the left dome of the diaphragm to be ill-defined[1,2]. So, if the left dome is ill-defined on a bedside CXR and this is unexpected or does not fit with the findings on clinical examination, then the CXR should be repeated ensuring that the beam is perpendicular to the thorax. Alternatively, obtain a lateral CXR and check the appearance of the left lower lobe.

WHAT ARE THE LUNG ZONES?

It is common practice to define areas of the lung on the frontal CXR in terms of "zones". The purpose is to describe approximately where lesions are situated. Some experts attempt to define these zones very precisely by reference to specific ribs. Others are much more pragmatic, using the terms "upper", "mid" and "lower" zones informally, without feigning pseudo-scientific precision. We follow the latter course.

READING THE FRONTAL CXR

Many different schemes have been proposed for reading CXRs. There is no single correct or best system. In general it does not matter what your system is provided that you:

- always address—first and foremost—the clinical question

- analyse the CXR whilst adopting an inquisitive approach

- are aware of the areas where mistakes are made

- look for the hidden abnormality

- feel comfortable with your system

THE FRONTAL CXR: A TEN-POINT CHECKLIST

1. Is it a PA or AP radiograph?
   - ❏ Pitfall. AP radiographs magnify the heart and mediastinum (Fig. 1.11).
2. Is it a satisfactory inspiration?
   - ❏ If the anterior end of the left sixth rib reaches or is projected above the level of the dome of the diaphragm—then a good inspiration is likely.
   - ❏ Pitfall. A small inspiration can cause: (a) the heart to appear enlarged; and (b) vessel crowding at the bases mimicking infection (Fig. 1.12).
3. Is the patient rotated?
   - ❏ The medial end of each clavicle should be equidistant from a vertical line drawn through the spinous processes of the T1–T5 vertebral bodies.
   - ❏ Pitfalls. Rotation can distort the mediastinal and hilar appearances and lead to the erroneous suggestion of a mediastinal or hilar mass. One lung may appear blacker than the other (see p. 257). Always interpret rotated films with caution.
4. Is the heart enlarged?
   - ❏ In an adult, the cardio-thoracic ratio (CTR) should be less than 50% on a PA radiograph (see p. 148).
5. Are both domes of the diaphragm clearly seen and well-defined?
   - ❏ If part of a dome is obscured—suspect pathology in the adjacent lower lobe (Fig. 1.13).
6. Are the heart borders clearly seen and well-defined?
   - ❏ If not, then there is a high probability of pathology (Fig. 1.14) in the immediately adjacent lung (see pp. 45–48).
7. Are the hila normal…position, size and density?
   - ❏ **Rule of thumb**: The left hilum should be at the same level or higher than the right…never lower than the right (Fig. 1.15).
   - ❏ **Rule of thumb**: The hilar density on each side should be similar.
8. Are the bones normal? (e.g. Fig. 1.16)
9. Check the *tricky hidden areas* (Fig. 1.17): lung apex, superimposed over the heart, around each hilum, below the diaphragm.
10. Finally, ask yourself once again—have I addressed this patient's *particular* clinical problem?

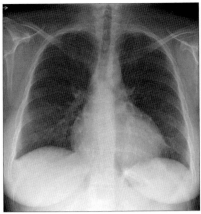

Figure 1.11   *The heart appears enlarged in this 25-year-old female... but this is an AP CXR. Magnification factors can mislead the unwary.*

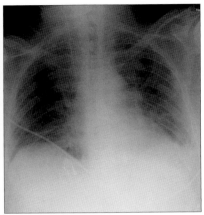

Figure 1.12   *Patient in ITU. Age 70. Shadowing at the bases suggests infection... but this is a poor inspiration. Crowding of vessels at the lung bases results from the inadequate inspiration.*

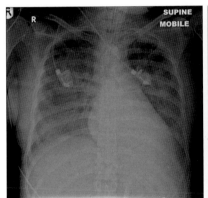

Figure 1.13   *ITU. Patient has adult respiratory distress syndrome (ARDS) and clinical deterioration. The normal, well-defined margin of the left dome of the diaphragm is absent...because of pneumonia in the adjacent left lower lobe.*

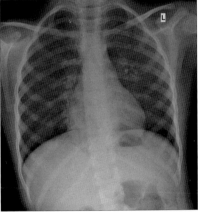

Figure 1.14   *Patient with cough and fever. The normal, sharply defined right heart border is lost...because of pneumonia in the adjacent middle lobe.*

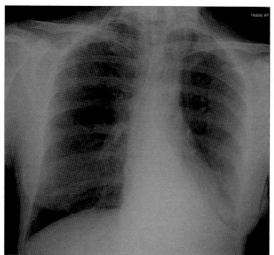

Figure 1.15 *Checking the hila. In this patient the left hilum has disappeared because there is collapse of the left lower lobe. (Hilar appearances, both normal and abnormal, are described in Chapter 6, pp. 70–79.)*

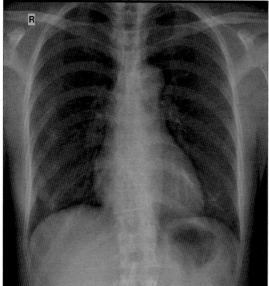

Figure 1.16 *Right-sided chest pain after an all-night party. No recollection of an injury. If you do not check the bones you will not see the several posterior rib fractures.*

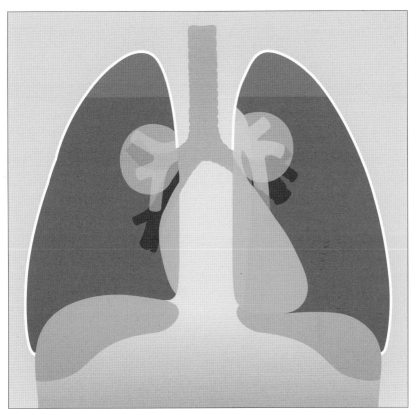

Figure 1.17 *Checking the four tricky hidden areas: apices (brown), superimposed over the heart (green), around each hilum (yellow), and below the domes of the diaphragm (blue). It has been shown that these are the four sites where small (and also large) lesions are most commonly overlooked.*

REFERENCES

1. Zylak CJ, Littleton JT, Durizch ML. Illusory consolidation of the left lower lobe: a pitfall of portable radiography. Radiology 1988; 167: 653–655.

2. Hollman AS, Adams FG. The influence of the Lordotic Projection on the interpretation of the Chest Radiograph. Clin Radiol 1989; 40: 360–364.

2 THE LATERAL CXR

A COMMON SCENARIO

Patient with a persistent cough. Normal clinical examination.

▪ An equivocal frontal CXR appearance.

▪ Physician unfamiliar with the normal appearances on a lateral CXR.

▪ Physician goes for the easy option — "let's get a CT".

However:

▪ CT = high dose of radiation. Lateral CXR = low dose.

▪ The lateral CXR will rapidly exclude or confirm most equivocal abnormalities seen on the frontal projection.

▪ The lateral CXR can be very, very useful provided you are familiar with the normal appearances.

"The man who is too old to learn was probably always too old to learn."[1]

The novice may feel that getting to grips with the lateral CXR is too much at this stage. Don't worry. Keep going on the other chapters and come back to the lateral CXR later on. Eventually, you will realise its importance. Also, analysing the lateral CXR is fun — Sherlock Holmes type fun.

Reference drawings of the normal lateral appearance are provided on p. viii.

WHEN IS A LATERAL CXR USEFUL?

1. To check whether an equivocal frontal CXR shadow is actually present.

2. To position an abnormality shown on the frontal CXR.

   ❏ Is it anterior or posterior?

   ❏ Which lobe is it in?

   ❏ Is it actually in a lobe?

3. To check the tricky areas when a patient has a particularly worrying symptom (e.g. haemoptysis). This projection is particularly good at showing:

   ❏ behind the heart

   ❏ behind and in front of the hila

   ❏ behind the domes of the diaphragm

RADIOGRAPHIC TECHNIQUE

In a fit individual the arms are held high and well away from the thorax (Fig. 2.1). In a frail or elderly patient the arms may have to be positioned in front of the chest. The resulting upper arm shadows can mislead the unwary (Fig. 2.2). The scapulae cannot avoid intruding on the image, but they should be easy to recognise (Figs 2.3 and 2.4).

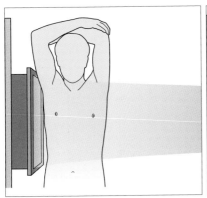

Figure 2.1   *Fit person. Arms up and out of the way.*

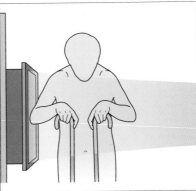

Figure 2.2   *Frail person. The upper arms often lie across the thorax.*

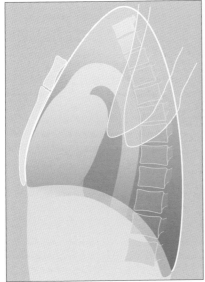

Figure 2.3   *The scapula shadows are usually projected over the thorax.*

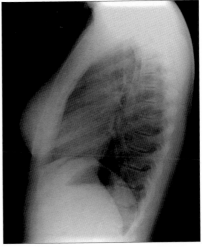

Figure 2.4   *Technically good CXR. The scapulae are visible, but do not cause a problem.*

UNDERSTANDING THE LATERAL CXR[2-6]

Figs 2.5–2.9 show how you can build up the main anatomical structures on a lateral CXR. Fig. 2.10 is the radiographic equivalent of the finished article.

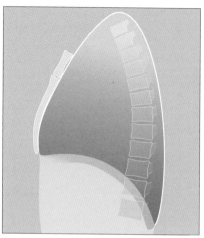

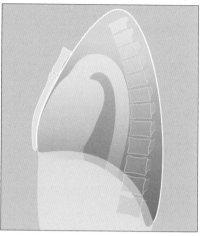

Figure 2.5 *Bare-bones lateral anatomy. Note that the lungs appear blacker inferiorly as compared with superiorly.*

Figure 2.6 *Add the heart, aorta and inferior vena cava…*

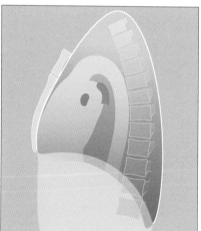

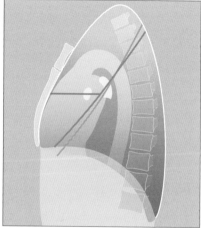

Figure 2.7 *…add the right (red) and left (blue) main pulmonary arteries (see Fig. 2.11)…*

Figure 2.8 *…add—in your mind's eye—the three fissures. Knowing their approximate position is important. They separate the three lobes of the right lung and the two lobes of the left lung. In practice, it is rare for much of either oblique fissure to be visualised on a normal lateral CXR.*

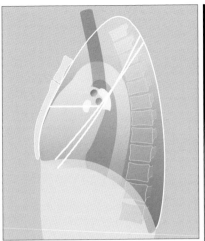

Figure 2.9 *Finally, add the trachea and the upper lobe bronchi (i.e. the two coloured circles). All the main structures are now in place.*

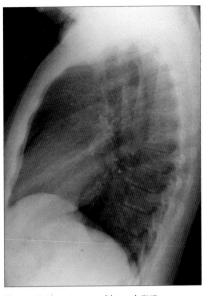

Figure 2.10   *A normal lateral CXR.*

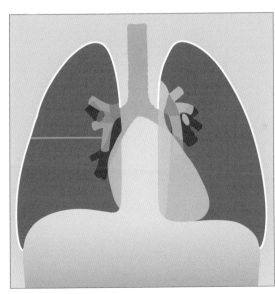

Figure 2.11   *Normal structures as seen on the frontal CXR, for comparison with Figs 2.5–2.10. Red = right main pulmonary artery; blue = left main pulmonary artery; purple = origin of right upper lobe bronchus; yellow = origin of left upper lobe bronchus.*

NORMAL LATERAL CXR—SPECIFIC APPEARANCES

DIAPHRAGM

The two domes are usually easy to separate from each other.

■ The right dome is visualised all the way from front to back.

■ The shadow of the left dome only extends from the costophrenic recess posteriorly to the back of the cardiac shadow anteriorly. This is because the heart obliterates the lung/diaphragm interface anteriorly.

Very occasionally the two domes are difficult to separate, because:

■ The domes may overlap each other precisely...coincidence.

■ If the base of the heart is very narrow then obliteration of the anterior aspect of the left dome is minimal and its shadow will extend almost all the way to the sternum—i.e. it can mimic the normal "seen all the way from front to back" right dome.

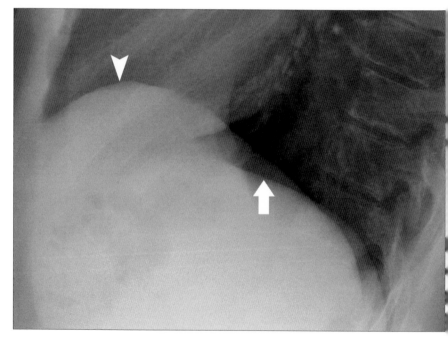

Figure 2.12 *Normal CXR. The right dome (arrowhead) is seen all the way from front to back. Note that the left dome (arrow) is not identified anteriorly. The outlines of both domes posterior to the heart are crisp and clean. The right dome is also crisp and clean anteriorly.*

HILA

The novice will find this a difficult area to assess. Bear these points in mind:

- Of the soft tissue density at each hilum, 95% is due solely to pulmonary artery and pulmonary veins.

- The main pulmonary artery on the right side passes anterior to the right main bronchus, whereas the main pulmonary artery on the left side passes posteriorly and hooks over the left main bronchus.

- There is summation of some of the left and right hilar densities (i.e. the vessels) on the lateral CXR.

You will be delighted to know that even the experts find this area difficult. However, the expert always evaluates the lateral view of a hilum together with the frontal projection. By taking the two views together it is much, much easier to answer a frequent question: "is this hilum enlarged or is it just prominent but normal?".

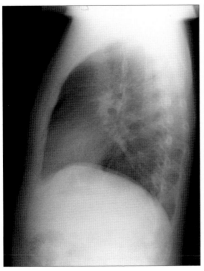

Figure 2.13 *Normal CXR. Fig. 2.14 explains the various components forming the hilar shadows.*

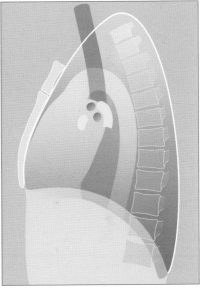

Figure 2.14 *Normal CXR. To show the location of the main pulmonary arteries (yellow). These arteries account for most of the hilar shadows. Remember—the right main pulmonary artery crosses in front of the right main bronchus and the left main pulmonary artery hooks over the left main bronchus.*

LUNG FISSURES

The horizontal fissure can be identified on most lateral CXRs (Fig. 2.15).

The oblique fissures are not aligned along a flat plane. Both have configurations similar to that of an aeroplane propeller (Fig. 2.16).

It is often stated that the right oblique fissure lies—at its most inferior position—about 4–5 cm posterior to the sternum, and that the left oblique fissure is positioned slightly more posterior. In practice, very slight rotation of the patient can project these fissures closer to, or further away from, each other on the CXR. The good news is that absolute certainty as to which oblique fissure is which is rarely important in clinical practice.

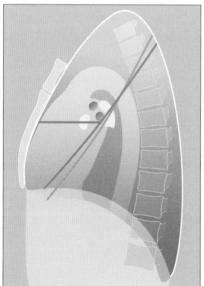 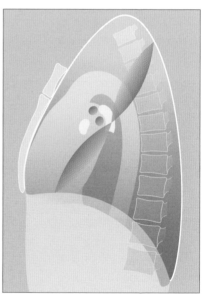

Figure 2.15 *The three fissures. Red = horizontal; green = right oblique; blue = left oblique. Visibility of the fissures varies from patient to patient—some, all, or none of a fissure may be evident. The fissures divide each lung into lobes. The right lung has three lobes—upper, middle and lower. The left lung has two lobes—upper and lower. (See p. viii.)*

Figure 2.16 *The normal configuration of an oblique fissure. Each oblique fissure resembles an aeroplane propeller.*

COSTOPHRENIC ANGLES (RECESSES, SULCI)

The posterior and inferior part of each lung occupies a well-defined gully created by the pleura reaching the posterior limit of each dome of the diaphragm. These two gullies—one on each side—are the costophrenic angles or sulci (Figs 2.15 and 2.16).

On the lateral radiograph, each costophrenic recess represents the most inferior aspect of the lung and pleura on an erect CXR. This is where most pleural effusions will collect.

LUNG APICES

The lateral CXR is not much help in assessing either lung apex, due to the overlying soft tissues, shoulders and chest wall.

RETROSTERNAL LINE

A soft tissue interface with the lung is visible immediately behind the sternum (Fig. 2.17). This is the retrosternal line.

The line is caused by the interface between the retrosternal soft tissues (mainly fat) and the anterior aspect of the right lung.

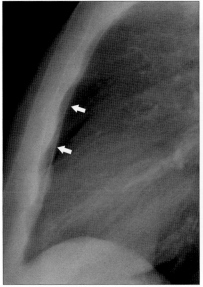

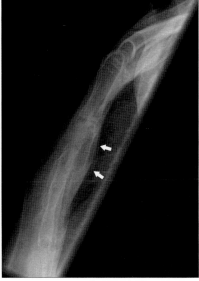

Figure 2.17 *This retrosternal line (arrows) is normal.*

Figure 2.18 *Road traffic accident. Sternal fracture. The retrosternal line (arrows) bulges posteriorly due to the adjacent haematoma.*

HEART

The heart occupies most of the mediastinum (Figs 2.19 and 2.20). The cardiac borders seen on the lateral CXR are formed as follows:

■ Anteriorly—right ventricle

■ Posteriorly immediately behind the hila—left atrium

■ Posteriorly below the hila—left ventricle

Important rule of thumb: On the lateral CXR there should not be any abrupt change in density across the shadow of the heart. If there is a change in density, you should suspect superimposed pulmonary pathology.

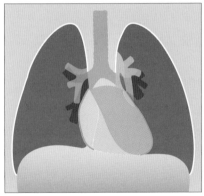

Figure 2.19 *Cardiac chambers. Frontal CXR allows correlation with the lateral CXR (Fig. 2.20). Pink = right atrium; blue = right ventricle; brown = left ventricle; green = left atrium.*

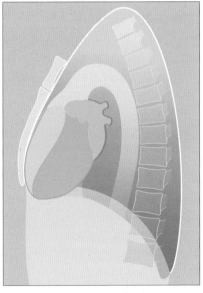

Figure 2.20 *The cardiac chambers. See colour coding in Fig. 2.19.*

INFERIOR VENA CAVA

On many lateral CXRs a short (1.5–2.0 cm) well-defined vertical shadow meets the posterior and inferior aspect of the heart. This shadow is the inferior vena cava. Its posterior wall is visible because it is outlined by air in the adjacent right lung (see Figs 2.21–2.23).

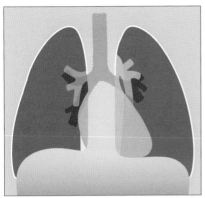

Figure 2.21 *Frontal view showing the shadow of the inferior vena cava (yellow) merging with the right atrium.*

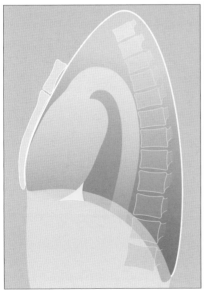

Figure 2.22 *Inferior vena cava shadow on the lateral CXR.*

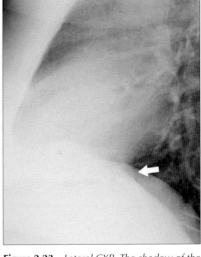

Figure 2.23 *Lateral CXR. The shadow of the inferior vena cava (arrow) is easily identified.*

TWO BRONCHIAL RINGS

Two circular rings are often projected over the hila or peri-hilar regions
(Figs 2.24–2.26). Sometimes only one ring is visible. Usually the higher ring is
the right upper lobe bronchus and the lower ring is the left upper lobe bronchus.

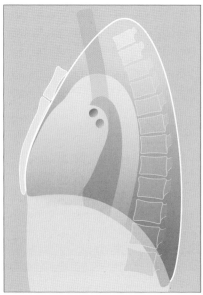

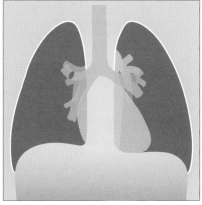

Figure 2.25 *The positions of each ring as shown on the frontal CXR.*

Figure 2.24 *Normal lateral CXR. Trachea = green; right upper lobe bronchus (seen end on) = purple; left upper lobe bronchus (seen end on) = brown.*

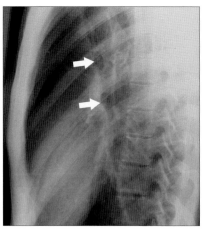

Figure 2.26 *The two rings (arrows) are visible in this patient. The rings represent—in almost all patients—the orifices of the upper lobe bronchi. Occasionally, they represent the main bronchi[2].*

BONES AND SOFT TISSUES

All lateral CXRs include part of the axial and appendicular skeleton. Bones will occasionally cause an overlap shadow. Familiarity with the normal skeletal appearances will prevent misunderstandings. Note:

■ The vertebrae and sternum are easy to see, and are not a problem (Fig. 2.27).

■ The ribs are also easy to see, and are rarely a problem.

■ The scapulae and upper arms are often visible, and are sometimes confusing.

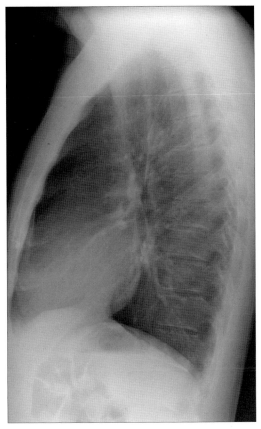

Figure 2.27 *Normal CXR. The lower vertebral bodies are blacker because there is less soft tissue (muscle) and no scapulae superimposed. Consequently, there is less absorption of the x-ray beam inferiorly, and thus more blackening on the radiograph. Whiteness inferiorly on the CXR invariably indicates pathology (e.g. collapse, consolidation, lung mass, paravertebral mass). Also, note that assessment of a lung apex is very difficult— usually impossible.*

NORMAL LATERAL CXR—THREE COMMON PITFALLS

1. Fake mass anteriorly. Sometimes the shadow of a high right dome of the diaphragm and the shadow of the posterior margin of the heart overlap and create a well-defined density that mimics an anterior mass (Fig. 2.28).

2. Age related aortic unfolding (Figs 2.29–2.31). In young people the descending aorta is situated posteriorly within the mediastinum and it is not visualised on the lateral CXR. In middle age the aorta unfolds and extends laterally to the left. Consequently its anterior and posterior walls are then outlined by the surrounding left lung. This produces a tubular opacity on the lateral CXR (Fig. 2.33).

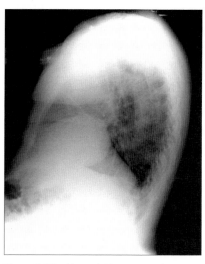

Figure 2.28 *Normal. Not an anterior mass.*

3. Another fake mass anteriorly. The apex of the heart and adjacent epicardial fat intrudes into the left hemithorax and displaces the most infero-medial and anterior aspect of the left lung. This often produces a shadow (Fig. 2.34) which can simulate a mass lesion. This appearance is often referred to as the cardiac incisura[6–8].

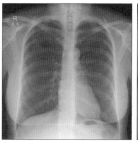
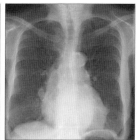
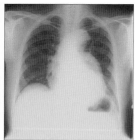

Figure 2.29 *Frontal CXR. Ascending and descending aorta, age 20.*

Figure 2.30 *Frontal CXR. Ascending and descending aorta, age 60.*

Figure 2.31 *Frontal CXR. Ascending and descending aorta, age 80.*

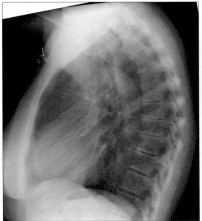

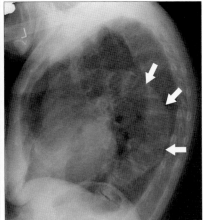

Figure 2.32 *Normal CXR. Age 20–40. The mid and distal part of the descending aorta is not visible.*

Figure 2.33 *Age 80. Age related aortic unfolding occurs in the middle-aged and elderly. The descending aorta is outlined by lung and is visible (arrows). (This is the same patient as Fig. 2.31.)*

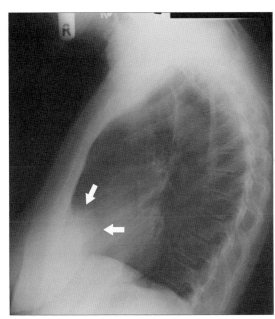

Figure 2.34 *The cardiac incisura. The anterior density (arrows) is caused by the normal cardiac apex and epicardial fat displacing the most infero-medial and anterior aspect of the left lung. The shape of the cardiac incisura will show considerable variation between patients. (Incidentally, a cardiac incisura shadow, with a somewhat different contour is also shown in Fig. 2.33, above.)*

READING THE LATERAL CXR

A lateral radiograph of the chest can be very valuable in helping to confirm, refute, position or characterise a suspected abnormality seen on the frontal projection. A checklist will help you to remember the important rules.

THE LATERAL CXR: A SIX-POINT CHECKLIST

1. Are the vertebral bodies becoming blacker from above downwards (Fig. 2.35)?

   ❏ If not (i.e. they are becoming whiter), then suspect disease in a lower lobe (Figs 2.36–2.38).

2. Are both domes of the diaphragm well-defined and clearly seen?

   ❏ If either dome is obscured, suspect disease in the adjacent lower lobe (Figs 2.36–2.38).

   ❏ Remember—the right dome should be visible from front to back; normally the anterior aspect of the left dome disappears (Fig. 2.35).

3. Are the hila normal (Fig. 2.35)?

   Two questions to ask:

   ❏ Does the overlapping/combination shadow of the two hila appear enlarged (Fig. 2.39)?

   ❏ Is the outline of the overlapping hila well-defined (i.e. normal vessels) or do the borders appear anarchic and irregular, or lumpy/bumpy?

4. Is there any abrupt change in density across the cardiac shadow?

   ❏ This is likely to be a lung abnormality (Fig. 2.40).

5. Are there any abnormal lung densities?

   Check:

   ❏ superimposed over the heart (Fig. 2.42)

   ❏ behind the heart

   ❏ posteriorly in a costophrenic recess

6. Always, always correlate the findings with the frontal CXR.

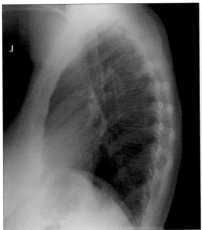

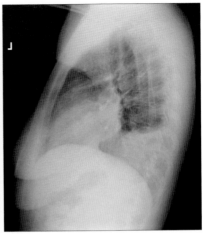

Figure 2.35   *Normal CXR. Note that the vertebral bodies become blacker from above downwards; the domes of the diaphragm are well-defined.*

Figure 2.36   *Cough and fever. Vertebrae whiter inferiorly. The outline of the left dome of the diaphragm is absent posteriorly. Left lower lobe pneumonia.*

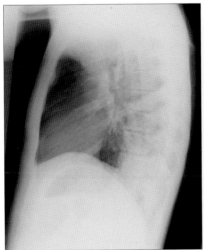

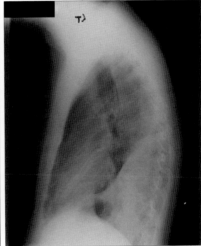

Figure 2.37   *Unwell, fever, chest pain. Vertebrae whiter inferiorly; the outline of the right dome of the diaphragm is absent posteriorly. Right lower lobe pneumonia.*

Figure 2.38   *Persistent cough and haemoptysis. The lower vertebrae are whiter than those above. Shadow of the left dome of the diaphragm is absent. The straight line of the oblique fissure is displaced posteriorly. Collapse of the left lower lobe (bronchial carcinoma).*

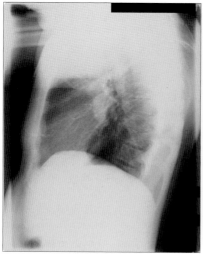

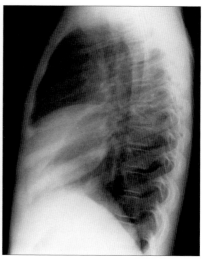

Figure 2.39 *The hilar shadows are enlarged. Lymphadenopathy. Compare this CXR with Fig. 2.35.*

Figure 2.40 *Abrupt change in density over the cardiac shadow. Middle lobe pneumonia with slight loss of volume.*

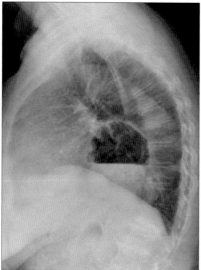

Figure 2.41 *A common finding in the middle-aged and elderly. Hiatus hernia revealed by the air–fluid level.*

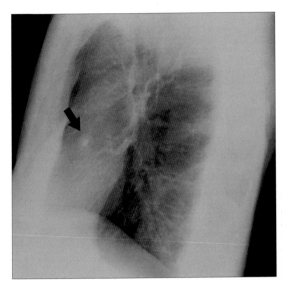

Figure 2.42 *Haemoptysis in a middle-aged smoker. Frontal CXR was unremarkable. Note the solitary pulmonary nodule (arrow) projected over the heart. Bronchial carcinoma.*

REFERENCES

1. Henry S Haskins. American author (b.1875).

2. Proto AV, Speckman JM. The left lateral radiograph of the chest. Part one. Med Radiogr Photogr 1979; 55: 30–74.

3. Proto AV, Speckman JM. The left lateral radiograph of the chest. Part two. Med Radiogr Photogr 1980; 56: 38–64.

4. Austin JHM. The lateral chest radiograph in the assessment of non-pulmonary health and disease. Radiol Clin North Am 1984; 22: 687–698.

5. Vix VA, Klatte EC. The lateral chest radiograph in the diagnosis of hilar and mediastinal masses. Radiology 1970; 96: 307–316.

6. Fraser RG, Muller NL, Colman NC, Pare PD. Fraser and Pare's Diagnosis of Diseases of the Chest. 4th ed. Philadelphia, PA: WB Saunders, 1999.

7. Heitzman ER. The Mediastinum. St Louis, MO: Mosby, 1977.

8. Hyson EA, Ravin CE. Radiographic features of mediastinal anatomy. Chest 1979; 75: 609–613.

3 ALVEOLAR DISEASE *VERSUS* INTERSTITIAL DISEASE

An area of diffuse shadowing on a CXR requires careful analysis. In large part the analysis depends upon relating the shadowing to the clinical details obtained from the history and the physical examination. However, on occasion this will not be enough on its own and it is the evaluation of the shadow pattern which will allow a particular diagnosis or group of diagnoses to be considered.

This chapter aims to help you to recognise two common disease patterns: alveolar and interstitial. There are aspects of alveolar disease, interstitial disease, consolidation and pneumonia which are all closely related. Please read this chapter and Chapter 4 together.

THE ALVEOLI AND THE INTERSTITIUM

Figure 3.1 illustrates the normal relationship between the alveoli and the interstitium.

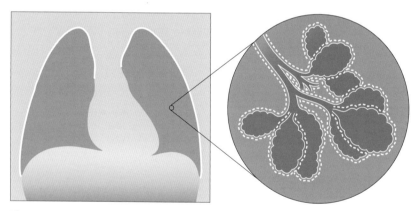

Figure 3.1 *Normal lung. The terminal bronchioles give rise to alveolar ducts which terminate in small air sacs (alveoli). The millions of thin walled alveoli are responsible for gas exchange...carbon dioxide out of the capillaries, oxygen into the capillaries. The interstitium of the lung surrounds both the alveoli and the terminal bronchioles. The interstitium has a most important mechanical function: it acts as a scaffold supporting the alveolar walls. It also has a dynamic function: fluid, cells and nutrients pass into and out of the interstitium.*

ALVEOLAR AND INTERSTITIAL LUNG DISEASE[1,2]

Alveolar disease = Air space disease (NB: these terms are often used interchangeably)

Alveolar disease: The filling of alveolar air spaces with abnormal material. That material may be blood, pus, water, protein, cell debris—or a combination of two or more of these.

Interstitial disease: Affects the supporting tissues of the lung parenchyma (i.e. the interstitium) including the alveolar walls.

Some disease processes affect mainly the alveoli, or mainly the interstitium. Some diseases involve the alveoli and the interstitium just about equally.

The pathological process consequent on most lung injuries can be summarised as follows: the insult causes the cellular lining of the alveolar walls and/or the capillaries in the interstitium to become leaky. The oedema that leaks out accumulates in the alveoli or in the interstitium. Sometimes the injury continues to progress and causes extensive necrosis with the production of fibrin and cell debris. These necrotic products fill the alveolar air spaces or thicken the tissues in the interstitium.

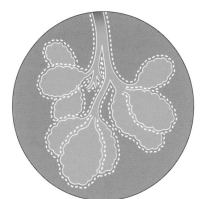 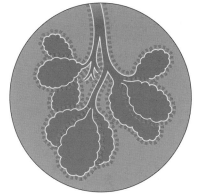

Figure 3.2 *Alveolar disease. The air in the alveoli has been replaced by blood, pus, water, protein or cell debris.*

Figure 3.3 *Interstitial disease. The scaffolding surrounding the alveoli is abnormal. The abnormal change can be due to oedema, inflammation or fibrotic thickening.*

THE CXR: ALVEOLAR VERSUS INTERSTITIAL DISEASE[1-4]

When a CXR shows an area of diffuse shadowing—whether localised or widespread—then the shadow pattern needs to be analysed carefully. It is worth emphasising: the CXR shadow pattern represents the underlying pathological process. The CXR features to look for are listed in Table 3.1.

Table 3.1 CXR features to look for.

	Alveolar changes	Interstitial changes
Usual shadows	■ Fluffy or blobby	■ Small nodules
	■ Ill-defined margins	■ Linear/reticular
	■ Coalescing/merging	■ Linear/reticular with septal lines
	■ Segmental/lobar	■ Reticulo-nodular
Sometimes ...additonally	■ Air bronchogram (see p. 227)	■ Reduced lung volume (extensive disease)
		■ Honeycomb pattern (end-stage disease)

Table 3.2 Descriptive terms.

■ Fine or small nodules = tiny opacities.

■ Reticular = mesh or basket-like. A pattern comprising fine or coarse lines.

■ Reticulo-nodular = a combination of small nodules and basket-like linear opacities.

■ Septal lines = fine thread-like lines produced by fluid or thickening of the septa between the lobules of the lung. Several different types of septal lines have been described[1,2,4], but much the most common are those referred to as Kerley B lines.

■ Kerley B lines = fine horizontal lines approximately 1 cm long, situated perpendicular to the lateral pleural surface. They are most commonly seen just above the costophrenic angles on a frontal CXR (see pp. 158–159).

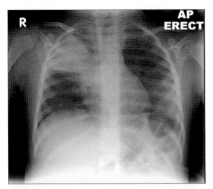

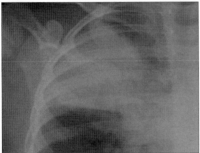

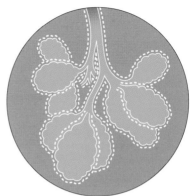

Figure 3.4 *Alveolar disease. The alveoli are (in this case) stuffed with pus, giving a fluffy homogeneous pattern which has coalesced. (Pneumonia.)*

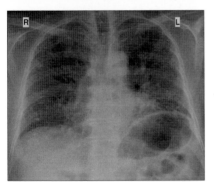

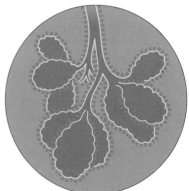

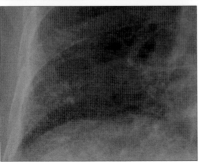

Figure 3.5 *Interstitial disease. The interstitium is fibrotic and thickened. (Sarcoidosis.)*

INTERSTITIAL SHADOWING—ARE YOU SURE?

A regular problem when evaluating a CXR is determining whether the lungs are actually clear and normal. Sometimes the lung markings (i.e. the normal vessels) are rather prominent and the question is raised—is there anything else there? Could some of these markings be fine linear interstitial shadows? This usually relates to a lower zone.

Normal lungs on the CXR should show nothing other than vessels and occasionally a lung fissure. Normal bronchial walls are only visualised if they are seen end on. Normal alveoli, normal interstitium, normal lymphatics—none of these are visible.

So, is there anything there? When in doubt apply these two rules:

Rule 1 Look at the lung immediately adjacent to the costophrenic angle— it should be clear. If this particular part of the lung shows prominent markings then interstitial disease at the lung base is likely. This rule is particularly helpful in females when part of the lung projects just lateral to the overlying breast shadow because the breast density sometimes mimics lung pathology.

Rule 2 Take all of the lung markings and throw them away. Remember, it is just the vessels that you should throw away. In most cases this can be done, metaphorically speaking, fairly easily.

 ❏ Vessels thrown away: nothing left = clear lungs

 ❏ Vessels thrown away: fine shadows remain = interstitial disease likely

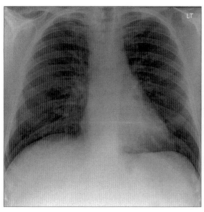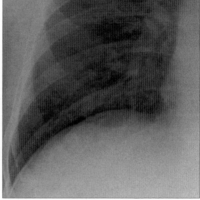

Figure 3.6 *The CXR raises the possibility of increased interstitial shadows. This equivocal appearance is a common dilemma. Careful scrutiny and applying the "throw away the vessels" rule (see the magnified image) shows that the lung is clear.*

THE CXR: NOT ALWAYS EASY TO ASSESS

Sometimes there is an "emperor's new clothes" approach to the implied ease with which the distinction can be made between alveolar disease and interstitial disease on a CXR. Take such claims with a pinch of salt. In a number of instances you will find that it is very difficult to decide whether the classic features (Table 3.1) are actually present (Figs 3.9 and 3.10). All the same it is often possible, following a careful analysis, to recognise a particular pattern. If a particular pattern can be identified then a legitimate differential diagnosis can be suggested (Table 3.3).

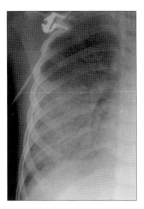

Figure 3.7 *Pneumonia. Classic alveolar pattern. Fluffy shadowing.*

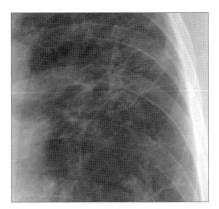

Figure 3.8 *Interstitial fibrosis. Classic interstitial pattern. Reticulo-nodular shadowing.*

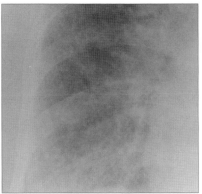

Figure 3.9 *The pattern is difficult to categorise. Neither classically alveolar nor classically interstitial. We are not able to pigeonhole the shadow pattern in this case.*

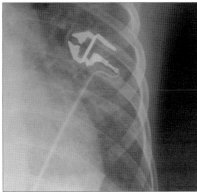

Figure 3.10 *The pattern is neither classically alveolar nor classically interstitial.*

DIFFERENTIAL DIAGNOSIS[1–4]

Frequently, a classical alveolar or interstitial CXR pattern is dominant (Table 3.3). A dominant pattern allows a selective differential diagnosis to be considered. When linked to the clinical history, physical examination, and laboratory tests, then the likely diagnosis usually emerges (Figs 3.11–3.14).

Table 3.3   Differential diagnosis.

Dominant alveolar/airspace pattern	Dominant interstitial pattern
Adults:	■ Pulmonary oedema
■ Pulmonary oedema:	■ Pneumonia:
❏ cardiac	❏ viral
❏ non-cardiac	❏ *Pneumocystis carinii*—early
■ Lobar pneumonia	■ Tuberculosis
■ Haemorrhage	■ Sarcoid
■ Lymphoma	■ Idiopathic pulmonary fibrosis
■ Bronchioloalveolar cell carcinoma	■ Rheumatoid lung
■ Adult respiratory distress syndrome (early)	■ Sclerodema
	■ Lymphangitis carcinomatosa
■ Aspiration pneumonia	■ Crack smoking
Infants:	
■ Hyaline membrane disease	
■ Transient tachypnoea of the newborn	

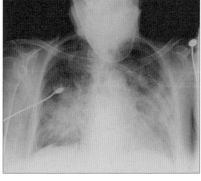

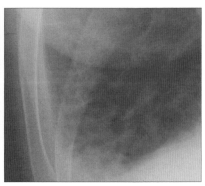

Figure 3.11 *Alveolar pulmonary oedema.*   **Figure 3.12** *Interstitial pulmonary oedema.*

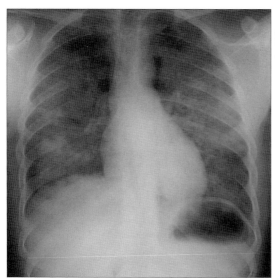

Figure 3.13 *Alveolar pattern. Pulmonary oedema. Patient using intravenous heroin.*

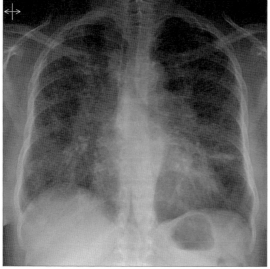

Figure 3.14 *Interstitial pattern. In this patient... sarcoidosis.*

CONFUSION: INTERSTITIAL FIBROSIS & ALL THOSE ACRONYMS

"What is it?"

BOOP? IIP? UIP? COP?

NSIP? DIP? AIP? LIP? RB-ILD?

BIF? BANG?

■ Very often the cause of a chronic interstitial pattern (or a honeycomb appearance) on the CXR will be obvious because of a particular clinical history and the age-old principle: common things occur commonly.

■ When the diagnosis remains obscure then CT will frequently suggest the probable cause[5-11]. In some patients a lung biopsy will still be necessary.

The CXR

Various classifications/descriptions of interstitial fibrosis are in use. The numerous acronyms can be very confusing. The confusion started after the histopathologists separated out several of the different disease processes. Chest physicians and CT radiologists then sought to match and mirror the microscopic findings with the CT patterns. Some of the acronyms are those used by histopathologists, some are those used by radiologists, and some are used incorrectly.

Remember, the CXR is a plain, simple, and very modest examination. It recognises its limitations and leaves the sophisticated separation of the BIFs from the BANGs to CT or to a lung biopsy.

In a patient with dyspnoea and a chronic interstitial CXR pattern, we use the following approach. The CXR shadows will represent either (A) or (B):

(A) True interstitial fibrosis.

Either: A complication or residuum of an already known disease or consequent on an extrinsic stimulus. Examples include: granulomatous diseases (tuberculosis, sarcoid); collagen-vascular diseases (rheumatoid arthritis, progressive systemic sclerosis); gastro-intestinal disease (aspiration pneumonitis); iatrogenic—radiotherapy or drug-related (Amiodorone, Nitrofurantoin, Methotrexate, Bleomycin); occupational disease (asbestosis, silicosis); extrinsic allergic alveolitis (bird fancier's lung, farmer's lung).

Or: Aetiology unknown, i.e. cryptogenic fibrosing alveolitis (idiopathic pulmonary fibrosis). The histopathologists call this usual interstitial pneumonia (UIP).

(B) Lung disease that can mimic the CXR appearance of interstitial fibrosis.

This includes: lymphangitis carcinomatosa; eosinophilic pneumonia; Langerhan's cell histiocytosis; bronchiolitis obliterans with organising pneumonitis (BOOP); lymphangioleiomyomatosis.

REFERENCES

1. Felson B. Chest Roentgenology. Philadelphia, PA: WB Saunders, 1973.

2. Reed JC. Chest Radiology: Plain Film Patterns and Differential Diagnosis. 5th ed. Philadelphia, PA: Mosby, 2003.

3. Schapiro RL, Musallam JJ. A radiologic approach to disorders involving the interstitium of the lung. Heart Lung 1977; 6: 635–643.

4. Collins J, Stern EJ. Chest Radiology: The Essentials. Philadelphia, PA: Lippincott Williams and Wilkins, 1999.

5. Padley SPG, Hansell DM, Flower CDR et al. Comparative accuracy of high resolution computed tomography and chest radiography in the diagnosis of chronic diffuse infiltrative lung disease. Clin Radiol 1991; 44: 222–226.

6. Green SJ, Khan SS, Desai SR. "Aunt Minnies" of thoracic high-resolution CT. Radiology Now 2004; 21: 20–24.

7. Travis WD, King TE and the multidisciplinary core panel. American Thoracic Society/European Respiratory Society international multidisciplinary consensus classification of idiopathic interstitial pneumonias. Am J Respir Crit Care Med 2002; 165: 277–304.

8. American Thoracic Society. Idiopathic pulmonary fibrosis: diagnosis and treatment. International consensus statement. American Thoracic Society (ATS) and the European Respiratory Society (ERS). Am J Respir Crit Care Med 2000; 161: 646–664.

9. Screaton NJ, Hiorns MP, Lee KS et al. Serial high resolution CT in non-specific interstitial pneumonia: prognostic value of the initial pattern. Clin Radiol 2005; 60: 96–104.

10. Flaherty K, Toews G, Travis W et al. Clinical significance of histological classification of interstitial idiopathic pneumonia. Eur Respir J 2002; 19: 275–283.

11. Mueller-Mang C, Grosse C, Schmid K et al. What every radiologist should know about idiopathic interstitial pneumonias. Radiographics 2007; 27: 595–615.

4 PNEUMONIA AND THE SILHOUETTE SIGN

The CXR is excellent for detecting the presence and extent of most pneumonias. All the same, on the CXR some pneumonias are furtive and secretive and do their best to hide. Fortunately there is help at hand—the silhouette sign. If you look for the silhouette sign then you will be able to detect these hidden pneumonias.

PNEUMONIA

"Words, like eyeglasses, blur everything that they do not make clearer" [1]

Bronchitis: Acute or chronic inflammation of the lining of a bronchus.

Pneumonia: An inflammation, usually due to infection, involving the alveoli.

Lobar pneumonia: Pneumonia involving a large part of a lobe. Sometimes the entire lobe is involved.

Bronchopneumonia: Pneumonia plus bronchitis. The involvement of the bronchi and bronchioles dominates over the alveolar inflammation [2]. The pathological process occurring in bronchopneumonia is frequently unappreciated.

Lung consolidation: The term "consolidation" is often used to describe pneumonic changes on a CXR. This can lead to misunderstandings because consolidation refers not only to infection, but to any pathological process that fills the alveoli with either pus, blood, fluid, cells...even lunch or pondwater.

Pneumonia is by far the commonest cause of an area of CXR consolidation. Consequently, some physicians use the two words—pneumonia and consolidation—synonymously but incorrectly. You need to be aware of this tendency. We favour using the word "consolidation" only when its generic meaning is implicit.

Alveolar shadowing: The generally accepted term when describing the CXR appearances of lung consolidation (see Chapter 3, pp. 32–35). Air space shadowing = alveolar shadowing. The two terms are used synonymously.

(a)

(b)

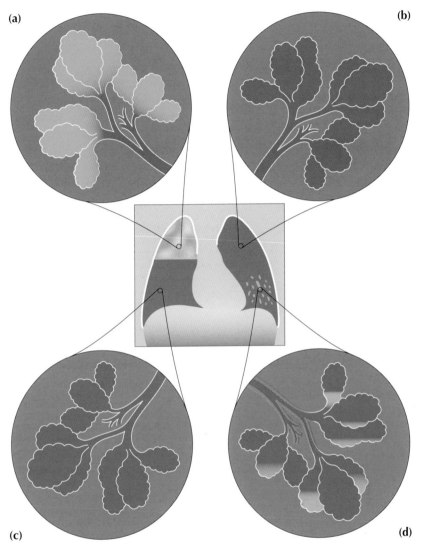

(c)

(d)

Figure 4.1   *(a) Lobar pneumonia; right upper lobe. The alveoli are stuffed full of pus. (b) and (c) Normal lung; the alveoli are healthy and full of air. (d) Bronchopneumonia; left lower lobe. The bronchial walls, bronchioles, and the alveolar walls are inflamed and some pus has accumulated in the alveoli. Note: with bronchopneumonia it is the inflammation involving the bronchi and the bronchioles that predominates.*

THE CXR AND PNEUMONIA

Three rules of thumb:

■ The CXR appearances of a lobar pneumonia, essentially an alveolar filling process, are usually obvious.

■ A very early bronchopneumonia, when the inflammation is mainly affecting the bronchi and bronchioles, can be difficult to detect.

■ Making a precise distinction between a lobar pneumonia and a bronchopneumonia on the CXR will sometimes be difficult. Ill-defined shadows in the context of an acute infection can then only be described as…pneumonia.

Table 4.1 CXR features: lobar pneumonia versus bronchopneumonia[3,4].

Pneumonia	CXR shadows	Occasional additional features	Likely organisms
Lobar	Homogeneous throughout much or most of a lobe Or	May show an air bronchogram Pleural effusion	*Streptococcus pneumoniae* (pneumococcus)
	Non-segmental* —i.e. patchy but confined to a lobe	May produce swelling or expansion of the affected lobe May cavitate	*Klebsiella pneumoniae*
Broncho-pneumonia[5,6]	A spectrum of appearances varying from near normal to grossly abnormal Mild—peribronchial thickening causing small, ill-defined, nodules In general, the nodular and linear opacities are scattered and diffuse When severe—the nodules enlarge and coalesce	Mucus plugging and inflammatory narrowing of the bronchi can result in some moderate volume loss in the affected lobe/lobes Pleural effusion	Numerous, including: ■ *Klebsiella pneumoniae* ■ *Escherischia coli* ■ *Pseudomonas* ■ *Staphylococcus aureus* ■ *Streptococcus pneumoniae* (pneumococcus) ■ Anaerobes

*A lung segment is an anatomical subdivision of a lobe of the lung. Each segment is served by a major branch of the lobar bronchus. There are 10 segments in the right lung and 9 segments in the left lung.

PNEUMONIA CAN HIDE: THE SILHOUETTE SIGN

BEN FELSON'S SILHOUETTE SIGN[7,8]

Silhouette: the outline of a solid object. Also the representation of such an outline, but filled solely with black or colour and used as a picture. It is often claimed that the word owes its origin—because of the lack of any filling—to Etienne de Silhouette, a notoriously miserly finance minister to King Louis XV of France.

Silhouette sign: an intrathoracic lesion touching a border of the heart, aorta, or diaphragm will obliterate that border on the CXR. An intrathoracic lesion not anatomically contiguous with a border will not obliterate that border.

Misnomer: The term "silhouette sign" is a deliberate misnomer—convenient shorthand. The silhouette sign principle actually refers to the loss of part of the silhouette.

Ben Felson: a ground-breaking twentieth-century American radiologist and a wonderful teacher. He was not the first person to describe the silhouette sign but the description is invariably associated with his name.

On a normal CXR the well-defined borders of the heart and the domes of the diaphragm are visualised because the adjacent normal lung provides a flawless interface. If a pneumonia (i.e. pus-filled alveoli / inflamed bronchioles) abuts one of these interfaces then the sharp margin (heart or diaphragm) is lost. The CXR appearance of a blurred or missing interface is referred to as the silhouette sign[7,8].

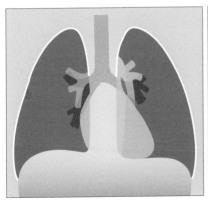

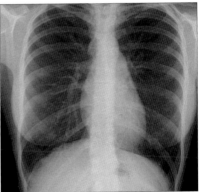

Figure 4.2 *Normal appearances. Note the clean, well-defined margins of the heart and domes of the diaphragm. The left lateral margin of the descending aorta is also well-defined.*

Figure 4.3 *Normal CXR. There is neither blurring nor effacement of any part of the silhouette of the heart or domes of the diaphragm.*

CLINICAL APPLICATIONS OF THE SILHOUETTE SIGN

APPLICATION 1

Whenever infection is suspected it is essential that evaluation of the CXR always includes checking whether a silhouette sign is present. Loss of part of the silhouette of the heart border or of the diaphragm may be the only abnormal feature on the CXR. This allows the precise position of the abnormality to be deduced (Fig. 4.4).

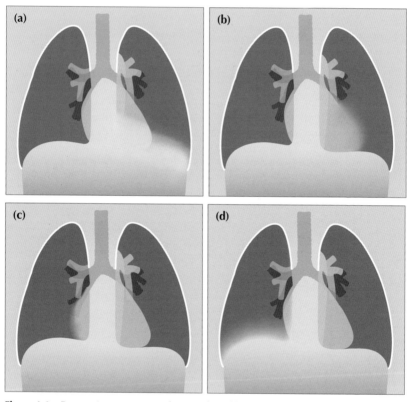

Figure 4.4 *Four patients present with a cough and fever. The silhouette sign tells us that there is consolidation (pneumonia) in: (a) the left lower lobe—because the left dome of the diaphragm is blurred; (b) the lingular segments of the upper lobe—because the left heart border is blurred; (c) the middle lobe—because the right heart border is blurred; (d) the right lower lobe—because the right dome of the diaphragm is blurred.*

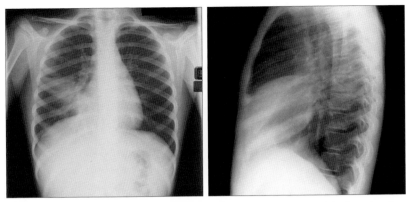

Figure 4.5 *Cough and fever. Right mid zone shadow and effacement of the heart border. The frontal CXR indicates middle lobe pneumonia. The lateral view confirms the diagnosis.*

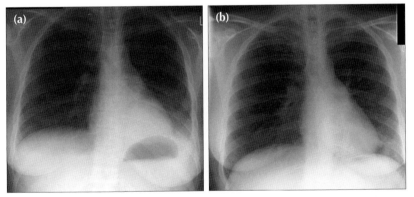

Figure 4.6 *Cough and fever. (a) The left dome of the diaphragm is ill-defined…and so is the lateral margin of the descending aorta. These features indicate left lower lobe pneumonia. (b) Following treatment, a repeat CXR obtained six weeks later shows that all of the normal sharp borders and margins have returned.*

APPLICATION 2

The silhouette sign is not solely applicable to pneumonia. It can be applied to any water density lesion that is in contact with the mediastinum or the diaphragm. Examples: lobar collapse, lung tumour, mediastinal mass.

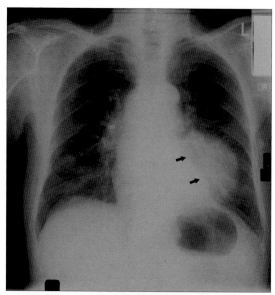

Figure 4.7 *Middle-aged patient with a chronic cough. The CXR shows an ill-defined left dome of the diaphragm but a normal left border of the heart (arrows). In addition, note the increased density projected over the left side of the heart. These features indicate pathology in the left lower lobe. The lateral view showed a large lower lobe mass. Bronchial carcinoma.*

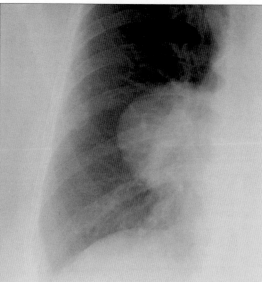

Figure 4.8 *Another example of the silhouette sign. A mass lesion overlies the right hilum. The right border of the heart is obliterated—i.e. it is not sharply defined. Note that the right dome of the diaphragm remains well-defined. These findings indicate that the lesion is intimately related to the margin of the heart. This was a benign mass—a pericardial cyst.*

Caution: some common pitfalls[8]

1. A well-defined and clearly identifiable right heart border will only be seen if it projects beyond the thoracic vertebrae. In a small percentage of normal individuals the heart does not do so.

2. A depressed sternum can produce loss of the right heart border, an appearance which mimics middle lobe pneumonia (Fig. 4.9). This is because: (a) the depressed sternum pushes the heart posteriorly and to the left; and (b) bunching of the soft tissues of the deformed chest wall causes an increase in density.

3. Some normal people have pulmonary vessels or fat closely applied to a heart border. Either may result in a false positive silhouette sign. Fat as a cause of blurring of the right heart border may be present in as many as 4% of patients aged 50 and over (see Chapter 16, p. 238).

4. A large amount of fat (prosperous middle age) can be situated between the pericardium, lung, and dome of the diaphragm. Occasionally this fat will blur part of a dome.

5. Be careful with some bedside radiographs[9,10]. If the x-ray beam is angled upwards it can project extrapleural fat over the base of the left lung. This technical effect can cause loss of definition of the left dome of the diaphragm[10].

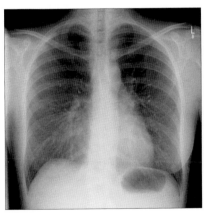

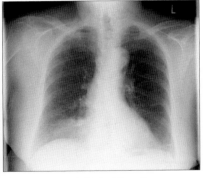

Figure 4.10   *Pitfall. The blurred area on the right heart border is caused by adjacent epicardial fat. This is not a pneumonia.*

Figure 4.9   *Pitfall. The indistinct right heart border and the right mid zone shadowing are caused by a depressed sternum.*

APPLICATION 3

The absence of a silhouette sign can tell you where a shadow (consolidation or mass) is not situated (Fig. 4.11).

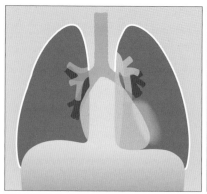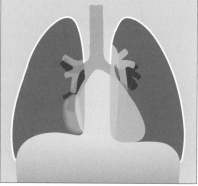

Figure 4.11   *The patient on the left has consolidation in the left lung…but the left heart border remains sharp and clear. This consolidation must be in the lower lobe; it is not in a lingular segment of the upper lobe. The patient on the right has consolidation in the right lung…but the right heart border remains sharp and clear. This consolidation must be in the lower lobe; it is not in the middle lobe.*

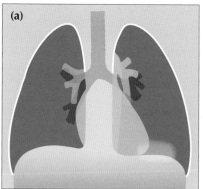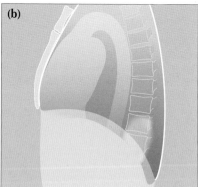

Figure 4.12   *Silhouette sign…not infallible. Sometimes consolidation will be seen on the frontal CXR and the dome of the diaphragm remains sharp and clear (a). Yet a lateral CXR (b) shows that the consolidation is situated in the lower lobe. This can occur when the consolidation is situated far posteriorly—well below the highest point of the dome of the diaphragm.*

PNEUMONIA — A SIX-WEEK RULE

Sometimes an important question will be raised — could there be an underlying bronchial carcinoma in this patient who has CXR evidence of pneumonia? If there are no specifically worrying social (e.g. smoking), clinical, or radiological features then the following approach is recommended:

■ There is no need to rush to repeat the CXR if the patient is clinically well or improving. In approximately 73% of patients with a community acquired pneumonia the CXR will be clear at six weeks[5]. Some simple pneumonias take even longer to clear[6].

■ *Adopt the six-week CXR rule:* following the initial CXR in a patient who is now well, do not repeat the CXR before six weeks. If the CXR is not clear at six weeks then: (a) If the patient is still well and there are no worrying features, obtain CXRs at four-weekly intervals in order to ascertain that clearing is continuing; (b) For all smokers older than 40 years, and for any patient with another risk factor or clinical feature for lung cancer, then arrange bronchoscopy[6] or CT.

REFERENCES

1. Joseph Jonbert. French essayist and moralist (1754–1824).

2. Glossary of terms for thoracic radiology: recommendations of the Nomenclature Committee of the Fleischner Society. AJR 1984; 143: 509–517.

3. Reed JC. Chest Radiology: Plain Film Patterns and Differential Diagnosis. 5th ed. Philadelphia, PA: Mosby, 2003.

4. Itoh H, Tokunaga S, Asamoto H, et al. Radiologic–pathologic correlations of small lung nodules with special reference to peribronchiolar nodules. AJR 1978; 130: 223–231.

5. Mittl RL, Schwab RJ, Duchin JS et al. Radiographic resolution of community-acquired pneumonia. Am J Respir Crit Care Med 1994; 149: 630–635.

6. Johnson JL. Slowly resolving and nonresolving pneumonia. Postgraduate Medicine 2000; 108: 115–122.

7. Felson B, Felson H. Localization of intrathoracic lesions by means of the postero-anterior roentgenogram: The silhouette sign. Radiology 1950; 55: 363–374.

8. Felson B. Chest Roentgenology. Philadelphia, PA: WB Saunders, 1973.

9. Hollman AS, Adams FG. The influence of the lordotic projection on the interpretation of the chest radiograph. Clin Radiol 1989; 40: 360–364.

10. Zylak CJ, Littleton JT, Durizch ML. Illusory consolidation of the left lower lobe: a pitfall of portable radiography. Radiology 1988; 167: 653–655.

5 LOBAR COLLAPSE

It is very important to recognise the CXR appearances indicating lobar collapse. The inexperienced observer will not find this easy as some of the five lobes produce subtle changes on the CXR. For example, in Fig. 5.1 do you recognise which lobe is collapsed? What is your diagnosis in Fig. 5.2?

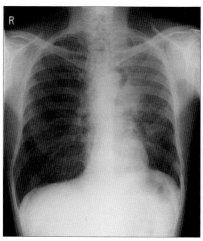

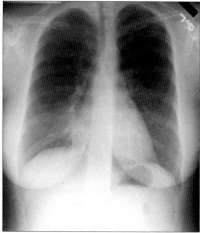

Figure 5.1 *Male. Age 55. Recent onset of shortness of breath and a cough. Diagnosis on p. 68.*

Figure 5.2 *Female. Age 48. Unexplained loss of weight. Recent coughing episodes. Diagnosis on p. 68.*

BASIC TERMINOLOGY[1-3]

Occasionally the words "consolidation" and "collapse" are used interchangeably. This is careless, incorrect, and leads to confusion.

Consolidation: An essentially homogeneous opacity in the lung characterised by little or no loss of volume…applicable only in an appropriate clinical setting when the opacity can with reasonable certainty be attributed to replacement of alveolar air by exudate, transudate, or cell debris.

Atelectasis: A synonym for collapse (i.e. volume loss). Atelectasis is the favoured term in the USA. Very small areas of collapse/atelectasis may produce a linear shadow, which is often, but not always, horizontal. This is usually referred to as "plate-like", "linear", or "subsegmental" atelectasis. Derivation of "Atelectasis" from the Greek: Ateles = incomplete, Extasis = expansion.

Lobar and total lung atelectasis (collapse) also occur. These larger varieties of atelectasis are usually associated with increased density in the affected part of the airless lung. To diagnose lobar atelectasis there must be specific evidence of volume loss such as displacement of a fissure, mediastinum or hilum. Elevation of a hemidiaphragm or a decrease in the spacing between the ribs can also be signs associated with atelectasis.

Collapse: Precise use of language differs between physicians in different countries. In the USA the word "collapse" generally connotes total atelectasis (i.e. total loss of volume of a lung or lobe). In everyday practice, North American physicians refer to all degrees of collapse—whether large or small—as "atelectasis". In the UK the word "collapse" has a more general meaning and is utilised however large or small the amount of volume loss.

WHITE AREA ON THE CXR—CLARIFICATIONS

■ Lung consolidation appears as a white (an extra dense) area on the CXR. The most common cause is pneumonia. A simple pneumonia will not be associated with any major loss of volume in the affected lobe.

■ Lobar collapse: the affected lobe is also usually white…but volume loss will be evident. The whiteness is because: (a) the affected lung tissue occupies a smaller volume, (b) it has no air within it, and (c) mucus secretions back up and collect in the alveoli.

■ Exceptions: sometimes lobar collapse is very rapid and the lobe collapses to a paper thin structure/slice. When this occurs the collapsed lobe will not necessarily be very white. Similarly, longstanding (i.e. chronic) lobar collapse can lead to scarring and contraction of the lobe. The shrivelled lobe may become a small remnant of lung tissue and may not be very white at all.

■ When lung consolidation (i.e. a white area) is associated with lobar collapse then this often signifies very bad news. Obstructive collapse is common and it is always worrying (Table 5.1).

Table 5.1   Likely cause of a collapsed lobe by presentation.

Patient	Likely cause
Middle-aged smoker	Bronchial carcinoma
Two days after surgery/ in the intensive therapy unit	Mucus plug or incorrect position of an endotracheal tube
Asthmatic	Mucus plug
Toddler/young child	Inhaled foreign body

TYPES OF COLLAPSE / ATELECTASIS

Three different disease processes represent the most common causes of volume loss (Table 5.2). A fourth type of collapse/atelectasis is also recognised. This is termed adhesive collapse, and occurs in neonatal surfactant deficiency, in adult respiratory distress syndrome, and as a complication of smoke inhalation.

Table 5.2 The common mechanisms causing volume loss.

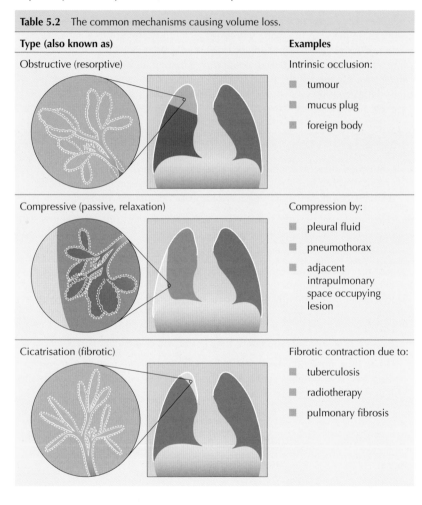

Type (also known as)	Examples
Obstructive (resorptive)	Intrinsic occlusion: ■ tumour ■ mucus plug ■ foreign body
Compressive (passive, relaxation)	Compression by: ■ pleural fluid ■ pneumothorax ■ adjacent intrapulmonary space occupying lesion
Cicatrisation (fibrotic)	Fibrotic contraction due to: ■ tuberculosis ■ radiotherapy ■ pulmonary fibrosis

COLLAPSE ANALYSIS: BASIC ANATOMY

THE NORMAL FISSURES

We need to understand where the normal fissures are positioned.

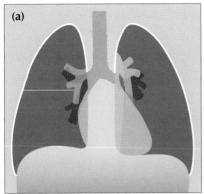

Figure 5.3 *Normal fissures. (a) The horizontal fissure in normal position. The fissure is only visible in part or in whole on 67% of normal CXRs (see p. 241). (b) The horizontal and right oblique fissure. (c) The left oblique fissure. (d) Sometimes the horizontal fissure appears as two lines on the frontal CXR (see p. 241). The explanation is shown in (e); the fissure is single but not perfectly horizontal—it has taken a small step, or undulation, in the horizontal plane.*

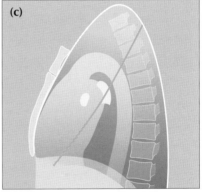

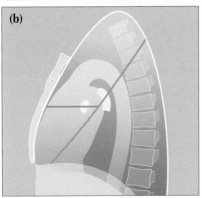

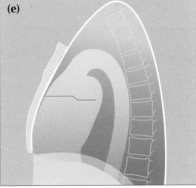

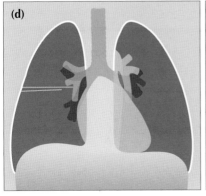

THE NORMAL HILA

When a lobe collapses this frequently alters the position of the hilum. The one exception is collapse of the middle lobe. So we need to understand how to assess the position of each hilum. Hilar anatomy and position are described in Chapter 6 (pp. 70–73). Figs 5.4–5.6 illustrate the normal hilar appearances. These figures can be used as baseline normals as you evaluate the various examples of lobar collapse that now follow.

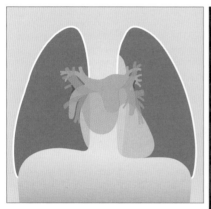

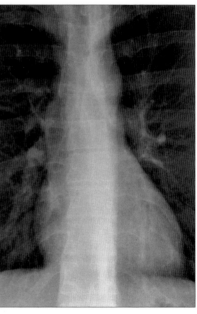

Figure 5.4 *The normal hilar shadows. The left hilum is higher than the right in 95% of normal CXRs. In 5% the hila are at the same level. The right hilum is never higher than the left on a normal CXR (see p. 240). The horizontal hila vees (red arrowheads) are explained in Chapter 6, p. 73.*

Figure 5.5 *Normal hila. The left hilum is higher than the right. Both lower lobe main pulmonary arteries are identified (see Chapter 6, p. 71).*

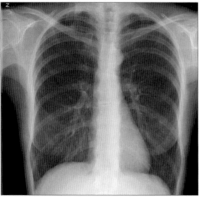

Figure 5.6 *Normal hila and lower lobe pulmonary arteries. The "little finger" analogy: the right lower lobe pulmonary artery is clearly visible as a "little finger". The left lower lobe pulmonary artery shows the "proximal part of a little finger". This analogy is described in Chapter 6, pp. 71–73.*

LOBAR COLLAPSE—GENERAL FEATURES

We will concentrate on the most common type of lobar collapse—obstructive.

Collapse of a lobe:

- Will show evidence of volume loss (e.g. displacement of a fissure, hilum, trachea, or mediastinum). Sometimes there will also be elevation of a dome of the diaphragm and/or decreased spacing between the ribs.

- May show evidence of over-inflation of the adjacent unaffected lobe(s). This compensatory over-inflation can cause hypertransradiancy (i.e. increased blackness) of the ipsilateral hemithorax. Also, the vessels in the over-expanded lobe(s) may be more widely separated compared with the opposite normal lung (Fig. 5.7).

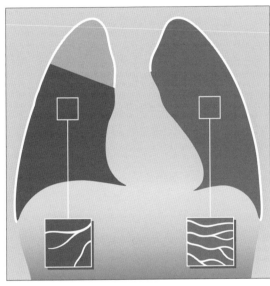

Figure 5.7 *Lobar collapse will affect the other lobe(s). The right upper lobe shows partial collapse. The middle and lower lobes over-inflate and as a result often appear slightly blacker than the normal opposite lung. Also, the normal vessels in the over-inflated middle and lower lobes frequently appear more spread out than in a matching area in the opposite normal lung…as shown in the two boxes.*

LOBAR COLLAPSE — SPECIFIC FEATURES

COLLAPSE OF THE RIGHT LOWER LOBE

On the frontal CXR:

- Oblique fissure moves posteriorly and medially. The medial displacement of this fissure causes it to be seen in profile and it forms the lateral edge of a triangular density projected over the heart.
- Right hilum is depressed.
- Right lower lobe pulmonary artery is not visualised.
- Medial aspect of the right dome of the diaphragm is obscured.
- Lateral margin of the adjacent vertebrae is effaced.

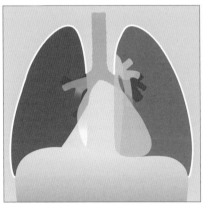

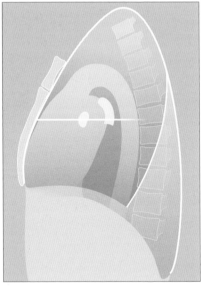

Figure 5.8 *Collapsed right lower lobe. The triangular density of the collapsed lower lobe is easy to detect. When the collapse is more severe then it can be much more difficult to recognise because the lobe is tucked in behind the heart against the spine. However, hilar and lower lobe pulmonary artery changes (Fig. 5.12b) will be evident.*

Figure 5.9 *Collapsed right lower lobe. The oblique fissure has moved posteriorly and forms the anterior border of the collapsed lobe.*

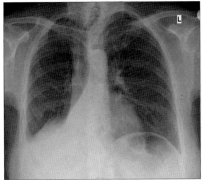

Figure 5.10 *Collapsed right lower lobe. Classic triangular shadow. Note the effacement of part of the dome of the diaphragm, and effacement of the adjacent vertebral margin.*

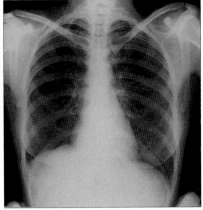

Figure 5.11 *Major collapse of the right lower lobe. Contrast this CXR with Fig. 5.10. The abnormal features are more subtle. Note that the right lower lobe main pulmonary artery has disappeared (it lies within the collapsed lobe). The remainder of the right lung is hypertransradiant (i.e. blacker than the normal left lung).*

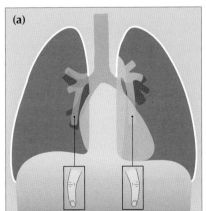
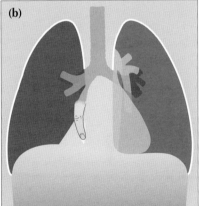

(a)

(b)

Figure 5.12 *The lower lobe pulmonary arteries on each side can be likened to a "little finger". This is explained on p. 71. When a lower lobe collapses the "little finger" disappears. (a) Normal CXR with "little finger" lower lobe pulmonary arteries visible. (b) Right lower lobe collapse. The right lower lobe pulmonary artery (the "little finger") is not visible—it is hidden behind the heart within the collapsed lobe.*

COLLAPSE OF THE LEFT LOWER LOBE

On the frontal CXR:

■ Oblique fissure moves posteriorly and medially. The medial displacement and rotation of the fissure causes it to be seen in profile and it forms the lateral edge of a triangular density superimposed over the heart.

■ Left hilum lies at a lower level than usual.

■ Left lower lobe pulmonary artery is not visualised.

■ Medial aspect of the left dome of the diaphragm is obscured.

■ Lateral margin of the adjacent vertebrae is effaced.

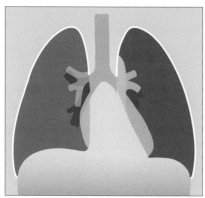

Figure 5.13 *Major collapse of the left lower lobe. A triangular density is superimposed over the heart. Note the hypertransradiancy of the overexpanded remaining lung (i.e. the left upper lobe) when compared with the normal right lung.*

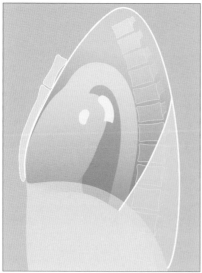

Figure 5.14 *Collapsed left lower lobe. The oblique fissure has moved posteriorly and forms the anterior border of the increased density overlying the vertebral column. Note that the posterior aspect of the left dome of the diaphragm has disappeared (see silhouette sign, p. 45).*

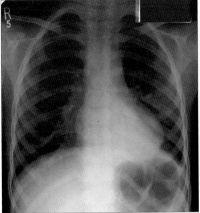

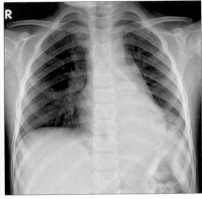

Figure 5.15 *Collapse of the left lower lobe. Triangular shadow superimposed over the heart. Left hilum abnormally low compared with the right hilum. The lower lobe pulmonary artery is not identified. Adjacent vertebral margin is indistinct.*

Figure 5.16 *Collapsed left lower lobe. Left hilum is abnormally low. Increased density overlies the left side of the heart. The lower lobe pulmonary artery is not identified. Part of the outline of the left dome of the diaphragm is effaced.*

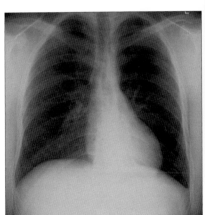

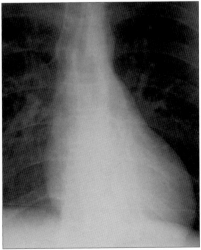

Figure 5.17 *Major collapse of the left lower lobe. Detection is more difficult than for Fig. 5.15 because the collapse is nearly total. The crucial signs to note: the left hilum is low and the left lower lobe pulmonary artery is not visible; increased density overlying the heart is evident but subtle.*

COLLAPSE OF THE MIDDLE LOBE

On the frontal CXR:

■ Horizontal fissure moves inferiorly.

   ❑ NB: this fissure is not always visible. In patients over 50 the fissure was visible in only 67% of normal CXRs (see data in Chapter 16, p. 241).

■ Blurring of the right heart border (Figs 5.18, 5.20 and 5.21). Incidentally the position of the hilum does not alter.

■ The density in the collapsed lobe may be obvious or very subtle.

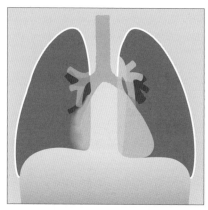

Figure 5.18 *Middle lobe collapse. Sometimes the associated increase in density is very obvious. On other occasions the horizontal fissure may be clearly depressed. Sometimes (as in this case) the only evidence raising the possibility of collapse is blurring of the right border of the heart.*

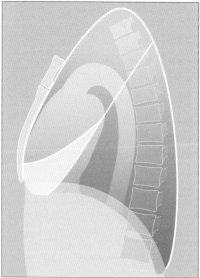

Figure 5.19 *Major collapse of the middle lobe. The horizontal fissure has moved inferiorly and the collapsed lobe is dense—it appears like a slice of cake.*

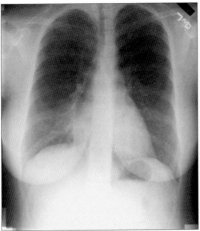
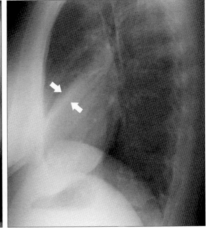

Figure 5.20   *Middle lobe collapse is evident when the two views are assessed as a pair. The subtle density (between the arrows) is the collapsed lobe.*

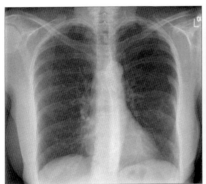
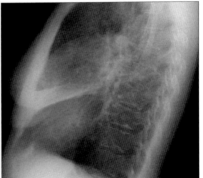

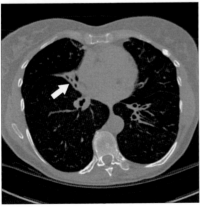

Figure 5.21   *Middle lobe collapse. Subtle change on the frontal CXR—a blurred heart border. The lateral CXR shows the white wedge (or slice of cake) of the collapsed middle lobe. The CT section also shows the collapsed lobe (arrow).*

COLLAPSE OF THE RIGHT UPPER LOBE

On the frontal CXR:

■ Horizontal fissure moves superiorly (Figs 5.22 and 5.23).

■ Right hilum is elevated.

■ Collapsed lung is dense (i.e. white).

■ In an adult, look for Golden's S sign (Fig. 5.22). This will sometimes be present when a tumour at the right hilum is the cause of the lobar collapse. See Chapter 10, pp. 147.

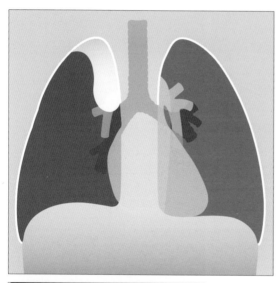

Figure 5.22 *Major collapse of the right upper lobe. The collapsed lobe is easy to identify. In this example there is a bulge overlying the elevated right hilum. This bulge is the tumour that has caused the collapse, and this overall appearance is often referred to as Golden's S sign or the reverse S sign of Golden. In clinical practice the tumour mass is not always evident and the appearance of right upper lobe collapse in Fig. 5.23 is more typical.*

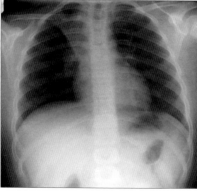

Figure 5.23 *Young patient. Asthmatic. A mucus plug has caused collapse of the right upper lobe.*

COLLAPSE OF THE LEFT UPPER LOBE

The pattern of collapse is very different to that seen with right upper lobe collapse. This is because there is no horizontal fissure on the left side. A most peculiar, but characteristic, appearance results.

On the frontal CXR:

■ A veil-like density covers much of the left hemithorax. This is due to the lack of aeration within the collapsed upper lobe.

■ Left heart border is obscured — in whole or in part.

■ Left hilum is elevated.

■ The Luftsichel sign may be present…i.e. a crescentic lucency around the left side of the aortic knuckle (Fig. 5.26). It is caused by the overexpanded apical segment of the left lower lobe positioning itself between the collapsed upper lobe and the aortic arch.

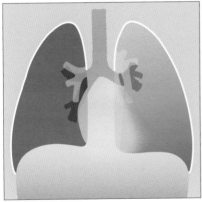

Figure 5.24 *Collapse of the left upper lobe. Note the classic features: veil-like opacity overlies the left lung and the left heart border is ill-defined.*

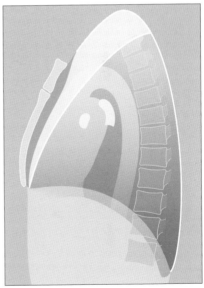

Figure 5.25 *Collapse of the left upper lobe. The oblique fissure has moved far anteriorly.*

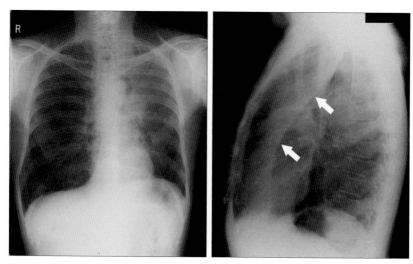

Figure 5.26 *Collapse of the left upper lobe. The lateral CXR confirms the diagnosis. The oblique fissure (arrows) is displaced anteriorly. Note: this is the same frontal CXR as Fig. 5.1. The underlying lesion was a bronchial carcinoma. On the frontal CXR the Luftsichel sign is present. On the lateral CXR a lucent (black) area is present. Although it appears to outline the anterior margin of the collapsed lobe, this is a common misconception. This well-defined margin is actually the anterior wall of the ascending aorta outlined by part of the right upper lobe which has herniated across the midline[4].*

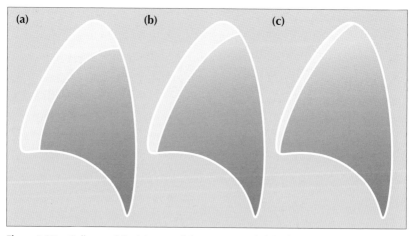

Figure 5.27 *Collapse of the left upper lobe can cause slightly different appearances on the lateral CXR. In effect there is a race between the degree of collapse and the build up of secretions in the collapsed lobe. If the collapse occurs slowly then the lobe becomes full of secretions or pus and the collapse is not total—patients (a) and (b). If the bronchial obstruction is nearly complete and occurs quickly, e.g. a mucus plug and some bronchial carcinomas, then the lobe collapses very swiftly and the collapse is total—patient (c).*

PITFALLS: BEWARE OF IMPOSTERS

There are various benign appearances that can superficially mimic some of the changes of lobar collapse on the frontal CXR (Table 5.3). Whenever you are in any doubt, always obtain a lateral CXR. The lateral radiograph will confirm whether or not pathology is present.

Table 5.3 Benign appearances which can occasionally be mistaken for lobar collapse.

Collapse	Imposters
Right upper lobe	▦ Azygos fissure (Fig. 5.28)
	▦ Unfolded neck vessels in the elderly— usually only on a supine CXR
Middle lobe	▦ Depressed sternum
	▦ Normal vessel (or fat) touching the heart border
Right lower lobe	▦ Epicardial fat pad
	▦ Accessory fissure (developmental variant)
Left lower lobe	▦ Unfolded aorta
	▦ Hiatus hernia
Left upper lobe	…is unique—no impersonators!

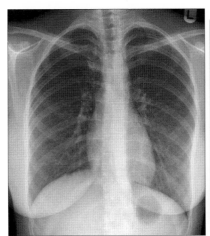
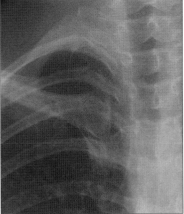

Figure 5.28 *An azygos fissure is a common normal variant. It should not be confused with an elevated horizontal fissure. This fissure is formed when the azygos vein crosses the apex of the lung as it passes anteriorly to enter the superior vena cava. As a result of this minor congenital anomaly four layers of pleura are pulled down into the lung by the vein, which creates an azygos fissure.*

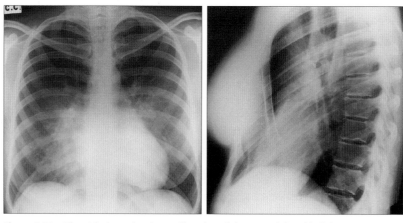

Figure 5.29 *The right heart border is effaced, and there is subtle added density suggesting middle lobe consolidation. The lateral CXR shows the depressed sternum which is causing the appearance on the frontal CXR.*

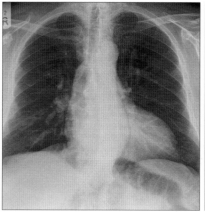

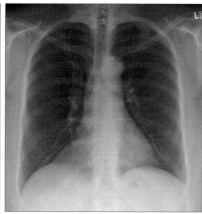

Figure 5.30 *Unfolded descending aorta…the unwary might confuse this with left lower lobe collapse.*

Figure 5.31 *A large epicardial fat collection could be misinterpreted as consolidation— or collapse—within the right lower lobe.*

Answers to Figs 5.1 and 5.2 on p. 52:

Fig. 5.1: Collapse of the left upper lobe.

Fig. 5.2: Shadowing in the middle lobe…a lateral CXR showed collapse (i.e. fissure displacement) of the lobe.

Both patients had an underlying bronchial carcinoma.

AN INTERESTING CONDITION—
ROUND (OR ROUNDED) ATELECTASIS[5,6]

Aetiology / pathology

Occurs in patients who have long-standing pleural thickening. It represents an infolding of the visceral pleura around an area of collapsed lung tissue.

Clinical features

Usually an incidental CXR finding. Some, but not all, patients have been exposed to asbestos in the past[5]. The appearance may be mistaken for a lung tumour.

The CXR

■ A mass in contact with a pleural surface, 2.0–5.0 cm in diameter. It may be almost round, or oval, or lobulated, or irregular or even wedge-shaped.

■ Adjacent pleural thickening.

■ May become visible when a pleural effusion starts to absorb. Easily confused with a peripheral bronchial carcinoma.

■ A benign lesion. It can remain unchanged for years. Sometimes, it resolves completely. CT characteristics can help to distinguish round atelectasis from a carcinoma[5,6].

■ NB: not to be confused with round pneumonia (see p. 199).

REFERENCES

1. Glossary of terms for thoracic radiology: recommendations of the Nomenclature Committee of the Fleischner Society. AJR 1984; 143: 509–517.

2. Proto AV, Tocino I. Radiographic manifestations of lobar collapse. Semin Roentgenol 1980; 15: 117–173.

3. Woodring JH, Reed JC. Types and mechanisms of pulmonary atelectasis. J Thorac Imaging 1995; 11: 92–108.

4. Hansell DM, Armstrong P, Lynch DA, McAdams HP. Imaging of Diseases of the Chest. 4th ed. St Louis, MO: Mosby, 2005.

5. Schneider HJ, Felson B, Gonzalez LL. Rounded atelectasis. AJR 1980; 134: 225–232.

6. Carvalho PM, Carr DH. Computer tomography of folded lung. Clin Radiol 1990; 41: 86–91.

6 HILA AND HILAR ABNORMALITIES

Assessing the hilar shadows can be difficult. Accurate assessment requires a basic understanding of the normal anatomy.

BASIC ANATOMY[1,2]

- Components:
  - ❑ 99% of each hilar shadow is due to vessels— pulmonary arteries and to a lesser extent veins.
  - ❑ There is a very minor contribution from fat, lymph nodes, and bronchial walls.
- Size:
  - ❑ There is wide variation between normal individuals.
  - ❑ Unusual prominence of a hilum is frequently due to a technical factor (e.g. rotation) or to a skeletal abnormality (e.g. scoliosis).
- Shape:
  - ❑ There are no lumpy, bumpy elements to a normal hilum.
  - ❑ The vessel margins are smooth, and the vessels have branches.

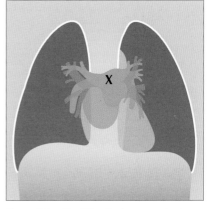

Figure 6.1 *The hilar shadows are due to pulmonary arteries and pulmonary veins. X marks the main pulmonary trunk. Blue = pulmonary trunk and pulmonary arteries; brown = pulmonary veins; pink = part of left atrium...atrial appendage not shown.*

- Position:
  - ❑ The superior margin of the left hilum is normally higher than the right. This is because the left main pulmonary artery passes over the left main bronchus whereas the right main pulmonary artery passes in front of the right main bronchus[1,2]. The hila are at the same level in 5% of normal CXRs (see p. 240).
  - ❑ **The important rule:** The left hilum should never be lower than the right.

RELATED ADJACENT ANATOMY

■ The lower lobe pulmonary arteries extend inferiorly from the hilum. Each is the size of a little finger[3].

■ On the right side: either the whole of a little finger (Fig. 6.2) or at least a (metaphorical) proximal phalanx will be visible in 94% of normal CXRs.

■ On the left side: the lower lobe pulmonary artery takes a sharp posterior course and is not always clearly identified. All the same, it appears as a little finger (or a proximal phalanx) in 62% of normal people. See Chapter 16, p. 239.

Useful rule: A little finger shadow should always be looked for on both sides. If it is not identified then you should check whether there is any evidence to suggest collapse of a lower lobe (pp. 58–61).

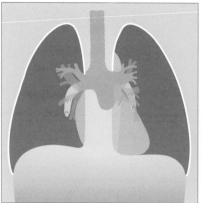

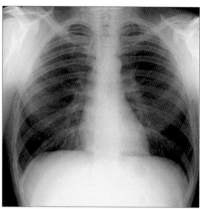

Figure 6.2 *The main lower lobe pulmonary arteries can be likened to a little finger pointing downwards. Sometimes—particularly on the left side—this arterial shadow comprises only the proximal phalanx of the finger. We should see these little fingers (or at least their proximal phalanges) on virtually all normal CXRs.*

Figure 6.3 *Normal CXR. Both little fingers—i.e. the lower lobe arteries—are clearly seen.*

THE HILUM—IS IT TOO HIGH OR TOO LOW?

When making this assessment, two approaches are available. In effect, both identify a similar position or site to look for, but the descriptions differ slightly. We have termed these the purist's approach and—the one we use—the pragmatist's approach.

PURISTS IDENTIFY THE HILAR POINT ON EACH SIDE[4]

On a CXR the pulmonary veins and arteries are indistinguishable from each other in the outer two-thirds of the lung. In the inner third they can be separated because of their different directions of travel. Specifically:

■ Arteries radiate out from the hilum and this particular direction of travel allows them to be distinguished from the pulmonary veins. The veins run towards the left atrium.

■ The main upper lobe vein converges on the left atrium and can be identified as it crosses the descending pulmonary artery. The latter is directed inferiorly and medially. This crossing position is referred to as the hilar point. The left hilar point is approximately 1 cm higher than the right.

■ Our problem: in everyday practice we find that distinguishing this vein from an artery can be difficult. Because of this difficulty we have developed a pragmatic approach when defining the level of each hilum.

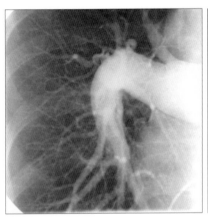

Figure 6.4 *Normal pulmonary angiogram. Right lung. Showing the large, finger-like, descending lower lobe pulmonary artery.*

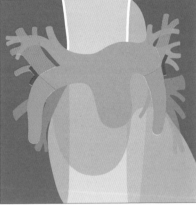

Figure 6.5 *The hilar point (red arrowhead) on each side.*

PRAGMATISTS CHECK THE HILAR HORIZONTAL VEES

We have always found the purist's description of the hilar point just a little bit confusing. So we adopt a more practical approach. We look for the vee on each side as follows. First, identify the lower lobe pulmonary artery. Each lower lobe artery curls gently downwards and medially and has the approximate diameter of your little finger. Now look for the site where the most superior upper lobe vessel—either vein or artery—crosses the lateral margin of the little finger. The point of crossing forms a horizontal vee. The apex of the vee at the left hilum should be higher than the apex of the vee at the right hilum (Fig. 6.6). Occasionally, the two vees will be at the same level.

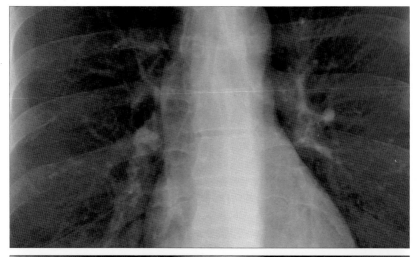

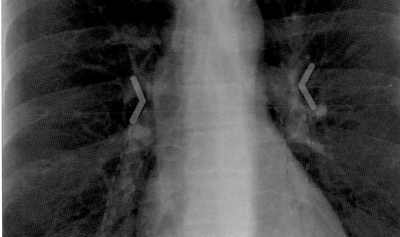

Figure 6.6 *Normal horizontal vees (green) and descending pulmonary arteries (red).*

APPLIED ANATOMY—MAINLY LOBAR COLLAPSE[1,2,5,6]

■ Firstly, always look for the horizontal vee on each side.

■ Whenever a left hilum appears lower than the right hilum—check whether there is other evidence suggestive of:

❏ collapse of either the left lower lobe or of the right upper lobe; or

❏ enlargement of the right hilum (e.g. tumour or nodes).

■ If the little finger shadow of the right lower lobe artery is not seen then you must check for evidence suggesting collapse of the right lower lobe.

■ The silhouette sign. On the frontal CXR the principle of the silhouette sign (p. 45) can be applied to any mass lesion projected over a hilum. If the mass is at the hilum then it will obscure the adjacent soft tissues (i.e. the margins of the arteries at the hilum). On the other hand, if the mass is situated anterior or posterior to the hilum then the margins of the arteries at the hilum will not be obscured.

■ For descriptions of the hilum overlay sign and the hilum convergence sign see Chapter 16, p. 233).

■ For descriptions of lobar collapse see pp. 52–69.

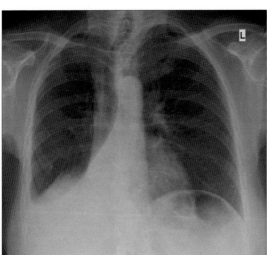

Figure 6.7 *The right lower lobe is collapsed. The hilar vee site on the right side is not identified because the lower lobe pulmonary artery is now lost within the collapsed and unaerated lobe.*

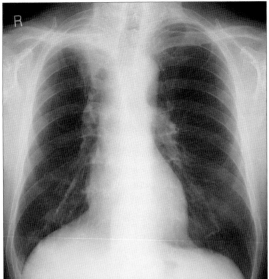

Figure 6.8 *The right hilum is higher than the left hilum. This is an abnormal finding. Also there is shadowing at the right lung apex. Diagnosis: major collapse of the right upper lobe. Subsequently, proven bronchial carcinoma.*

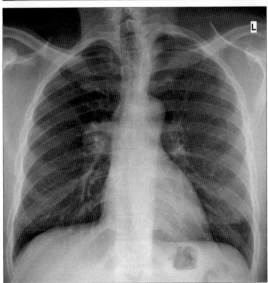

Figure 6.9 *Enlarged right hilum due to lymph nodes. The hilum has a lumpy, bumpy outline. Subsequently, proven primary tuberculosis.*

THE EQUIVOCAL HILUM — IS IT ENLARGED?

First — make sure that rotation is not causing one hilum to appear more conspicuous than the other. This is a very common explanation for a seemingly enlarged hilum. All the same, deciding whether a hilum is abnormal is a common problem. Even the experts have the occasional difficulty.

Second — always enquire if a previous CXR is available for comparison. If a previous CXR is not available, then ask yourself three questions. If the hilum is normal then the answer to all three questions will be "yes".

Question 1   Is the left hilum in a normal position? The left hilum must never be lower than the right hilum.

Question 2   Do the branches of the pulmonary artery clearly originate from the site of concern? Normal arteries can be prominent and give an initial impression that enlarged lymph nodes are present.

Question 3   Are the densities of the two hila approximately equal? Anything more than a slight difference in density always raises the suspicion that there is abnormal tissue at the hilum — e.g. a hilar mass.

If the answer to any of these three questions is in the negative, then an experienced observer should be asked to give an opinion.

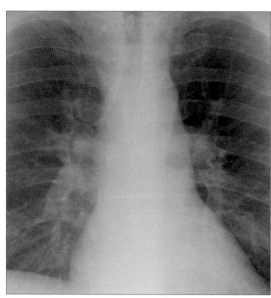

Figure 6.10   *Both hila appear prominent. However, the hilar vee sites have a normal relationship to each other, normal arteries branch from both right and left pulmonary arteries, and the density of each hilum is equal and within normal limits. Normal CXR.*

WHY IS THE HILUM ENLARGED?

An enlarged hilum may be due to large nodes, tumour infiltration, or enlarged arteries (Table 6.1). These are the features to assess:

- Nodes are lumpy, bumpy.

- Arterial enlargement:

  - Arteries will be seen to be emerging from the hilar "mass"; i.e. the arteries can be traced into and are seen to be part of the "mass".

  - Vessels always have smooth margins.

  - In pulmonary arterial hypertension the arteries in the outer two-thirds of each lung are disproportionately smaller (diameter) than those at the hila.

- Compare with previous CXRs. Lack of change, or obvious interval change, will often favour a particular diagnosis.

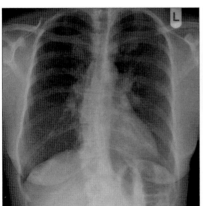

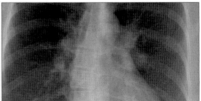

Figure 6.11 *Both hila are prominent. They show a lumpy, bumpy outline. Lymphoma.*

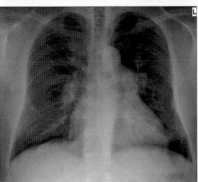

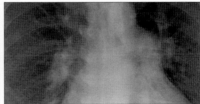

Figure 6.12 *Both hila are prominent. The margins of the hilar vessels are smooth. Smaller arteries emerge and are continuous with the right and left pulmonary arteries. Pulmonary arterial hypertension.*

Table 6.1 Synopsis: causes of hilar enlargement[2,5,7,8].

Unilateral	Bilateral
■ Infection	■ Sarcoidosis
❏ tuberculosis	■ Tumour
❏ viral infection in children	❏ metastases
■ Vascular	❏ lymphoma
❏ pulmonary artery stenosis	■ Vascular
❏ pulmonary artery aneurysm	❏ pulmonary arterial hypertension (chronic obstructive pulmonary disease; mitral valve disease; left-to-right shunt; recurrent pulmonary embolism)
■ Tumour	
❏ lymph nodes (metastases; lymphoma; bronchial carcinoma)	■ Infection
	❏ tuberculosis (occasionally)

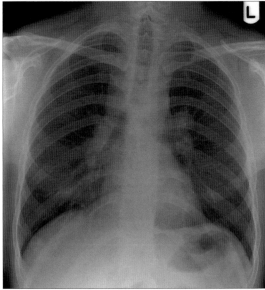

Figure 6.13 *Both hila are enlarged and lumpy, bumpy. Additional right paratracheal shadowing. Lymphadenopathy. This pattern of lymph node enlargement (both hila and right paratracheal) is highly suggestive of sarcoidosis.*

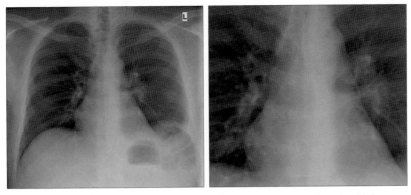

Figure 6.14 *Enlarged left hilum. It has a lumpy bumpy appearance. Associated left pleural effusion. Primary tuberculosis.*

REFERENCES

1. Felson B. Chest Roentgenology. Philadelphia, PA: WB Saunders, 1973.

2. Fraser RG, Muller NL, Colman NC, Pare PD. Fraser and Pare's Diagnosis of Diseases of the Chest. 4th ed. Philadelphia, PA: WB Saunders, 1999.

3. Armstrong P. Personal communication and discussion, 2007.

4. Ryan S, McNicholas M, Eustace S. Anatomy for Diagnostic Imaging. 2nd ed. Philadelphia, PA: WB Saunders, 2004.

5. Hansell DM, Armstrong P, Lynch DA, McAdams HP. Imaging of Diseases of the Chest. 4th ed. St Louis, MO: Mosby, 2005.

6. Collins J, Stern EJ. Chest Radiology: The Essentials. Philadelphia, PA: Lipincott, Williams & Wilkins, 1999.

7. Nunes H, Brillet PY, Valevre D et al. Imaging in sarcoidosis. Semin Respir Crit Care Med 2007; 28: 102–120.

8. Haramati LB, Choi Y, Widrow CA et al. Isolated lymphadenopathy on chest radiographs of HIV infected patients. Clin Radiol 1996; 51: 345–349.

7 PLEURAL ABNORMALITIES

In this chapter we address several different processes that affect the pleura. The main emphasis is on pleural effusion and pneumothorax.

> Pleura = singular;   Pleurae = plural;   Derivation from the Greek (pleura: side or rib)

BASIC ANATOMY

The pleura can be likened to a sac enveloping the lung. This sac has two membranous walls—the inner visceral and the outer parietal.

The pleura is not visible on a normal CXR except where it forms part of a lung fissure or where the two lungs abut each other in the midline (p. 114).

The pleural space is a closed cavity between the layers of the visceral and parietal pleura (Fig. 7.1). A small amount of lubricating fluid lies within the cavity. The lung fissures extend between the lobes of each lung and are lined by two layers of visceral pleura (Figs 7.3–7.5).

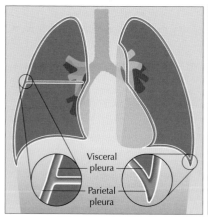

Figure 7.1 *The pleural sac, showing the visceral and parietal pleural membranes. The visceral pleura extends into and lines both sides of the horizontal fissure.*

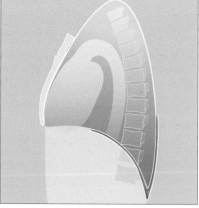

Figure 7.2 *The inferior extent of the posterior pleural space is well shown on the lateral projection. This posterior depth is considerable and not obvious from the frontal CXR.*

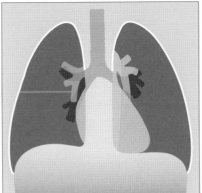

Figure 7.3 *Horizontal fissure. As with all the lung fissures it is formed by two layers of visceral pleura. There is a potential space between the two closely opposed layers.*

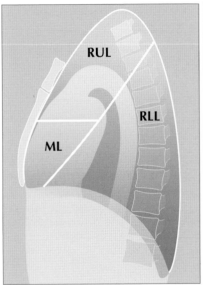

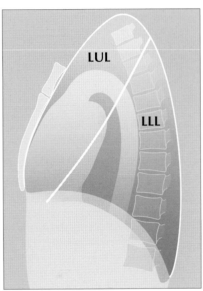

Figure 7.4 *The oblique fissure and the horizontal fissure separating the three lobes of the right lung. RUL = right upper lobe; ML = middle lobe; RLL = right lower lobe. Three anatomical points to note: (1) This lung differs from the left lung primarily because the fissures divide it into three lobes. (2) The high position of the apical segment of the lower lobe is often not appreciated. (3) A sliver of the middle lobe touches the anterior aspect of the right dome of the diaphragm.*

Figure 7.5 *The oblique fissure separating the two lobes of the left lung. LUL = left upper lobe; LLL = left lower lobe. Three anatomical points to note: (1) The single fissure divides this lung into two lobes only. (2) The high position of the apical segment of the lower lobe is often not appreciated… particularly when only a frontal CXR is obtained and a lesion is present in this lower lobe segment. (3) A sliver of the upper lobe touches the anterior aspect of the left dome of the diaphragm.*

PLEURAL EFFUSION

The pleura is composed of a dynamic membrane of mesothelial cells and a deeper layer of connective tissue containing vessels, nerves and lymphatics. This membrane responds actively to adjacent inflammation and to accumulations of fluid (e.g. from heart failure) within its space.

RECOGNISING THAT A PLEURAL EFFUSION IS PRESENT

Fluid in the pleural space can adopt several different appearances on both erect and supine CXRs[1–3].

On the erect frontal CXR

■ The commonest appearance is an opaque meniscus at a costophrenic angle. It requires approximately 200–300 ml pleural fluid to efface the normal sharp recess between the diaphragm and the ribs (Fig. 7.6a).

■ If the effusion is very large, then the entire hemithorax may be opaque (Chapter 19) and the heart may be pushed towards the normal side (Fig. 7.6c).

■ There are other patterns:

❏ Lamellar. A linear (lamellar) shadow (Fig. 7.7) paralleling the lateral aspect of the lung.

❏ Encysted. Loculation within a fissure or elsewhere (Fig. 7.8).

❏ Subpulmonary. Pooling within the pleural space below the lung. This is a subpulmonary effusion and is a relatively common occurrence. A subpulmonary effusion is usually easier to detect on the left side, where the pool can cause the gastric air bubble to appear widely separate from the (apparent) superior margin of the diaphragm (Fig. 7.11). The normal distance between the dome of the diaphragm and the air in the stomach does not normally exceed 7 mm in 98% of people aged 50 years and over (see Chapter 16, p. 242).

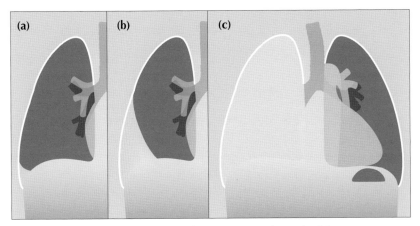

Figure 7.6 *From the frontal CXR a rough assessment can be made of the volume of pleural fluid. (a) Approximately 200–300 ml. (b) Approximately 2 litres. (c) Approximately 5 litres.*

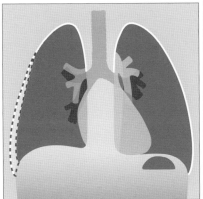

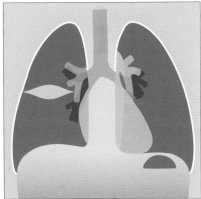

Figure 7.7 *A lamellar pleural effusion on the right side.*

Figure 7.8 *An encysted pleural effusion. The fluid has collected between the two layers of the pleura lining the horizontal fissure. The oval or rounded shadow can sometimes be mistaken for a lung tumour.*

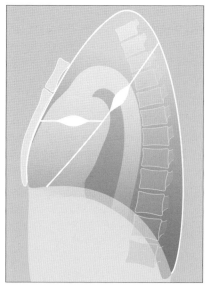

Figure 7.9 *Two separate encysted effusions. One is in the horizontal fissure. The other is in the right oblique fissure. Encysted effusions can occur anywhere in the pleural space. They occur most commonly in patients who are in heart failure.*

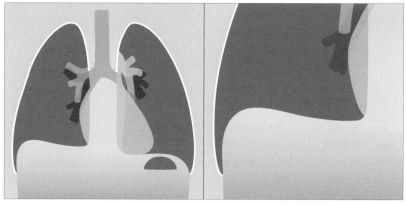

Figure 7.10 *Subpulmonary effusion on the right side. This puddle of fluid is often difficult to distinguish from a high dome of the diaphragm. A helpful characteristic: whereas the highest point on a normal dome is invariably central, the highest point on the (apparent) dome is situated laterally when a subpulmonary effusion is present.*

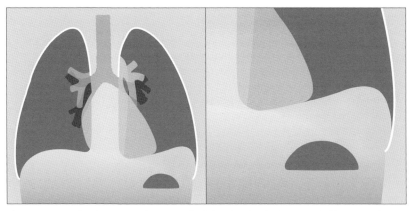

Figure 7.11 *Subpulmonary effusion on the left side. The fluid has pooled between the visceral and parietal pleura at the base of the lung. It simulates an elevated dome of the diaphragm. Note the low position of the pushed down gastric air bubble; also, the highest point of the "dome" is situated laterally.*

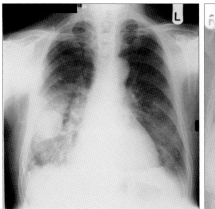

Figure 7.12 *Encysted fluid in the horizontal fissure. Patient in heart failure. Alveolar pulmonary oedema is evident.*

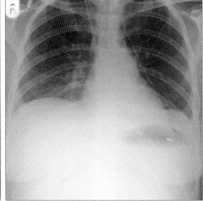

Figure 7.13 *Left subpulmonary effusion. The pool of fluid is displacing the gastric air bubble inferiorly.*

On the supine CXR

When the patient is supine, pleural fluid layers out in the posterior part of the pleural space. This causes the hemithorax to appear whiter or paler grey than the normal side. In most instances the normal lung vessels will be seen through this shadowing. Approximately 200 ml of fluid needs to be present before an abnormal pale grey appearance is produced[2,3].

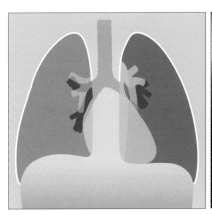

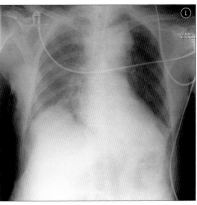

Figure 7.14 *The appearance of a (right) pleural effusion on a supine CXR. The pleural space needs to contain approximately 200 ml fluid before the abnormal hemithorax appears paler than the opposite normal side.*

Figure 7.15 *Patient in ITU. A right-sided pleural effusion has layered out posteriorly. The right hemithorax is paler than the left hemithorax. Lung vessels are visible on the right side and this supports the diagnosis of pleural fluid rather than lung consolidation… but this distinction can sometimes be difficult.*

A frequent puzzle: A patient is very ill, e.g. in the intensive therapy unit (ITU). The CXR shows basal shadowing. Is it mainly fluid or mainly consolidation?

■ In practice, most of these patients have some pleural fluid and some lung consolidation.

■ On a supine CXR it can be very difficult (usually impossible) to determine if the shadowing is predominantly fluid. If thoracocentesis is considered as a therapeutic option then an ultrasound examination will confirm or exclude a significant volume of pleural fluid. Alternatively, a lateral decubitus CXR (p. 231) will usually clarify.

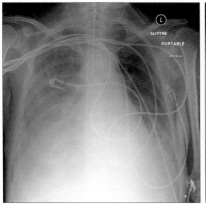

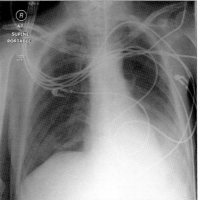

Figure 7.16 *Supine CXR. A large right pleural effusion has layered out posteriorly.*

Figure 7.17 *Supine CXR. This is the same patient as in Fig. 7.16—on the same day after the large right effusion had been drained. Incidentally, some pleural fluid is also evident on the left side.*

A "WHITE OUT" CAUSED BY A MASSIVE PLEURAL EFFUSION

A completely white hemithorax, often referred to as a "white out", may be caused by a large volume (5–7 litres) of pleural fluid (Fig. 7.18). There are other causes for a CXR white out. These are described in Chapter 19, pp. 264–267.

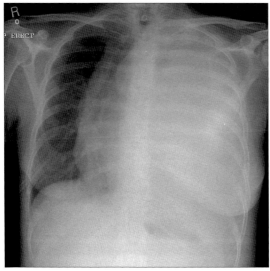

Figure 7.18 *A large left-sided pleural effusion has produced a white out and displaced the trachea and mediastinum to the right side.*

EMPYEMA

■ Pus in the pleural space. Most commonly due to pneumonia. Other causes include trauma, infection outside the thorax, thoracic surgery.

■ The appearance on the CXR is essentially the same as that of an uninfected pleural effusion. The diagnosis is usually arrived at by combining evidence of sepsis, pleural fluid on the CXR, and organisms found on needle aspiration.

■ Sometimes an organised empyema will form a walled-off collection, seen as a round or oval shape indenting the lung (Figs 7.19 and 7.20).

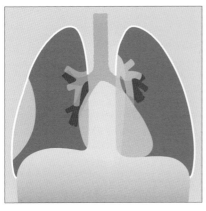

Figure 7.19 *The right-sided shadow represents an encysted pleural collection; the collection may be sterile or it may represent an empyema.*

PLEURAL FIBROSIS / THICKENING

ORDINARY PLEURAL THICKENING

This thickening usually occurs at one of two sites:

■ At a costophrenic angle as a result of a previous pleural infection. Occasionally it is consequent on a haemorrhagic effusion following trauma. The appearance of fibrotic blunting of a costophrenic angle may be very similar to a small (300 ml) pleural effusion. The overall clinical picture or previous clinical history or a previous CXR will usually help to make the distinction. If there is doubt whether blunting might be fluid, a lateral decubitus radiograph (p. 231) or ultrasound will clarify.

■ Over the apex of one or both lungs. The cause: either old lung infection (e.g. tuberculosis) or due to compression of lung and pleural tissue by small apical bullae. The concern: if the appearance is unilateral then it can appear identical to a flat apical (Pancoast) carcinoma. See Chapter 10, p. 142. Comparison with a previous CXR often provides reassurance.

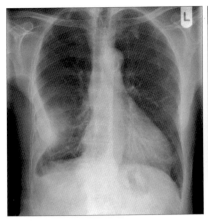

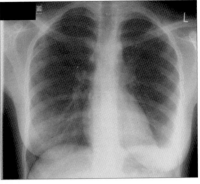

Figure 7.21   *Chest infection. A small (approximately 500 ml) left-sided pleural effusion. Note that a lamellar component, or configuration is also present.*

Figure 7.20   *Encysted pleural effusion. The collection contained organisms…an empyema.*

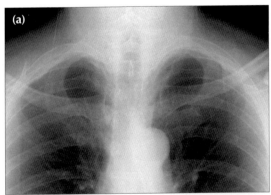

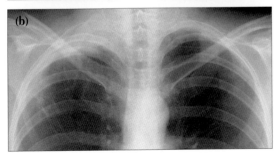

Figure 7.22   *Lung apices can be difficult. Patient (a): normal left apex; benign apical pleural thickening on the right side. Patient (b) shows a right apical appearance which is very similar to patient (a). This proved to be a flat apical carcinoma (Pancoast tumour).*

PLEURAL PLAQUES[4]

Plaques are focal areas of thickening of the parietal pleura due to previous exposure to asbestos. Characteristically they appear as scattered islands of well circumscribed pleural densities (Figs 7.23–7.25). Plaques:

■ Are most commonly seen posteriorly and laterally, predominantly affecting the lower third of the thorax.

■ Do not involve the costophrenic angles.

■ May be calcified; sometimes extensively.

■ Are unilateral in 25% of cases.

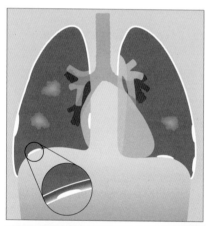

Figure 7.23 *To show the various appearances of asbestos related pleural plaques. Seen en face the plaques (two on the right side, one on the left side) appear as islands of low density projected over the lung. In profile, when calcified, they appear as areas of high density against the lateral margins of the thorax, heart, vertebrae and over the domes of the diaphragm. The inset shows that the plaques represent areas of thickening of the parietal pleura.*

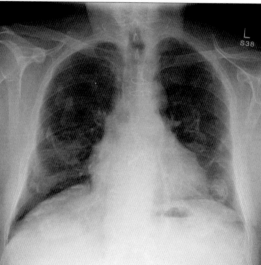

Figure 7.24 *Bilateral mid and lower zone pleural plaques. Some are calcified. The characteristic very high density of the calcified plaques is well-shown in profile. Where seen en face (mid and lower zones of both lungs), the plaques appear ill-defined and of low density.*

PLEURAL CALCIFICATION

When it is due to asbestos:

■ The parietal pleura covering the domes of the diaphragm is most commonly affected.

■ Plaque calcification can be very extensive; usually bilateral.

■ Non-calcified plaques may also be present.

Other causes of pleural calcification include haemorrhagic effusion, pleural infection +/− empyema (including tuberculosis), and talc inhalation. Usually these causes result in unilateral calcification.

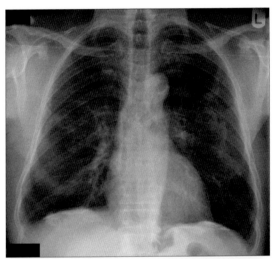

Figure 7.25 *Asbestos related pleural plaques. Some of these plaques are calcified. In this patient they mainly involve the parietal pleura overlying the domes of the diaphragm.*

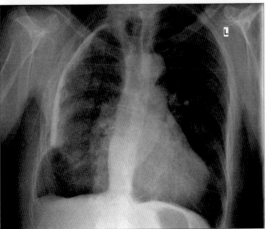

Figure 7.26 *Extensive unilateral pleural calcification. Previous tuberculosis.*

PLEURAL TUMOURS

A pleural tumour, whether a primary pleural neoplasm or a secondary deposit from (say) a breast carcinoma, will commonly present with an accompanying effusion (Fig. 7.27).

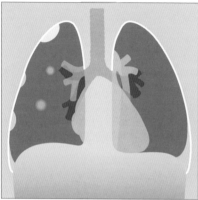

Figure 7.27 *Pleural metastases. Nodular metastatic deposits (right hemithorax). Note the small pleural effusion. On the left side no focal lesion is seen other than the pleural effusion. The left pleural appearance is more typical of metastatic disease to the pleura—i.e. the CXR usually shows a pleural effusion only.*

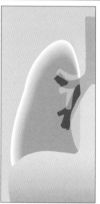
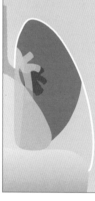

Figure 7.28 *To illustrate some of the various features that can be seen on a CXR in a patient with a mesothelioma. An extensive pleural mass, sometimes creating an encasement or "peel" surrounding the lung[5]. A smaller or shrunken ipsilateral hemithorax. A pleural effusion.*

An occasional dilemma

A frontal CXR shows a discrete mass hard up against a pleural surface. Is it in the lung, e.g. bronchial carcinoma? Is it arising from the pleura, e.g. breast deposit? Is it a rib lesion indenting the pleura and the lung, e.g. a rib metastasis? Table 7.1 indicates the CXR features that you should look for.

Table 7.1 Pulmonary mass vs Pleural mass vs Extrapleural mass.

Origin	Characteristic CXR features
Intrapulmonary lesion abutting a pleural surface	■ Margins clear and well-defined. ■ Interface between the pleura and the lesion forms an acute angle.

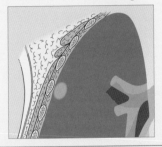 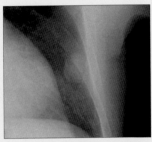

| Intrapleural mass indenting the lung | ■ Viewed *en face* its margins appear ill-defined.
■ Viewed in profile—only one border is sharply defined.
■ Interface between the pleura and the lesion forms an obtuse angle. |

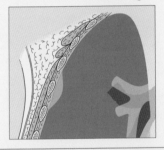 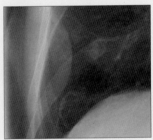

| Extrapleural mass but intruding on to or into the lung | ■ As for an intrapleural mass. And…
■ Almost always an abnormal rib. Most extrapleural lesions arise in a rib (e.g. metastatic deposit; simple fracture with haematoma). |

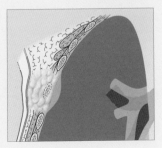 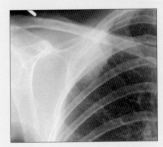

PNEUMOTHORAX[6-13]

Pneumothoraces are common and the erect CXR is usually definitive. Sometimes the CXR appearances are subtle. There are multiple aspects that we need to be familiar with when assessing erect or supine CXRs.

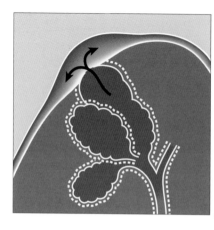

Figure 7.29 *Primary spontaneous pneumothorax. An apical pleural bleb thins the visceral pleural membrane. The alveolar wall and the visceral pleura "pop" and air passes from the alveolar bleb into the pleural space.*

PNEUMOTHORAX—RULES

You need to bear in mind the following:

■ Small can be difficult…"you only see what you look for".

■ Erect or supine…"you must look in the correct place".

■ On a supine CXR…"you only look for what your know".

■ Tension pneumothorax can kill…quickly.

■ Beware the regular imposters…skin fold, clothing artefact, tubes, lines.

PNEUMOTHORAX—CAUSES

The groups of individuals who are most at risk of developing a pneumothorax are indicated in Table 7.2.

Table 7.2   Causes of pneumothorax.

Spontaneous—primary	Spontaneous—secondary	Traumatic/iatrogenic/other
Healthy young adults	Pre-existing lung disease	■ Blunt trauma
■ Age 20–40 years	■ Chronic obstructive pulmonary disease	■ Penetrating trauma
■ Male:Female 6:1		■ Placement of central line
■ No known lung disease	■ Cavitating pneumonia	■ Lung biopsy
	■ Pleural metastases	■ Aspiration of pleural fluid
■ Rupture of a subpleural bleb. A bleb (Fig. 7.29) is an outpouching of the alveolar wall; it bulges and thins the visceral pleural membrane. In general, blebs are present at the lung apices only.		■ Thoracic surgery
		■ Mechanical ventilation
		■ Acute asthma
		■ Smoking cocaine or marijuana

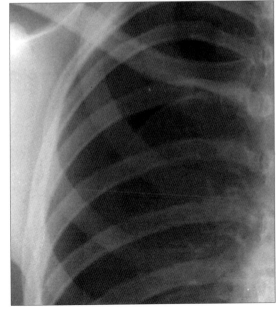

Figure 7.30 *Large pneumothorax. The diagnosis is easy.*

PNEUMOTHORAX—DETECTION

The erect CXR

Three principles:

1. You must exclude a pneumothorax in any patient with pleuritic chest pain or unexplained breathlessness.

2. You must hunt for the evidence. A brief glance at the CXR and you will miss a small pneumothorax.

3. You must know where to hunt—always, always double check the lung apices.

Three cardinal features:

1. A clearly defined line (i.e. the visceral pleura) is visible in profile. It parallels the chest wall.

2. The upper part of the line is curved at the lung apex...i.e. it parallels the internal contour of the thorax. Overlapping ribs can be a problem—keep looking through and between the ribs.

3. An absence of lung markings, i.e. vessels, between the lung edge and the chest wall.

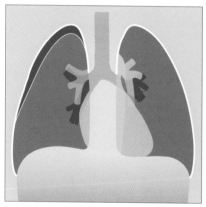 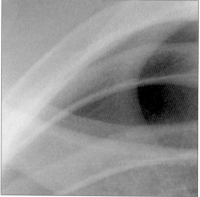

Figure 7.31 *Erect CXR. A shallow pneumothorax. Curved visceral pleural membrane at the lung apex and no vessels lateral to the visceral pleural line.*

Figure 7.32 *Erect CXR. Shallow pneumothorax. The visceral pleural line is visible.*

Three tricks — if in doubt:

1. An erect CXR obtained in full expiration. This can assist in making the pneumothorax easier to see because lung density increases on expiration.

   Or

2. A lateral decubitus CXR (p. 231) with the suspect side raised. Even a very small volume of intrapleural air will rise and outline the visceral pleura along the lateral margin of the lung.

   Or

3. CT. The ultra-sensitive test.

The supine CXR — a pneumothorax can be very subtle[8,9]

A severely injured patient or a patient in ITU will not be able to sit up. The patient may have extensive lung pathology, e.g. haemorrhage, pneumonia, adult respiratory distress syndrome (ARDS). These factors can affect the position and appearance of air in the pleural space. Remember, an unrecognised pneumothorax may develop into a life-threatening tension pneumothorax in a patient treated with positive pressure ventilation.

Intrapleural air may accumulate in several different positions when a patient is supine. Two areas need to be inspected particularly carefully.

1. Lung base inspection (Figs 7.33–7.37).

■ In the supine position the highest part of the pleural space is at the lung base under the inferior surface of the lung. The lowermost part of the CXR will hold the evidence (Fig. 7.33).

■ Look for:

   ❑ A hyperlucent (i.e. blacker) upper quadrant of the abdomen…blacker because air collecting at the base of the lung overlies the liver (Fig. 7.34).

   ❑ Air situated in the lateral costophrenic sulcus (the most lateral and inferior aspect of the pleural space)…the so called "deep sulcus sign" (Fig. 7.34).

   ❑ A sharply outlined dome of the diaphragm (Fig. 7.37). This appearance may be particularly prominent if there is adjacent lower lobe pulmonary disease (e.g. pneumonia or ARDS).

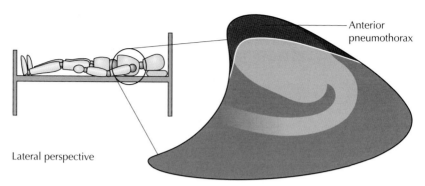

Anterior
pneumothorax

Lateral perspective

Figure 7.33 *Pneumothorax. On a supine CXR the air rises to the highest point in the pleural space — i.e. anteriorly.*

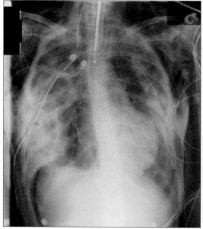

Figure 7.34 *Supine CXR. Right-sided pneumothorax showing: (a) a hyperlucent right upper quadrant of the abdomen; and (b) a deep sulcus sign (i.e. intrapleural air collected in the lateral costophrenic sulcus).*

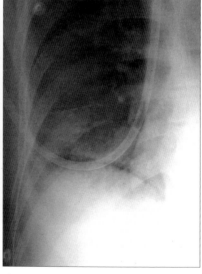

Figure 7.35 *Supine CXR. Right-sided pneumothorax revealed by the very sharply defined margin to the dome of the diaphragm. It is sharply defined despite the immediately adjacent lower lobe lung consolidation.*

2. Medial inspection

■ In the supine position the pleural air may collect anteromedially against the heart.

■ Look for:

  ❏ A deep and well-defined anterior cardiophrenic sulcus (Figs 7.36 and 7.37). The anterior cardiophrenic sulcus is the most medial part of the pleural space, lying hard up against the inferior margin of the heart. If it appears deep and well-defined, this may be the earliest sign of a small pneumothorax.

  ❏ A sharply defined cardiac border...clear and crisp.

  ❏ A sharply defined pericardial fat pad.

  ❏ A sharply defined margin of the anterior junction line. This line may also be displaced away from the midline. (See Chapter 8, p. 114).

A PROBLEM SOLVED

ITU patient has ARDS. CXR—equivocal pneumothorax.

Confirm or refute:

■ With a lateral decubitus bedside CXR with the suspect side raised and utilising a horizontal x-ray beam (p. 231).

■ Or by leaving the patient supine and obtaining a horizontal beam lateral CXR.

■ Or by taking the patient to CT.

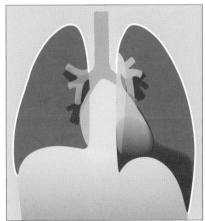

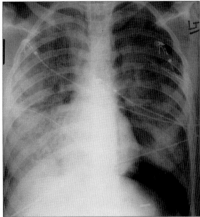

Figure 7.36 *Supine radiograph. Left pneumothorax. The left dome of the diaphragm is sharply defined, and the left cardiac border has a fine black margin compared with the right side.*

Figure 7.37 *ARDS. Supine CXR. A left pneumothorax is revealed by the well-defined dome of the diaphragm and the sharply defined left heart border.*

TENSION PNEUMOTHORAX[10,11,13]

A medical emergency. As air enters the pleural space the normal negative intrapleural pressure (approximately –5 mmHg) becomes atmospheric. Sometimes a valve-like effect occurs and air continues to enter but cannot exit the pleural cavity. The pressure then rises above atmospheric. This build up of tension can cause compression of the inferior vena cava and obstruction to the venous return to the right side of the heart. This is potentially—and rapidly—lethal.

In most instances, the recognition of a tension pneumothorax is primarily a clinical diagnosis. Immediate treatment without recourse to a CXR is mandatory.

Underlying pulmonary or pleural disease (e.g. a patient with a stiff lung) can cause clinical confusion because some of the typical clinical findings—dyspnoea, chest pain, cough, tracheal deviation, diminished breath sounds, cyanosis—may not be present. Therefore it is essential to be familiar with the CXR findings indicating a tension pneumothorax. Two cardinal features to look for:

1. The ipsilateral dome of the diaphragm is nearly always depressed and flattened.

2. The mediastinum and heart are usually—but not always—pushed to the opposite side.

Recognition on an erect CXR

The visceral pleura is visible, and no vessels are seen beyond the visceral pleural line; the dome of the diaphragm, in most instances, is depressed, flattened or inverted, and the mediastinum is usually displaced towards the opposite side.

ACTION: Urgent placement of a cannula anteriorly. Ideally in the triangle of safety (Fig. 7.40)[14,15].

Recognition on a supine CXR

Findings as for the erect CXR, but stiff or diseased lung (e.g. extensive pneumonia or ARDS) will sometimes produce a deceptive appearance. Deceptive because the lung may be too solid to collapse or the mediastinum may not be displaced. However, the dome of the diaphragm will usually be flattened/inverted by the raised intrapleural pressure.

ACTION: Urgent placement of a cannula.

The important clinical rule

If the CXR shows evidence of a pneumothorax but the radiographic findings of a tension are equivocal then manage clinically. In other words, if tension is suspected on the clinical findings—then treat as for tension.

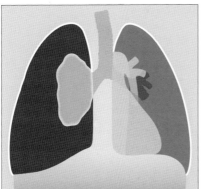

Figure 7.38 *Tension pneumothorax with total collapse of the right lung. Note the displacement of the mediastinum to the left side and the flattened (in this case inverted) dome of the diaphragm.*

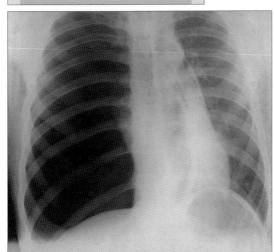

Figure 7.39 *Tension pneumothorax. Note that the dome of the diaphragm is flattened and the mediastinum is displaced to the left side.*

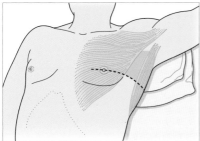

Figure 7.40 *Pneumothorax. Safe insertion of an intercostal drain—within the triangle of safety[14,15]. The margins of the triangle are: the anterior border of the latissimus dorsi, the lateral border of the pectoralis major, a horizontal line at the level of the nipple defining the base of the triangle, and the apex of the triangle just below the axilla. This triangle is the optimum position for insertion of a drain in a non-emergency situation. It is also the preferred site for drain insertion in an emergency when a tension pneumothorax is diagnosed.*

An occasional pitfall—mediastinal displacement

A simple pneumothorax—not under tension—can cause mediastinal displacement towards the opposite, normal, side (Fig. 7.41). This can occur when the underlying lung is completely collapsed. The elastic recoil of the lung is no longer counterbalanced by the normal negative pressure in the pleural space. As a consequence the mediastinum moves towards the normal side[5].

A useful guideline: if the ipsilateral dome of the diaphragm is not depressed or flattened do not rush to judgement. A flattened dome is almost always evident when tension is present in the pleural space—though this does not occur in 100% of cases[5].

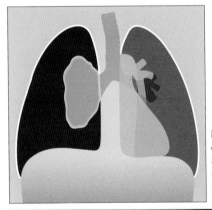

Figure 7.41 *Mediastinal displacement—but not a tension pneumothorax. Note that the ipsilateral dome of the diaphragm is neither flattened nor depressed.*

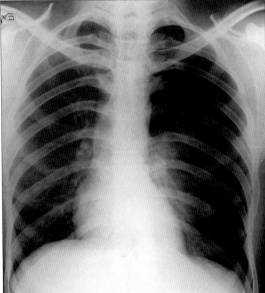

Figure 7.42 *Large left pneumothorax. Note the displacement of the mediastinum towards the right side—but the left dome of the diaphragm is neither depressed nor flattened. This was not a tension pneumothorax.*

HAEMO- OR HYDRO-PNEUMOTHORAX

Many patients with a spontaneous pneumothorax, whether primary or secondary, will show a little fluid in the pleural space. Usually this is a small amount of blood resulting from a tear of a pleural adhesion.

If a moderate size haemo- or hydro-pneumothorax is present, then an air–fluid level, i.e. a straight line, will be seen at the air–fluid interface (Figs 7.43 and 7.44).

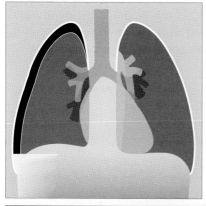

Figure 7.43 *The air–fluid level within the pleural space indicates the presence of a haemo- or hydro-pneumothorax.*

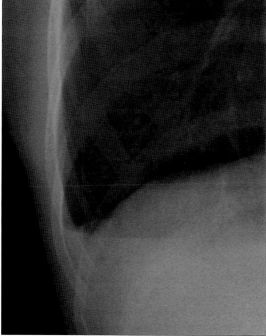

Figure 7.44 *Haemo-pneumothorax. The straight line represents an air–fluid interface.*

AN OCCASIONAL PUZZLE

Clinically a patient has a pneumothorax, but air is also seen elsewhere in the mediastinum or chest wall. How did it get there? There are two possibilities[5]:

1. A ruptured alveolus

   In some patients (e.g. an asthmatic or treatment with positive pressure ventilation) a pneumothorax does not result from rupture of the visceral pleural membrane. Instead an increase in intra-alveolar pressure causes rupture of an alveolus or a bronchiole, and air dissects through the lung parenchyma along the sheaths of the pulmonary vessels to the hilum and thence into the mediastinum. This mediastinal air can then rupture through the mediastinal parietal pleura and so produce a pneumothorax. Because the mediastinal tissue planes are contiguous with those of the neck and the retroperitoneum the dissecting air from the ruptured alveolus can also cause extensive mediastinal and surgical emphysema (Fig. 7.45).

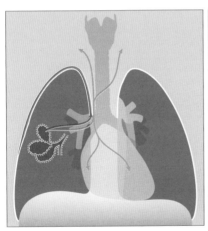

Figure 7.45 *To illustrate the mechanism underlying the development of both a pneumothorax and mediastinal emphysema in a patient with asthma. The ruptured alveolus has caused pulmonary interstitial emphysema (PIE) and the air has dissected through the lung to reach the hilum. The air then dissects into the mediastinum and it also crosses the parietal pleura adjacent to the mediastinum to enter the pleural space.*

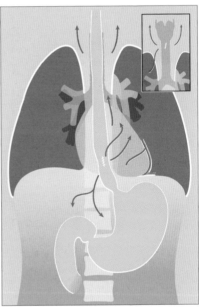

Figure 7.46 *(a) Vomiting. A tear has developed in the oesophagus. Swallowed air escapes and dissects through the surrounding soft tissues to cause mediastinal emphysema. This may extend laterally and rupture the parietal pleura, causing a pneumothorax. (b) Trauma. A tear of the trachea.*

2. Rupture of the trachea or oesophagus

If either of these structures rupture (e.g. external trauma or an oesophageal tear due to vomiting) then air can dissect along the mediastinal tissue planes. The air may then rupture through the mediastinal parietal pleura and enter the pleural space (Fig. 7.46). Occasionally it is the pneumothorax which is the dominant CXR finding, not the surgical emphysema.

PNEUMOTHORAX SIZE—IMPACT ON TREATMENT[10–12,15]

▪ Some physicians regard the CXR as a poor tool for measuring the size of a pneumothorax, and they emphasise that it is the clinical status of the patient not the radiographic size of a pneumothorax that should influence the decision as to the appropriate treatment[11].

▪ Other physicians utilise the CXR to estimate the size of a pneumothorax in order to help choose between treatment options. Approximate measurements can be made (Fig. 7.47). These descriptive terms are in common usage:

❑ **A small pneumothorax** is one in which the distance (i.e. the rim) between the visceral pleura and the internal chest wall is less than 2 cm.

❑ **A large pneumothorax** is one in which this distance (or rim) measures more than 2 cm.

Why are rim measurements regarded as useful? A rim with a diameter of 2 cm equates to a pneumothorax which occupies approximately 50% of the volume of the hemithorax. At this size, and if clinically indicated, the pneumothorax can be treated safely by aspiration[12,15].

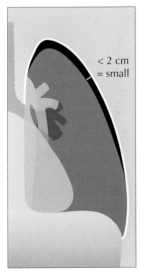
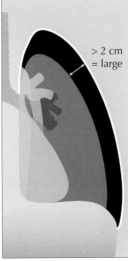

< 2 cm = small

> 2 cm = large

Figure 7.47 *Erect CXR. Pneumothorax. Measurement of the rim allows a pneumothorax to be classified as either small or large.*

PNEUMOTHORAX: SOME IMPOSTERS

■ Common: a white line on the CXR may be misread as the visceral pleural line. These spurious shadows include clothing artefacts, hair plaits, skin wrinkles (Fig. 7.48), venous lines or tubing, an overlying scapula margin.

■ Uncommon: the Great Pretender...a large bulla (Fig. 7.49).

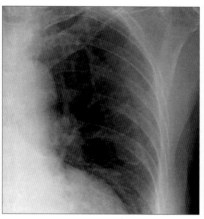

Figure 7.48   *Not a pneumothorax. The fine line crossing the left hemithorax is a wrinkle, or fold, of the skin.*

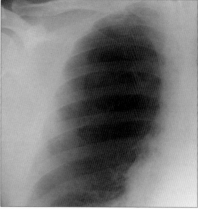

Figure 7.49   *Not a pneumothorax. A large bulla. Note that there is no evidence of a visceral pleural line. On an erect CXR a pleural line is almost always evident when a pneumothorax is present.*

AN INTERESTING CONDITION— CATAMENIAL PNEUMOTHORAX[16]

Aetiology / pathology

Recurrent pneumothorax occurring only in relation to menstruation. Pathogenesis remains speculative. One suggestion is that air enters the peritoneal cavity via the unplugged cervix during menstruation. The air then enters the pleural space via a leaky diaphragm. It is of interest that some patients do have pelvic or diaphragmatic endometriosis.

Clinical features

Recurrent pneumothoraces occurring within 48–74 hours of onset of a menstrual period. Women aged 30–40 years are most commonly affected.

The CXR

The pneumothorax is usually on the right side and is small.

REFERENCES

1. Raasch BN, Carsky EW, Lane EJ et al. Pleural effusion: explanation of some typical appearances. AJR 1982; 139: 899–904.

2. Woodring JH. Recognition of pleural effusion on supine radiographs: how much fluid is required? AJR 1984; 142: 59–64.

3. Emamian SA, Kaasbol MA, Olsen JF et al. Accuracy of the diagnosis of pleural effusion on supine chest x-ray. Eur Radiol 1997; 7: 57–60.

4. Schwartz DA. New developments in asbestos related pleural disease. Chest 1991; 99: 191–198.

5. Fraser RG, Muller NL, Colman NC, Pare PD. Fraser and Pare's Diagnosis of Diseases of the Chest. 4th ed. Philadelphia, PA: WB Saunders, 1999.

6. O'Connor AR, Morgan WE. Radiological review of pneumothorax. BMJ 2005; 330: 1493–1497.

7. Seow A, Kazerooni EA, Pernican, PG et al. Comparison of upright inspiratory and expiratory chest radiographs for detecting pneumothoraces. AJR 1996; 166: 313–316.

8. Tocino IM. Pneumothorax in the supine patient: radiographic anatomy. Radiographics 1985; 5: 557–586.

9. Cummin ARC, Smith MJ, Wilson AG. Pneumothorax in the supine patient. BMJ 1987; 295: 591–592.

10. Baumann MH, Strange C, Heffner JE et al. Management of spontaneous pneumothorax. An American College of Chest Physicians Delphi consensus statement. Chest 2001; 119: 590–602.

11. Baumann MH, Strange C. Treatment of spontaneous pneumothorax: a more aggressive approach? Chest 1997; 112: 789–804.

12. Henry M, Arnold T, Harvey J. BTS guidelines for the management of spontaneous pneumothorax. Thorax 2003; 58(suppl ii): 39–52.

13. Teplick SK, Clark RE. Various faces of tension pneumothorax. Postgraduate Medicine 1974; 56: 87–92.

14. Laws D, Neville E, Duffy J. BTS guidelines for the insertion of a chest drain. Thorax 2003; 58(suppl): 55–59.

15. Griffiths JR, Roberts N. Do junior doctors know where to insert chest drains safely? Postgrad Med J 2005; 81: 456–458.

16. Carter EJ, Ettensohn DB. Catamenial pneumothorax. Chest 1990; 98: 713–716.

8 MEDIASTINUM: ANATOMY, MASSES AND AIR

The mediastinum is situated between the pleurae covering the medial aspects of the right and left lungs. Its borders are the thoracic inlet (superiorly), the diaphragm (inferiorly), the parietal pleurae (laterally), the vertebral column (posteriorly) and the sternum (anteriorly).

At the root of each lung the lateral parietal pleural boundary is absent.

ANATOMICAL COMPARTMENTS

Anatomists and surgeons use various classifications to define the mediastinal compartments. Felson[1] and Zylak[2] have pointed out that, in terms of CXR diagnosis, a simple longitudinal division is most relevant.

We like Felson's description[1]. He divided the mediastinum into three compartments — anterior, middle and posterior — there being no need to refer to a superior compartment.

The anatomical compartments are best understood with reference to the lateral CXR (Figs 8.1 and 8.2).

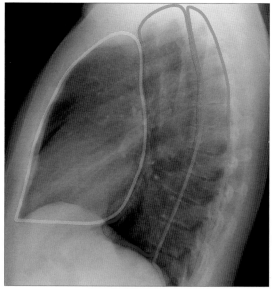

Figure 8.1 *The anterior, middle and posterior compartments of the mediastinum are easy to identify on the lateral CXR.*

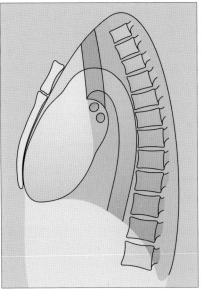

Figure 8.2 *The three anatomical compartments: anterior, middle and posterior—as described by Felson[1].*

Table 8.1 Mediastinal boundaries.

Compartment	Anteriorly	Posteriorly
Anterior	Sternum	Anterior aspect of trachea and posterior margin of heart
Middle	Anterior aspect of trachea and posterior margin of heart	A vertical line drawn along the thoracic vertebrae 1 cm behind their anterior margins
Posterior	Vertical line drawn along the thoracic vertebrae 1 cm behind their anterior margins	Costovertebral junctions

Table 8.2 Mediastinal contents.

Compartment	Main structures / tissues
Anterior	Fat, lymph nodes, thymus/thymic remnant, heart, ascending aorta
Middle	Trachea, bronchi, lymph nodes, oesophagus, descending aorta
Posterior	Paravertebral soft tissues

CXR APPEARANCES — NORMAL

FRONTAL CXR

In adults the normal mediastinal shadow is in effect the cardiac outline, the thoracic aorta, the superior vena cava, and the vessels arising from the aortic arch.

In young adults neither the aortic arch nor its vessels are prominent and they contribute very little to the outline of the mediastinum. In middle age unfolding of the aortic arch occurs. As we get even older, other vessels become tortuous and the mediastinal contour continues to widen and alter (Fig. 8.3).

Some normal mediastinal appearances on the frontal CXR may be confusing or puzzling; particularly fat collections (Figs 8.4 and 8.5) and various interface lines (Figs 8.6–8.13).

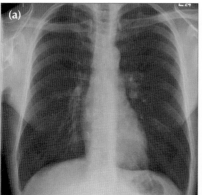

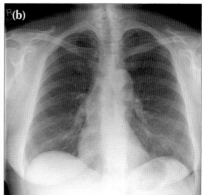

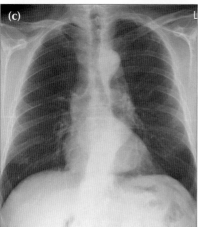

Figure 8.3 *The normal mediastinal outline can change with age. In particular, the ascending and descending aorta unfolds and becomes more prominent from middle age onwards. (a) Age 30. (b) Another patient, age 50. (c) An elderly patient, age 80.*

Fat collections[3]

Visible pads of fat are present at the right and/or left cardiophrenic angles in approximately 50% of patients aged 50 or older (see Chapter 16, p. 239). If a large fat collection is present it may:

- Cause part of the well-defined margin of the heart to be blurred.
- Mimic a mass lesion.

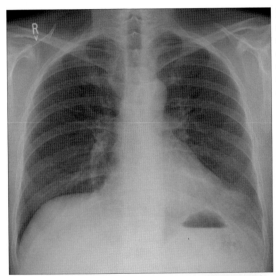

Figure 8.4   *The mediastinum often contains small or large collections of fat. In this patient a large fat collection (or pad) is situated at the left cardiophrenic angle.*

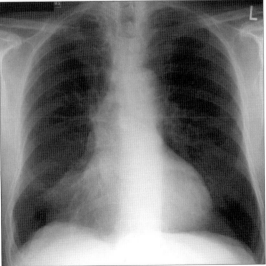

Figure 8.5   *A prominent fat pad blurs part of the right cardiac border. Sometimes this blurring is mistaken for middle lobe disease (see pp. 49 and 238).*

Interface lines and stripes

The air in the lung abuts various mediastinal structures. Where the interface is long and vertical it results in a longitudinal or slightly angled line on the CXR. These normal shadows can baffle the novice. Their occurrence on a CXR varies from individual to individual.

There are six mediastinal lines (stripes) that are regularly seen on normal CXRs. Two of these stripes can be helpful in detecting an abnormality. Specifically:

■ The right paratracheal stripe:

   ❑ Is formed where the right lung abuts the right side of the trachea.

   ❑ Is visible on approximately 60% of normal CXRs[1]. Also see our data in Chapter 16, p. 242).

NB: the left side of the trachea does not interface with the lung, so there is no matching stripe on the left side.

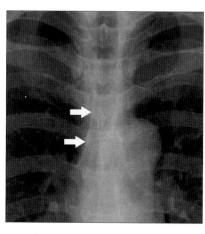

Figure 8.6 *A normal right paratracheal stripe (arrows). The stripe represents the right wall of the trachea outlined by the air in the trachea and the air in the adjacent right lung. The thickness of this stripe should not exceed 2.5 mm (see data on p. 242).*

■ The paravertebral stripes[4,5]:

   ❑ The left paravertebral stripe is visualised on almost all well-penetrated CXRs. This is because the descending aorta displaces the adjacent lung laterally. This displacement causes the pleural surface and lung edge to be seen tangentially as they pass lateral to the paravertebral soft tissues from front to back.

   ❑ A right paravertebral stripe is not visualised until middle age, when age related osteophytes are often present and may displace the adjacent pleura laterally (Fig. 8.8).

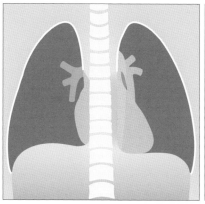

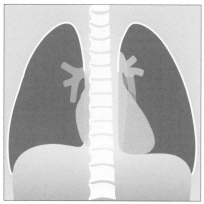

Figure 8.7 *Normal left paravertebral stripe (blue). Compare this with the CXR appearance in Fig. 8.9.*

Figure 8.8 *A right paravertebral stripe (blue) is rarely seen on a normal frontal CXR—unless age related osteophytes are present.*

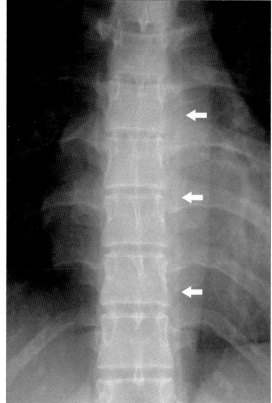

Figure 8.9 *Normal left paravertebral stripe (arrows). This is the interface between the lung and the paravertebral soft tissues. Note that a right paravertebral stripe is not evident.*

Four other lines or stripes also occur.

- Azygo-oesophageal line:
  - ❑ Formed where the right lung abuts the right side of the oesophagus and the azygos vein.
  - ❑ Extends below the aortic arch to the diaphragm (Fig. 8.10)
- Anterior junction line:
  - ❑ Formed where the two lungs abut each other anteriorly below the level of the manubrium (Fig. 8.11).
  - ❑ The line is made up of four layers of pleura (i.e. the parietal and visceral layers covering both lungs).
- Posterior junction line:
  - ❑ Formed where the two lungs abut each other posteriorly. It extends from above the clavicles to the level of the arch of the aorta (Fig. 8.12).
  - ❑ This line is also made up of four layers of pleura.
- Aorto-pulmonary stripe:
  - ❑ In some people a segment of mediastinal pleura does not blend with the outline of the mediastinum but is reflected as a straight line between the main pulmonary artery and the aortic arch (Fig. 8.13).

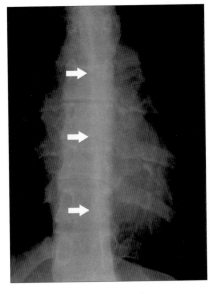

Figure 8.10 *Normal azygo-oesophageal line (arrows). This lung–soft tissue interface is visible on many CXRs.*

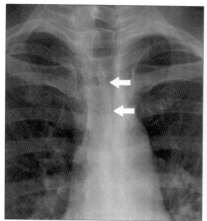

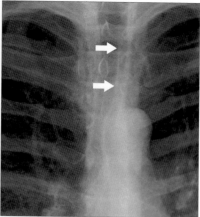

Figure 8.11 *The anterior junction line (arrows). An occasional normal finding.*

Figure 8.12 *The posterior junction line (arrows). Another normal appearance.*

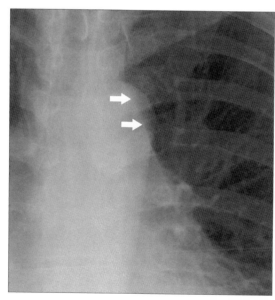

Figure 8.13 *The aorto-pulmonary stripe (arrows). A normal, but uncommon, appearance. It alters the usual configuration seen between the main pulmonary artery and the arch of the aorta. This normal variant (a pleural reflection) may cause confusion.*

LATERAL CXR

Mediastinal shadows show age related differences due to progressive unfolding of the ascending and descending thoracic aorta (see Chapter 2, Figs 2.32 and 2.33).

Fat collections and the cardiac incisura

Fat at the cardiophrenic angles (often a feature of middle-aged prosperity) are superimposed over each other on the lateral CXR. In addition, the apex of the heart intrudes onto and displaces part of the left lung. This combination of epicardial fat and the cardiac apex (the latter creating the cardiac incisura) sometimes produces a fairly dense shadow situated anteriorly (see Chapter 2, Figs 2.33 and 2.34).

Lines and stripes

Two stripes are visible on most lateral CXRs.

- The posterior tracheal stripe. This is produced by the interface between the posterior wall of the trachea and the adjacent lung (Fig. 8.14).

- The retrosternal soft tissue margin (or stripe). A small amount of fat and connective tissue lies between the parietal pleura and the sternum. On the lateral CXR this narrow soft tissue interface (it is only occasionally referred to as a stripe or a line) is readily visualised (Fig. 8.14).

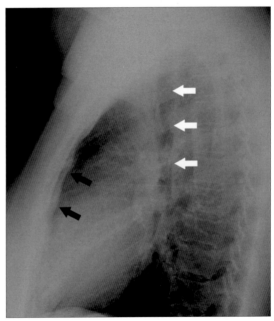

Figure 8.14 *The posterior tracheal stripe (white arrows). This stripe represents the posterior wall of the trachea outlined by air within the trachea and air in the adjacent lung. Part of the retrosternal soft tissue (stripe) is also visible (black arrows).*

MEDIASTINAL MASSES

MASSES—OFTEN OBVIOUS...SOMETIMES SUBTLE

Obvious

Many mediastinal masses are large. Most of these will be readily apparent on the frontal CXR (Fig. 8.15). You should attempt to place the mass within a particular mediastinal compartment in order to create a helpful differential diagnosis. The key to doing this is to decide which particular structure(s) the mass lies against (see below).

Subtle

Small mediastinal masses may be difficult to detect. This occurs when the mass barely projects or does not project beyond the mediastinal boundaries— i.e. the normal mediastinal silhouette remains superficially or truly unaltered.

Three key features can help you to detect such a mass.

1. Increased density. The extra tissue created by a mass will make that part of the mediastinum appear more dense (white) on the CXR. A useful tip is to look at the density of the left and right sides of the cardiac shadow and compare them. They should be approximately equal. A mass can cause an asymmetrical increase in density (Fig. 8.16).

2. Minor alteration to the mediastinal contour. If a mass projects just beyond the normal mediastinal contour it will cause the mediastinum to become very slightly widened (Fig. 8.17). You will need to familiarise yourself with the normal range of mediastinal contours.

3. Displacement of a normal stripe. This is a particularly important feature for detecting a posterior mediastinal mass from the frontal CXR—because a paraspinal mass (Fig. 8.18) will often displace either or both paravertebral stripes laterally.

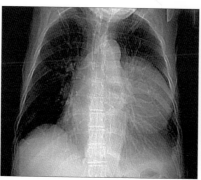 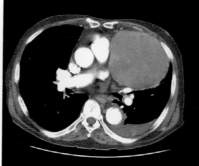

Figure 8.15 *The large anterior mediastinal mass is obvious.*

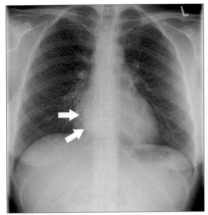

Figure 8.16 *Density alteration. Increased density (arrows) over the right side of the heart adds to the suggestion of a mediastinal mass. Bronchogenic cyst.*

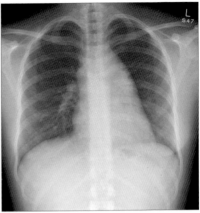

Figure 8.17 *Contour alteration. Widening of the mediastinum to the right and left sides is evident. Lymphoma. (Incidentally, this is a good example of the hilum overlay sign[1], described in Chapter 16, p. 233).*

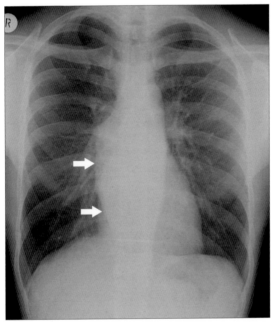

Figure 8.18 *Stripe alteration. Note the presence of a right paravertebral stripe. Actually, the stripe is bulging (arrows). This appearance indicates a posterior mediastinal mass. Subsequently proven vertebral column tuberculosis with a paravertebral abscess.*

CREATING A DIFFERENTIAL DIAGNOSIS

Table 8.3 Mediastinal masses.

Compartment	Common causes	Notes
Anterior	The Four Ts: ■ Thyroid mass ■ Thymoma ■ Teratoma ■ (Terrible) lymphoma	■ Lymphadenopathy from any cause can occur in the anterior mediastinum. It often has a lumpy, bumpy appearance.
Middle	■ Lymphadenopathy ■ Centrally situated lung tumours ■ Oesophageal lesions including duplication cysts	
Posterior	■ Spinal/paraspinal abscess ■ Neurogenic tumours	■ Look at the intervertebral discs and the vertebral bodies. ■ Look for rib splaying and / or vertebral body erosion

In order to create a helpful differential diagnosis, you should attempt to place the mass in a particular compartment. This can often be done reasonably accurately using the frontal CXR alone. The lateral CXR will almost always reinforce your frontal view assessment.

On the frontal CXR

The silhouette sign (p. 45) is the key.

■ An **anterior** mediastinal mass lies adjacent to the heart. It may efface a heart border or the margin of the ascending aorta. It will not efface the hila nor widen a paraspinal line (Fig. 8.19).

■ A **middle** mediastinal mass may splay the carina or efface a normal hilar shadow. It will not efface a heart border nor widen a paraspinal line (Fig. 8.20).

■ A **posterior** mediastinal mass will displace either or both of the paravertebral stripes laterally. It may also widen the space between adjacent ribs and may destroy or erode a vertebra or a rib. It will not efface a heart border or a hilar shadow (Fig. 8.21).

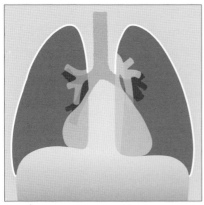

Figure 8.19 *The region of the right heart border is abnormal. The border is very prominent and it has a most unusual shape for an enlarged right atrium. Anterior mediastinal mass.*

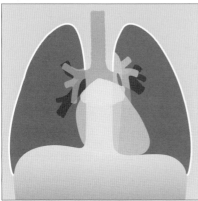

Figure 8.20 *The carina is splayed (i.e. its angle exceeds 100°). Middle mediastinal mass. An enlarged left atrium or very large subcarinal lymph nodes can cause this appearance.*

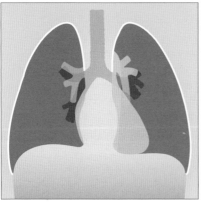

Figure 8.21 *The left paravertebral stripe is bulging. It normally has a straight margin. Posterior mediastinal mass. A paravertebral abscess, haematoma or vertebral tumour is the usual cause.*

On the lateral CXR

The lateral CXR will help to confirm or to modify the assessment that you have made from the frontal view. Trace Felson's mediastinal boundaries (Fig. 8.2) and place the main bulk of the mass in the appropriate compartment.

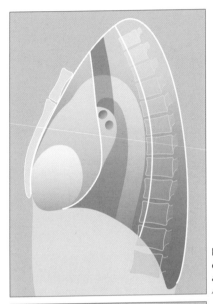

Figure 8.22 *An abrupt change in density is evident across the cardiac shadow. Anterior mediastinal mass.*

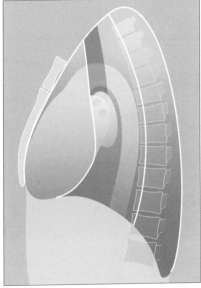

Figure 8.23 *Enlargement of the shadows at and around the region of the hila. Middle mediastinal mass.*

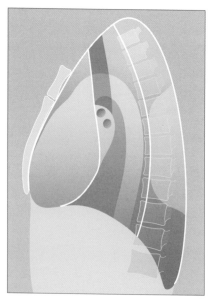

Figure 8.24 *Increase in density over the vertebral column. Posterior mediastinal mass.*

Some helpful hints—frontal and lateral CXRs

◼ The most common anterior mediastinal mass is an enlarged retrosternal thyroid. This mass will almost always displace or narrow the trachea. Its well-defined margins will fade out above the clavicles (the cervicothoracic sign—see Chapter 16, pp. 234–235).

◼ Linear calcification is often seen in vascular masses (e.g. an aneurysm). Occasionally a thymoma or a teratoma will also calcify.

◼ Lymphadenopathy can be seen in any compartment but is particularly common at or around the hila. Enlarged nodes tend to produce a lumpy, bumpy contour.

◼ An aortic aneurysm will follow the course of the aorta. Often a normal aortic knuckle will not be identified.

◼ A fixed hiatus hernia (middle mediastinum in position) can often be diagnosed from the frontal CXR. It shows an increased density overlying the heart. Usually it extends to the left of the midline. Classically, it will contain gas. An air–fluid level is often visible. See p. 320.

GAS IN THE MEDIASTINUM — PNEUMOMEDIASTINUM

Some aspects of pneumomediastinum are included on pp. 104–105 in Chapter 7; in particular, the causes for a co-existing pneumothorax and pneumomediastinum are explained.

The mediastinum communicates with extrathoracic sites via numerous fascial planes. Air in the mediastinum can dissect along these planes and may be seen in various positions outside the thorax. These extrathoracic sites include the:

- vascular sheaths in the neck

- retropharyngeal space

- submandibular space

- retroperitoneal space

PNEUMOMEDIASTINUM: CAUSES

The most common cause is rupture of an alveolus. There are other causes (Table 8.4). When an alveolus ruptures, the air dissects along vascular bundles within the lung to reach the root of the lung. From the lung root the air enters the mediastinal soft tissues (Fig. 8.25).

Table 8.4 Causes of pneumomediastinum.

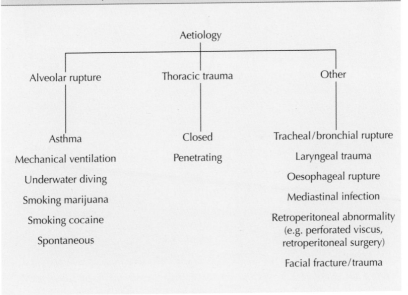

	Aetiology	
Alveolar rupture	Thoracic trauma	Other
Asthma	Closed	Tracheal/bronchial rupture
Mechanical ventilation	Penetrating	Laryngeal trauma
Underwater diving		Oesophageal rupture
Smoking marijuana		Mediastinal infection
Smoking cocaine		Retroperitoneal abnormality (e.g. perforated viscus, retroperitoneal surgery)
Spontaneous		Facial fracture/trauma

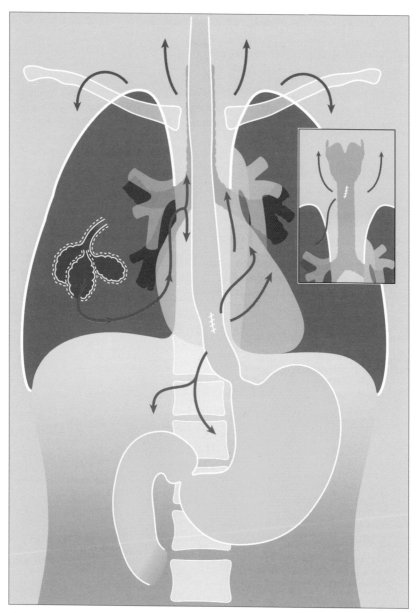

Figure 8.25 *Air or gas can enter the mediastinum as a result of different pathological processes. These include rupture of an alveolus, tracheal or bronchial rupture, or a tear in the wall of the oesophagus. The air commonly extends into the neck. Very occasionally the mediastinal air dissects inferiorly into the retroperitoneum.*

PNEUMOMEDIASTINUM: CXR APPEARANCES[2,6–9]

One, some, or all of these findings may be present:

- The "continuous diaphragm sign". Normally the central part of the diaphragm is not visualised on a frontal CXR because it is not in contact with lung. Mediastinal gas can dissect along this tissue plane. Consequently the entire surface of the diaphragm may be visible (Fig. 8.26).

- A lucent (black) halo surrounding the heart. This is air. It may elevate the mediastinal pleura away from the heart (Fig. 8.26).

- Streaks of gas in the neck or in the soft tissues of the chest wall (Fig. 8.26).

- Air around the pulmonary artery (and/or its main branches). This produces a black ring appearance.

- Air around the arteries arising from the aortic arch. Appearing as black rings and often referred to as the "ring around the artery sign", or the "tubular artery sign".

- The thymic "angel wing sign" (Fig. 8.27) in young children and neonates (see p. 210).

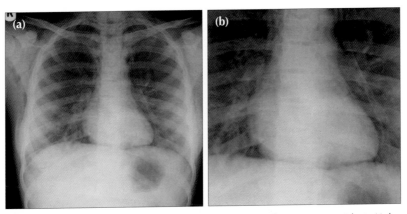

Figure 8.26 *Acute asthma (a). Very small bilateral pneumothoraces were evident. Air has also dissected into the mediastinum and resulted in surgical emphysema extending into the neck and the anterior chest wall. The blown-up image (b) shows: (1) the continuous diaphragm sign; and (2) a halo of air surrounding the heart.*

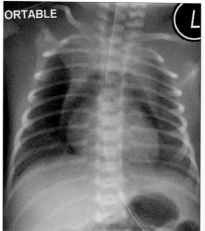

Figure 8.27 *Pneumomediastinum in a neonate. The angel wing sign. This represents the normal thymus surrounded by mediastinal air.*

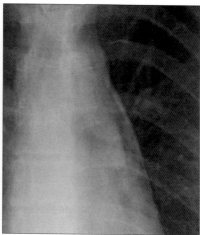

Figure 8.28 *Very subtle findings indicative of a pneumomediastinum. Air in the mediastinum is shown as black streaky lines in the soft tissues.*

PNEUMOMEDIASTINUM VERSUS OTHER GAS COLLECTIONS

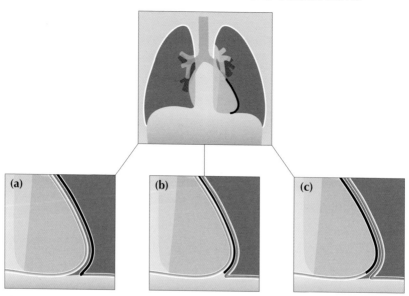

Figure 8.29 *A sharp black line around the cardiac margin may be due to: (a) air in the pleural space adjacent to the heart (pneumothorax); or (b) air in the mediastinal soft tissues (pneumomediastinum); or (c) air in the pericardial sac (pneumopericardium). Occasionally, this appearance is mimicked by a Mach effect (see p. 128).*

Pneumomediastinum versus pneumopericardium

- A pneumopericardium can mimic a pneumomediastinum. It usually results from penetrating trauma or immediately following thoracic surgery.

- Pneumothorax is common, pneumomediastinum is much less common, and pneumopericardium is very, very, rare.

- A useful **rule of thumb**: air in the pericardial sac stays in the sac and will not extend above the pericardial reflection—i.e. it will not extend above the ascending aorta. Air elsewhere in the mediastinum (i.e. a pneumomediastinum) is not constrained and will extend above the ascending aorta.

Pneumomediastinum versus pneumothorax

Sometimes air in the medial pleural space (pneumothorax) will outline the lateral margin of the heart and can be mistaken for a pneumomediastinum.

If you are in doubt as to where the air is situated—obtain a lateral decubitus CXR (see p. 231).

- Pneumopericardium…the air will move within the pericardial sac and will outline the side of the heart that is elevated.

- Pneumomediastinum…the air will remain in the same position. It will not move.

- Pneumothorax…the air will move to the lateral aspect of the pleural sac, i.e. adjacent to the chest wall.

POTENTIAL PITFALL: THE MACH EFFECT[10]

Sometimes a normal CXR will show a thin, well-defined, black line around one or both lateral margins of the heart. This is an optical illusion resulting from overlap of superimposed normal structures. This illusion is known as a Mach band or Mach effect.

Whenever a sharp black line is seen adjacent to a heart border the possibility of a pneumomediastium or a pneumothorax must be considered. Nevertheless, an unimportant Mach band must be kept in mind. Invariably, the clinical features will make a Mach band likely or unlikely. If uncertainty persists then a lateral decubitus CXR will clarify (see Chapter 16, p. 231).

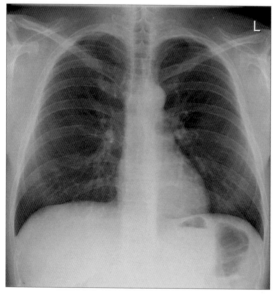

Figure 8.30   *A Mach effect[10] is responsible for the sharp black line adjacent to the left heart border. An occasional normal appearance which can be misinterpreted as a pneumomediastinum. In practice, the clinical features will usually distinguish between a Mach effect and air in the soft tissues.*

PNEUMOMEDIASTINUM IN AN INFANT

See Chapter 15, pp. 208–210.

AN INTERESTING CONDITION—
SPONTANEOUS PNEUMOMEDIASTINUM

Aetiology / pathology

Alveolar rupture. Thought to be linked to Valsalva's manoeuvre (e.g. athletic activity, defaecation, parturition, marijuana smoking, use of cocaine).

Clinical features

■ Chest pain and/or dyspnoea are common. Neck pain, dysphagia, back pain, shoulder pain, neck swelling also occur. Occasionally asymptomatic.

■ Physical signs may be absent. Hamman's sign (mediastinal systolic crunch heard over the precordium) occurs in less than 50% of cases.

The CXR

Air in the mediastinum. Air dissecting into the soft tissues of the neck is sometimes a particularly dominant feature.

REFERENCES

1. Felson B. Chest Roentgenology. Philadelphia, PA:. WB Saunders, 1973.

2. Zylak CM, Standen JR, Barnes GR et al. Pneumomediastinum revisited. Radiographics 2000, 20; 1043–1057.

3. Price JE, Rigler LG. Widening of the mediastinum resulting from fat accumulation. Radiology 1970; 96: 497–500.

4. Genereux GP. The posterior pleural reflections. AJR 1983; 141: 141–149.

5. Donnelly LF, Frush DP, Zheng JY et al. Differentiating normal from abnormal inferior thoracic paravertebral soft tissues on chest radiography in children. AJR 2000; 175: 477–483.

6. Rohlfing BM, Webb WR, Schlobohm RM. Ventilator related extra-alveolar air in adults. Radiology 1976; 121: 25–31.

7. Westcott JL, Cole SR. Interstitial pulmonary emphysema in children and adults; roentgenographic features. Radiology 1974; 111: 367–378.

8. Bejvan SM, Godwin JD. Pneumomediastinum: old signs and new signs. AJR 1996; 166: 1041–1048.

9. Han SY, McElvein RB, Aldrete JS et al. Perforation of the oesophagus: correlation of site and cause with plain film findings. AJR 1985; 145: 537–540.

10. Chasen MH. Practical applications of Mach band theory in thoracic analysis. Radiology 2001; 219: 596–610.

9 PATTERNS IN 21ST CENTURY LUNG INFECTIONS

In this chapter we describe CXR features that occur with:

■ different types of pneumonia

■ pulmonary tuberculosis

■ HIV-related opportunistic lung infection

PNEUMONIA[1,2]

Pneumonia:	An acute lower respiratory tract infection together with new radiographic shadowing[1].

■ See earlier descriptions in Chapters 3 and 4.

■ A patient who is diagnosed with pneumonia in primary care will receive antibiotic treatment. In most instances treatment of an uncomplicated community acquired pneumonia is relatively straightforward[1,2]. Amoxicillin is currently the antibiotic of choice because the causative organism is likely to be gram positive. The severity of the pneumonia will dictate whether a more complex antimicrobial regime is instituted.

■ A hospital acquired pneumonia is usually due to a gram negative organism and intravenous broad spectrum cephalosporins are usually recommended.

■ Sometimes the CXR appearances will raise the suspicion that the pneumonia may be caused by an unusual organism. This can alert the physician and may influence the choice of a particular antibiotic.

■ This chapter highlights a few selected points in relation to the value of a CXR—i.e. beyond confirming that pneumonic consolidation is present.

SOME GENERAL RULES

- Bronchopneumonia.
  - ❏ The CXR appearances cannot distinguish between causative organisms.
- Lobar pneumonia.
  - ❏ This is most commonly due to *Streptococcus pneumoniae* (pneumococcal pneumonia).
- Lobar pneumonia with evidence of expansion of the lobe.
  - ❏ The most likely organism is either *Klebsiella* or *Streptococcus pneumoniae.*

The typical CXR patterns of bronchopneumonia and lobar pneumonia are described on pp. 32–35 and 42–44.

MIGHT THE PNEUMONIA BE ATYPICAL?

This refers to an atypical organism—usually *Mycoplasma* or *Legionella*. If this is considered to be likely then a macrolide antibiotic will be introduced.

Table 9.1   Atypical pneumonia.

Clinical / laboratory	CXR
■ Prodromal illness ■ White cell count is often normal	■ Usually the CXR features are nonspecific ■ Sometimes there is just a hint— i.e. multilobar involvement and pleural effusion

STAPHYLOCOCCAL PNEUMONIA

This is usually acquired within the hospital. If the causative organism is *Staphylococcus aureus* then flucloxacillin is introduced. Several CXR features are not specific but are nevertheless suggestive of this organism:

- Patchy segmental consolidation which spreads rapidly and becomes confluent.
- Cavitation within an area of pneumonic consolidation.
- Development of a pneumatocoele. This occurs most commonly in children.
  - ❏ A pneumatocoele is a gas filled space in the lung adjacent to an area of consolidation. On the CXR it appears as a round lucent area (Fig. 9.3). A pneumatocoele is a transient CXR appearance.

ASPIRATION PNEUMONIA

This may result from inhalation of gastric or oropharyngeal fluids, pus from infected sinuses, or inhalation of external fluid. If aspiration is the likely cause of the pneumonia then intravenous cephalosporin/metronidazole is added to the antimicrobial treatment. The following are suggestive of aspiration:

■ Clinical: an episode of reduced level of consciousness.

■ CXR: patchy areas of consolidation in the dependent lobes of the lung. This will not necessarily be at a lung base. If aspiration occurs when supine, then the right apical lower lobe or posterior upper lobe segments are often involved.

BACTERIAL OR VIRAL?

■ In general the CXR shadows do not distinguish between a bacterial or viral aetiology.

■ An occasional helpful hint: a combination of obvious and widespread CXR consolidation with rather minor findings on clinical examination of the lungs suggests a viral pneumonia.

PNEUMONIA WITH CAVITATION

This can occur with an acute bacterial pneumonia. The most common causative organisms are *Staphylococcus aureus*, *Streptococcus pyogenes*, *Pseudomonas aeroginosa*, *Klebsiella*, *Escherichia coli*. (See pp. 134–137 for tuberculosis.)

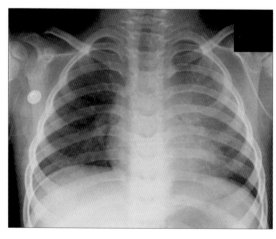

Figure 9.1 *Child with a chest infection. Fluffy/confluent homogeneous shadowing in the left upper lobe. Lobar pneumonia. See pp. 42–44.*

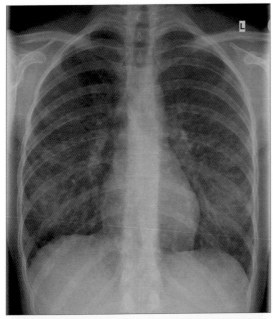

Figure 9.2 *Chest infection. The linear and nodular shadows in both lower zones represent the typical pattern of a bronchopneumonia (see pp. 42–44). This was a viral pneumonia.*

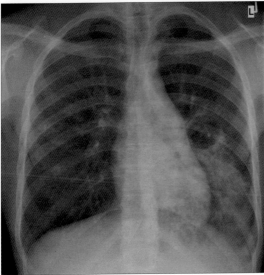

Figure 9.3 *Severe chest infection. The round lucent area adjacent to the left lower lobe consolidation is a pneumatocoele. Pneumatocoeles are distended air spaces that are characteristically transient— i.e. they disappear fairly quickly. Pneumatocoeles do not represent areas of cavitation. Staphylococcal pneumonia.*

PULMONARY TUBERCULOSIS[3]

CLASSIC PATTERNS

Pulmonary tuberculosis (PTB) is often suspected by the physician when a patient from a particular at-risk group (e.g. socio-economic/demographic) has minimal clinical symptoms and an abnormal CXR. If a patient is outside a generally accepted at-risk group then even a classic CXR PTB pattern may be misinterpreted and tuberculosis not considered.

It is important to recognise CXR patterns that raise the suspicion of PTB (Table 9.2). As a general rule, the distribution and position of PTB shadows differs between primary and post-primary disease.

Table 9.2   The most common CXR appearances.

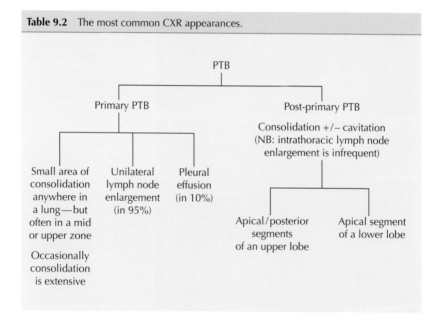

Pitfall. CXR changes in post-primary PTB have a strong predilection for the apical or posterior segments of the upper lobes and also for the apical segments of the lower lobes. Sometimes post-primary tuberculosis shadowing will occur in the anterior segment of an upper lobe or in a basal segment of a lower lobe. This distribution may lead to the assumption that the shadows are not due to PTB. However, an apparently atypical position for shadowing in post-primary disease is usually accompanied by shadowing in the classical segments. The message: if post-primary PTB is clinically possible you must always check out the classical segments on both the frontal and lateral CXRs[3].

MILIARY PTB

This represents haematogenous spread of the bacilli. It is most commonly associated with primary PTB but it can occur with post-primary PTB. The term "miliary" refers to the millet-seed appearance of the tiny nodules scattered throughout the lungs. To be truly miliary the small densities will all be of the same size (0.5–2.0 mm in diameter), sharply defined, and will usually involve the lung apices.

The visibility of these tiny nodules on the CXR is the result of superimposition of hundreds of the tiny foci one on top of another. If the number of foci are not yet in their hundreds and thousands then they will not be detectable. Consequently, a patient may have miliary PTB and yet the CXR may appear normal.

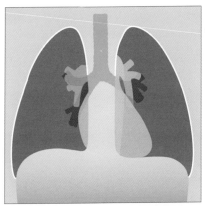

Figure 9.4 *A common pattern in primary PTB. Unilateral hilar lymph node enlargement.*

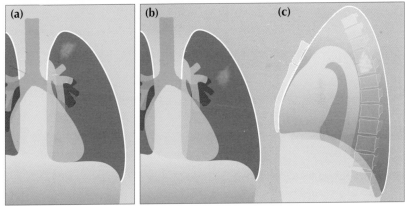

Figure 9.5 *Classic patterns in post-primary PTB. Lung shadowing that favours the apical or posterior segments of an upper lobe (a); or involving the apical segment of a lower lobe (b, c).*

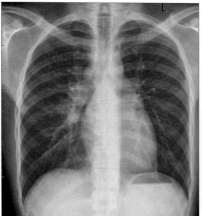

Figure 9.6 *Unilateral hilar lymph node enlargement (and, incidentally, the azygos node is also enlarged). Primary PTB.*

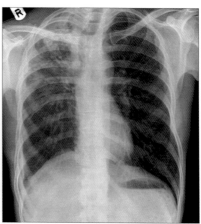

Figure 9.7 *Extensive shadowing, and some volume loss, in the right upper lobe. Post primary PTB.*

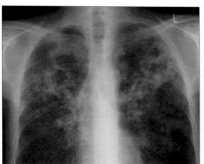

Figure 9.8 *Diffuse shadowing in both lungs with cavitation. A lateral CXR showed the apical segments of both lower lobes to be involved. Post-primary PTB. You might wish to remind yourself of the superior extent of both lower lobes on the reference images at the front of the book (p. viii.)*

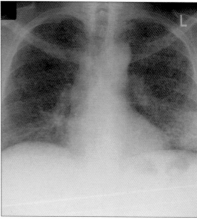

Figure 9.9 *Numerous fine nodules (0.5–2.0 mm in diameter) are present throughout both lungs. The lung apices are not spared. Miliary PTB.*

ARE THE CXR SHADOWS DUE TO ACTIVE OR INACTIVE PTB?

A recurring dilemma. A CXR shows PTB scarring—but are there any features to suggest that it could be active? Table 9.3 provides some guidelines which will help to make the assessment.

Table 9.3   Active or Inactive PTB?

Active	Probably inactive	Apply the precautionary principle:
■ Cavitation ■ Ill-defined shadows ■ Change from an earlier CXR (i.e. an increase in shadowing).	■ Considerable calcification with all shadows well-defined ■ No change on serial CXRs at least six months apart	■ Always…careful clinical assessment and sputum examination

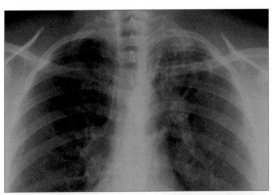

Figure 9.10   Note the well-defined ("hard") shadowing at the apex of the left lung with elevation of the left hilum. These features suggest old inactive PTB affecting the upper lobe.

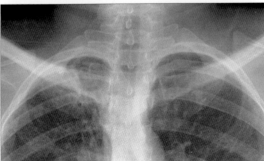

Figure 9.11   Ill-defined shadowing at the right lung apex. Active post-primary PTB. NB: the lung apices are where tuberculous shadows commonly occur…and they can hide behind the overlapping ribs and clavicle. On this CXR compare and contrast the appearance of the right lung apex with the entirely normal left apex.

HIV RELATED OPPORTUNISTIC LUNG INFECTIONS[4]

The Acquired Immune Deficiency Syndrome (AIDS) first appeared as a devastating epidemic during the 1980s. The cause of the syndrome is infection with human immunodeficiency virus (HIV). Affected patients are immunocompromised. Consequently they are vulnerable to secondary infection with other organisms. Debilitating and life-threatening lung infections (Table 9.4) are common.

Table 9.4 HIV-related lung infections.

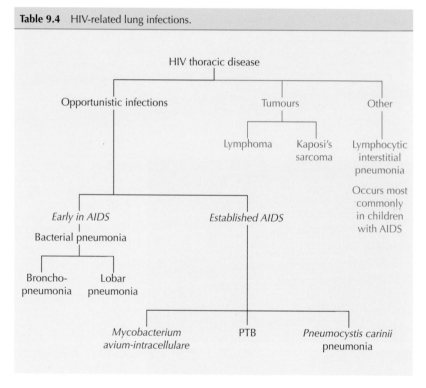

MYCOBACTERIUM AVIUM-INTRACELLULARE

The CXR appearances are non-specific. They include: hilar and mediastinal lymph node enlargement; and/or nodular lung shadows; and/or areas of alveolar consolidation.

PTB

The most common patterns on the CXR are:

■ Primary PTB...lymph node enlargement; or

■ Post-primary PTB...apical consolidation +/– cavitation.

PNEUMOCYSTIS CARINII PNEUMONIA (PCP)

■ With confirmed PCP infection the CXR is abnormal in the majority of cases. The reported incidence of a normal CXR varies in different series (5–30% of cases). The common CXR patterns:

    ❏ Initially...perihilar and basal fine reticular densities causing a ground glass or hazy appearance.

    ❏ These rapidly develop into extensive areas of alveolar consolidation.

■ Some uncommon patterns do occur:

    ❏ Thin walled cysts and cavities.

    ❏ Discrete focal areas of consolidation.

■ Very uncommon findings:

    ❏ Pleural effusion.

    ❏ Lymph node enlargement.

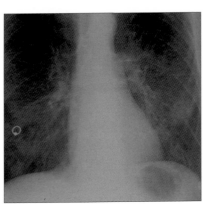

Figure 9.12 *Young male. Breathless. Lower zone reticular densities create a basal ground glass (i.e. a rather hazy) appearance. PCP. This is an early CXR finding and is often very subtle. Rapid progress to extensive areas of alveolar consolidation usually occurs. (Incidental body piercing artefact through the right nipple.)*

REFERENCES

1. Hoare Z, Lim WS. Pneumonia: update on diagnosis and management. BMJ 2006; 332: 1077–1079.

2. Woodhead M, Blasi F, Ewig S, et al. Guidelines for the management of adult respiratory tract infections. Eur Respir J 2005; 26: 1138–1180.

3. Woodring JH, Vandiviere HM, Fried AM, et al. Update: The radiographic features of pulmonary tuberculosis. AJR 1986; 146: 497–506.

4. O'Neil KM. The changing landscape of HIV-related lung disease in the era of highly active antiretroviral therapy. Chest 2002; 122: 768–771.

10 BRONCHIAL CARCINOMA

Every patient with an ominous symptom (e.g. smoker with recurrent haemoptysis) or with a less alarming symptom (e.g. a persistent cough in a man aged 65 years)—is thinking:

"Do I have cancer?"

Table 10.1 Basic information about bronchial carcinoma (USA/UK).

Histological type	% of all bronchial carcinomas	Relation to cigarette smoking	Usual position on the CXR	Notes
Adenocarcinoma (including bronchiolo-alveolar cell carcinoma)	45%	Strong Exception: bronchiolo-alveolar cell carcinoma has a weak association	Peripheral	May develop around a lung scar—a scar carcinoma.
Squamous cell	35%	Strong	Central* or peripheral	Cavitation recognised
Small cell (including oat cell carcinoma)	20%	Strong	Central or peripheral	Central adenopathy is often very bulky
Large cell	1%	Strong	Central or peripheral	Usually larger than 3 cm in diameter when it is a peripheral lesion.

* central = within a main or lobar bronchus.

CXR: MISSED LUNG CANCERS—IMPORTANT MESSAGES

- Most cancers (more than 70%) occur in the upper lobes[1].

- A carcinoma can be overlooked on the CXR because a superimposed structure (rib or vessel) makes it less conspicuous. This occurred in 71% of overlooked lesions in one series[2].

  - *Double check the lung areas covered by the ribs.*

  - *Always ask yourself: is that density really just rib and vessel overlap?*

OBVIOUS CXR ABNORMALITY

Many bronchial carcinomas are easy to detect—usually as a conspicuous mass peripherally or at a hilum (Figs 10.1–10.4).

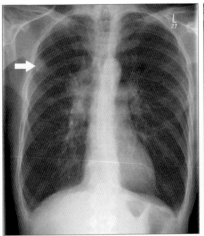

Figure 10.1 *Lung opacity (arrow) with an irregular outline. Enlarged right hilum. Peripheral bronchial carcinoma with metastatic spread to the hilar lymph nodes.*

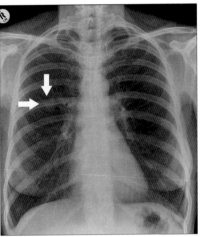

Figure 10.2 *Solitary nodule (arrows) in right mid zone. Bronchial carcinoma.*

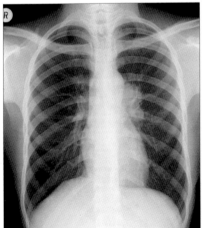

Figure 10.3 *The left hilum is (a) enlarged, and (b) denser than the opposite site. Centrally situated bronchial carcinoma.*

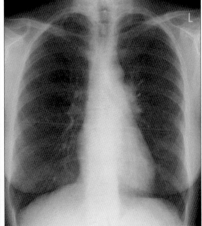

Figure 10.4 *The left hilum is enlarged and—importantly—is denser than the right hilum. Centrally situated bronchial carcinoma.*

SUBTLE CXR ABNORMALITY

TUMOURS WILL HIDE

Some carcinomas are difficult to detect because of their position or because they are overlapped by normal structures (Figs 10.5, 10.7 and 10.8). To locate a hidden mass you need to inspect four areas very carefully:

1. Superimposed on the heart.

   Make sure that the density of the heart on both sides of the spine is equal. Anything other than a very slight difference in density should raise the possibility of a lower lobe lesion/mass.

2. The lung apices.

   Some tumours begin as flat lesions and the CXR appearance may be dismissed as simple pleural thickening (Fig. 10.7). Overlap by the first and second ribs may compound the problem. A flat apical carcinoma can mimic a pleural cap (see box below and p. 230).

3. Below the horizon of each dome of the diaphragm.

   A large part of each lower lobe lies below the horizon of each dome of the diaphragm. Even so, if a lung mass is surrounded by air, then it is usually detectable on the frontal CXR (Fig. 10.8).

4. Around the hila.

   This does not refer to hilar enlargement. It refers to the lung parenchyma around, behind and in front of a hilum. Overlap by vessels entering or leaving the hilum can cause a nearby lung lesion to be overlooked.

BEWARE THE "BENIGN APICAL PLEURAL CAP"[3,4]

A flat apical carcinoma can mimic a pleural cap. Do not dismiss the appearance if:

- A cap has a depth greater than 5 mm.

- Bilateral caps are present and one is more than 5 mm deeper than the other.

Always assess the ribs adjacent to a presumed apical pleural cap for any evidence of bone involvement.

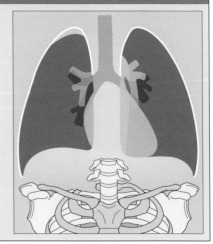

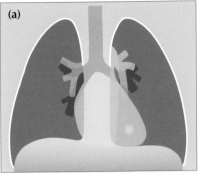
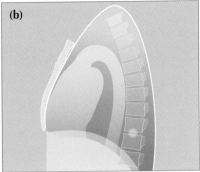

Figure 10.5 *A small nodule is situated in the left lower lobe. On the frontal projection it will be overlooked unless: (a) correct windowing is carried out; and (b) this "behind the heart" area is looked at very carefully.*

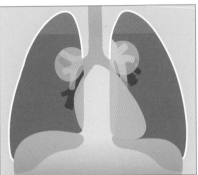

Figure 10.6 *The tricky hidden areas are shown in colour: behind the heart, at both lung apices, below the horizons of the domes of the diaphragm, and around the hila.*

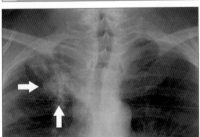

Figure 10.7 *The right apical lesion (arrows) should not be dismissed as benign apical pleural thickening or fibrosis. It is a bronchial carcinoma. The overlying ribs are partially obscuring the tumour.*

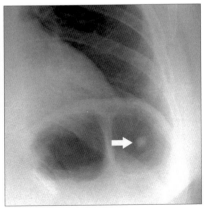

Figure 10.8 *A peripheral nodule (arrow) is situated below the horizon of the left dome of the diaphragm. Bronchial carcinoma.*

CENTRAL TUMOUR—NO LOBAR COLLAPSE

A tumour within a main bronchus which has not caused lobar collapse can be difficult to detect. Abnormal features may be subtle. Keep your eyes peeled for a dense hilum and/or an enlarged hilum.

Three questions to ask of the hila:

■ Are the hila of normal size? Yes = normal. So far so good. But...

■ Is either hilum lobulated (i.e. lumpy, bumpy)? Yes = abnormal.

■ Is either hilum denser than the opposite side? Yes = abnormal.

CENTRAL TUMOUR—WITH LOBAR COLLAPSE

Paradoxically, complete collapse of a lobe can often be more difficult to detect than partial collapse (see Fig. 10.10). The features indicating lobar collapse are described in detail in Chapter 5, pp. 52–69.

PERIPHERAL TUMOUR—WITH DISTAL CONSOLIDATION

Sometimes a carcinoma well away from the hilum will obstruct the distal airways. This can result in an area of consolidation merging with the tumour mass, making the overall appearance indistinguishable from a simple pneumonia (Fig. 10.11).

The clinical presentation will often help to distinguish between the patient with a simple infection and the patient who may be harbouring an underlying carcinoma. It is the overall clinical picture which dictates the next steps (Table 10.2).

Table 10.2   Peripheral consolidation on the CXR—the next steps.

Clinical presentation / impression	Recommended action
Simple community acquired infection	Treat as for infection. No need for a repeat CXR unless some other adverse feature is present.
Simple infection unlikely	Sputum cytology and bronchoscopy and/or CT
Indeterminate clinical features	Treat as for infection. CXR after six weeks to check that the CXR is now normal.
	NB: no need for early repeat CXRs—some simple pneumonias can take six or more weeks to clear. See: the six-week rule (Chapter 4, p. 51).

PERIPLEURAL TUMOUR—WITH A PLEURAL EFFUSION

A primary tumour may infiltrate the adjacent pleura and cause an effusion. The effusion can easily hide the carcinoma (Fig. 10.12).

EXTENSIVE NODAL DISEASE

Small cell carcinoma of the bronchus often presents with extensive mediastinal lymph node enlargement. Although the disease may be extensive it is possible for any mediastinal alteration on the CXR to be subtle. It is important not only to check that the mediastinal contour appears anatomical but also to check that no variation in density is present.

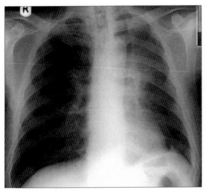

Figure 10.9 *A central tumour has obstructed the left main bronchus and caused collapse of the upper lobe. This classic, albeit peculiar, appearance is described in detail on pp. 65–66.*

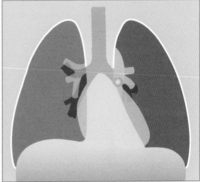

Figure 10.10 *A central tumour (pink circle) has caused major collapse of the left lower lobe. If the cardiac and retro-cardiac areas are not assessed then this CXR abnormality will be overlooked.*

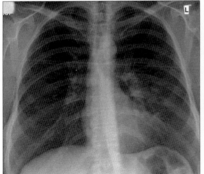

Figure 10.11 *Consolidation in a lingular segment of the left upper lobe. A central tumour is the underlying cause in this patient.*

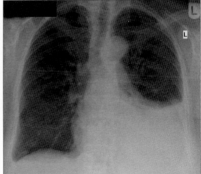

Figure 10.12 *The left pleural effusion hides the peripheral bronchial carcinoma. The effusion is caused by the tumour infiltrating the pleura.*

BEWARE—ONE CANCER IS THE GREAT IMPERSONATOR[5]

Bronchioloalveolar cell carcinoma (approximately 1–7% of all primary bronchial carcinomas) can adopt various disguises (Figs 10.13–10.15).

■ Most commonly it appears as a peripheral mass or nodule which is indistinguishable from any of the other primary carcinomas. The mass or nodule may cavitate.

■ Occasionally the CXR appearance mimics alveolar disease…similar to a pneumonia. The alveolar shadowing may extend to involve several lobes. An air bronchogram may also occur (see p. 227). A non-resolving pneumonia that is clinically puzzling should raise a warning flag: the pneumonic appearance might be tumour tissue—a bronchioloalveolar cell carcinoma.

■ Very occasionally it is multicentric, presenting as multiple discrete pulmonary nodules mimicking metastatic disease.

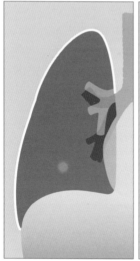 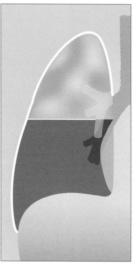 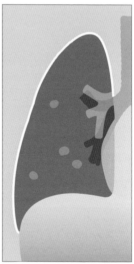

Figure 10.13 *Bronchiolo-alveolar cell carcinoma. The most common CXR finding—a peripheral solitary lung lesion.*

Figure 10.14 *Bronchiolo-alveolar cell carcinoma. An occasional CXR appearance—lobar consolidation mimicking a pneumonia.*

Figure 10.15 *Bronchiolo-alveolar cell carcinoma. Yet another CXR appearance: multiple discrete pulmonary nodules.*

FACTS AND FIGURES

Cavitation

15% of peripheral primary carcinomas cavitate. Most of these are squamous cell carcinomas.

Golden's S sign

A collapsed right upper lobe with a mass at the hilum results in a reverse S configuration. The reversed S is made up of an elevated horizontal fissure and a bulky tumour at the hilum. See p. 64.

Asbestos related bronchial carcinoma[6]

■ Lung cancer in asbestos workers usually occurs 20 years or more after the initial exposure.

■ The relative risk of developing a bronchial carcinoma in non-smoking asbestos workers varies in different series (1.4 to 4 times the risk as compared with non-smokers not exposed to asbestos).

■ Asbestos exposure and cigarette smoking have a synergistic effect—increasing the risk of developing a bronchial carcinoma. The risk is as high as 100 times greater than for non-smokers with no asbestos exposure.

■ It is uncertain whether the risk of developing lung cancer is increased in individuals with CXR evidence of asbestos related pleural plaques.

■ The risk of developing mesothelioma is increased in individuals exposed to asbestos whether or not they smoke.

REFERENCES

1. Kaneko M, Eguchi K, Ohmatsu H et al. Peripheral lung cancer: screening and detection with low-dose spiral CT versus radiography. Radiology 1996; 201: 798–802.

2. Lorentz GBA, Quekel MD, Kessels AGH et al. Miss rate of lung cancer on the chest radiograph in clinical practice. Chest 1999; 115: 720–724.

3. O'Connell RS, McLoud TC, Wilkins EW. Superior sulcus tumor: radiographic diagnosis and workup. AJR 1983; 140: 25–30.

4. Renner RR, Pernice NJ. The apical cap. Semin Roentgenol 1977; 12: 299–302.

5. Epstein DM. Bronchioloalveolar carcinoma. Semin Roentgenol 1990; 25: 105–111.

6. Aronchick JM. Lung cancer: Epidemiology and Risk Factors. Semin Roentgenol 1990; 25: 5–11.

11 CARDIAC DISEASE

The CXR has several important roles: alerting the physician that the heart is enlarged, sometimes revealing a complication resulting from cardiac disease, occasionally suggesting a specific cardiac diagnosis…frequently providing reassurance that all is well.

ACQUIRED CARDIAC DISEASE—WHAT TO LOOK FOR

HEART SIZE

Rules of thumb: Most normal adult hearts have a cardiothoracic ratio (CTR, Fig. 11.1) that does not exceed 50% when assessed on a PA CXR obtained in full inspiration[1]. Some people (perhaps as few as 5%) have an entirely normal heart and yet the CTR exceeds 50%.

In young children the normal CTR can be slightly larger than 50%[2].

■ The transverse cardiac diameter of a normal heart may vary from one PA CXR to another. In 200 normal adults having three CXRs at monthly/yearly intervals[3]:

   ❑ The average individual variation across the group was 0.5 cm

   ❑ A few individuals showed a variation of 1.0 cm

   ❑ One person in the 200 showed a variation of 2.0 cm

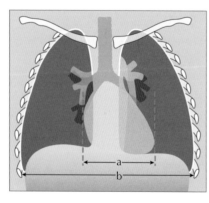

Figure 11.1 *Measuring the CTR. On a PA chest radiograph obtained in full inspiration, if a/b > 50% the heart is likely to be enlarged[1]. (a = maximum transverse diameter of the heart; b = maximum internal diameter of the thorax.)*

- On a PA radiograph variation in the transverse cardiac diameter or the CTR may be caused by:

  - Radiographic exposure during systole rather than diastole (this variation can be as much as 1.7 cm)[4].

  - Slight differences in patient rotation.

  - Difference in depth of inspiration. Be careful—a small inspiration may give a spurious impression of cardiac enlargement.

- A heart may have a CTR of less than 50% but it can still be enlarged—if its transverse diameter was very narrow to begin with. It may take some time before an enlarged heart reaches and exceeds a CTR of 50% (Fig. 11.2).

Rule of thumb: On interval PA CXRs, an increase in transverse cardiac diameter of more than 2.0 cm is significant.

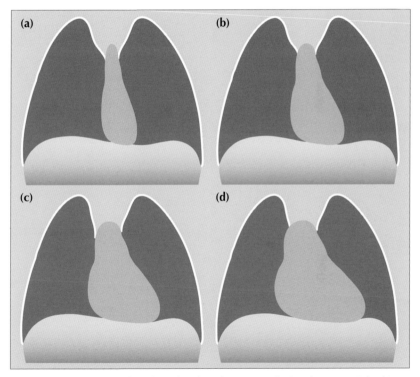

Figure 11.2   *A heart may be enlarged and yet the CTR can be less than 50%. Take this example. (a) The CTR is well within normal limits. The heart is very narrow. (b) Six months later, the heart has enlarged but the CTR remains at less than 50%. (c) After a further six months the heart has further increased in size but still remains less than 50%. (d) Eventually, additional enlargement occurs and the CTR exceeds 50%.*

CHAMBERS AND BORDERS

The margins of the cardiac silhouette are formed by the chambers of the heart. We need to be aware which chamber accounts for which particular border on both the frontal and the lateral CXR (Figs 11.3–11.6).

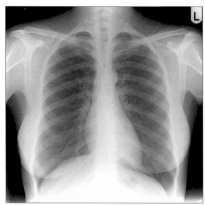

Figure 11.3 *Normal cardiac silhouette.*

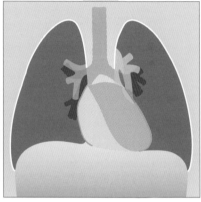

Figure 11.4 *The border-forming chambers: pink = right atrium; blue = right ventricle; brown = left ventricle.*

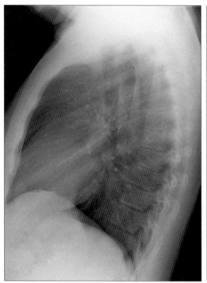

Figure 11.5 *Normal cardiac silhouette.*

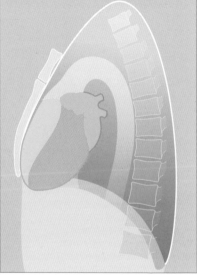

Figure 11.6 *The border-forming chambers: green = left atrium; blue = right ventricle; brown = left ventricle.*

Potential pitfalls:

Two incidental appearances on a frontal CXR are not pathological:

1. A confluence of normal veins entering the left atrium outlined by air in the right lung (Fig. 11.7). The appearance is of a density behind the right side of the heart[1,2]. This can be mistaken for an enlarged left atrium, or a mediastinal mass, or a paravertebral soft tissue swelling. This normal structure is not seen on the left side. Some regard this opacity as part of a normal left atrium rather than a confluence of veins. The distinction is a semantic one. The important point is that it can be detected in 10% of adult CXRs (Chapter 16, p. 239) and is a normal and clinically unimportant variant.

2. A very large fat collection (sometimes referred to as a fat pad) at either or both cardiophrenic angles (Fig. 11.8).

   ❑ These fat collections are commonplace as people become older and more affluent. The fat gives the apex of the heart or the inferior aspect of the right heart border a slightly ill-defined (blurred) appearance.

   ❑ **Rule of thumb**: If an apparent mass at the cardiac apex or adjacent to the right side of the heart: (a) is of low density; and (b) blurs the cardiac margin—then it is most likely to be a pad of fat.

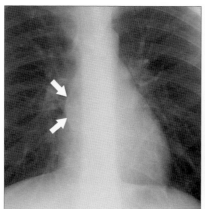

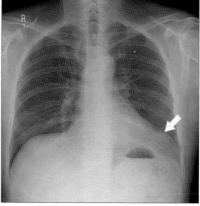

Figure 11.7 *Normal pulmonary venous confluence (arrows)[1,2]. Sometimes the structure is very prominent; in others it can be slight and subtle. On a PA CXR it can be identified in 10% of patients aged 50 or over (see Chapter 16, p. 239).*

Figure 11.8 *Fat collections can occur at either or both cardiophrenic angles. It is very common in well-fed people aged 50 or older (see Chapter 16, p. 239). In this 53-year-old male (who presented with lower abdominal pain) a large fat collection (arrow) causes a prominent shadow at the left cardiophrenic angle.*

CHAMBER ENLARGEMENT ON THE FRONTAL CXR[2,5,6]

The CXR can be very useful in suggesting whether or not a heart is enlarged. Echocardiography will determine whether enlargement is due to a pericardial effusion or to chamber enlargement.

The CXR appearance does not have the definitive role in the precise assessment of chamber enlargement. Echocardiography is definitive. All the same, it is worth being familiar with some of the features of specific chamber enlargement as deduced by analysing the CXR (Table 11.1 and Figs 11.9–11.12).

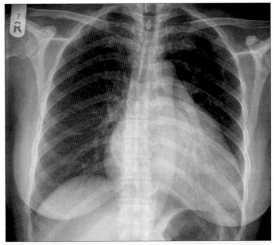

Figure 11.9 *Enlarged left ventricle and left atrium. Note the prominence (bulge) of the left atrial appendage just below and to the left of the main pulmonary trunk. Mitral stenosis and mitral incompetence.*

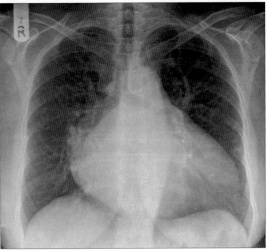

Figure 11.10 *Enlarged left ventricle and left atrium. In this patient the enlarged left atrium is evident because it is producing a distinctive double shadow seen through the heart and it is also pushing the right and left main bronchi apart. Mitral stenosis and mitral incompetence.*

Table 11.1 Chamber enlargement on the frontal CXR—some basic guidelines.

Enlarged	Features
Left ventricle	■ Prominent inferior aspect of the left heart border.
Right ventricle	■ May give a similar appearance to left ventricular enlargement …but often the upper part of the left heart border is most prominent and the cardiac apex is elevated.
Left atrium	■ A bulge of the left heart border just inferior to the main pulmonary trunk. This bulge is the left atrial appendage.
	■ Double shadow seen through the heart. This represents the enlarged atrium emerging posteriorly from the cardiac contour and consequently its left and right margins have become outlined by the air in the lungs.
	■ Gross enlargement can displace and separate the left and right main bronchi so that the carinal angle widens and exceeds 100°. The normal angle does not exceed 100°.
Right atrium	■ The right heart border becomes prominent. In practice… identifying enlargement of this particular chamber is really, really difficult.

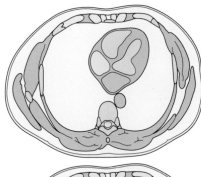

Figure 11.11 *Left atrium of normal size. Cross-sectional image. The atrium is not extending outside the normal cardiac shadow—i.e. its left and right margins are not prominent. Green = left atrium; brown = left ventricle; pink = right atrium; blue = right ventricle.*

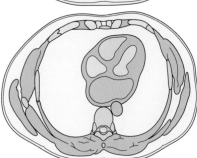

Figure 11.12 *An enlarged left atrium (green). Cross-sectional image. The posterior and side-to-side enlargement of this chamber causes it to emerge from the mediastinal silhouette and its borders become outlined by the air in the lungs. This air-around-the-atrium explains why a double shadow is seen on a frontal CXR.*

LEFT VENTRICULAR ANEURYSM

Aneurysmal dilatation results from myocardial infarction. On a frontal CXR the appearance is often highly characteristic (Figs 11.13 and 11.14).

- A localised bulge appears on the mid part of the left heart border.
- The bulge peaks upwards as well as laterally.
- A fine rim of calcification may be evident in the wall of the aneurysm.

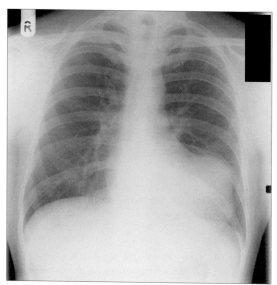

Figure 11.13 *Left ventricular aneurysm. The position and appearance of this bulge on the left border of the heart is fairly typical.*

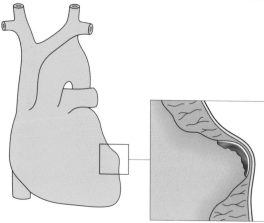

Figure 11.14 *Left ventricular aneurysm. Calcification on the endothelial lining of the aneurysm is a common CXR finding. Red = thrombus in the aneurysm. White = fine endothelial calcification.*

PERICARDIAL EFFUSION

The CXR appearance of fluid in the pericardial sac is very difficult to distinguish from simple chamber enlargement (Fig. 11.15). The distinction is rapidly and easily made using echocardiogaphy. The following[2] are worth noting:

■ The pericardial sac normally contains 15–30 ml fluid.

■ Change in cardiac size or shape only occurs once 250–500 ml of fluid has accumulated.

■ The claim that a pericardial effusion will produce a globular cardiac outline or a well-defined cardiac contour because of the tamponading effect of the effusion on cardiac motion is unsound[2].

■ **Rule of thumb**: The single most important sign of an effusion on a CXR is a rapid alteration in heart size or shape without any changes in the lungs[2].

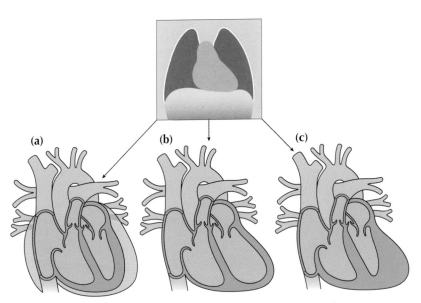

(a) (b) (c)

Figure 11.15 *An enlarged cardiac silhouette may be due to chamber enlargement, to a pericardial effusion, to inflammation/hypertrophy of the cardiac musculature...or to a combination of these possibilities. The CXR appearance of the cardiac shadow alone is insensitive in making a distinction between these causes of an enlarged heart. This is illustrated: (a) pericardial effusion; (b) ventricular dilatation (i.e. chamber enlargement with thin walls); (c) hypertrophy of the myocardium.*

VALVE CALCIFICATION[7,8]

Clinically important

- Aortic. Usually a complication of a bicuspid valve.

- Mitral leaflets. Usually consequent on rheumatic heart disease.

  ❏ The normal valve consists of a fibrous annulus (or ring), valve leaflets (or cusps), chordae tendinae and papillary muscles (Fig. 11.18).

  ❏ In rheumatic heart disease affecting the mitral valve it is the leaflets that are most commonly involved, and these thicken, calcify and retract. The calcification is variable—most comonly focal, blobby, or speckled. This is a very different appearance to age related calcification (see below).

Clinically unimportant

- Mitral ring. An age related phenomenon: calcification affects the ring around the mitral valve leaflets (Fig. 11.19). Clinically significant mitral stenosis resulting from this ageing process is very, very rare. This age related calcification is usually an incidental finding on a CXR. It has a very characteristic configuration—doughnut shaped (Fig. 11.20), circular, or a reverse C. This calcification is most commonly seen in elderly women.

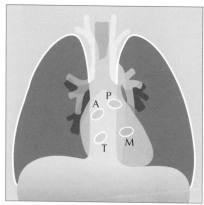

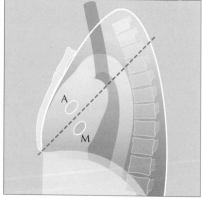

Figure 11.16 *The position of the valves on the frontal CXR.*
P = pulmonary; A = aortic;
M = mitral; T = tricuspid.

Figure 11.17 *The position of the aortic (A) and mitral (M) valves on the lateral CXR. The dotted line extends from the carina to the anterior costophrenic angle. A useful rule of thumb: calcification situated mainly above this line will lie in the aortic valve; calcification situated mainly below this line will lie in the mitral valve[2].*

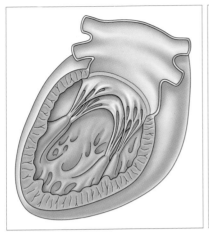

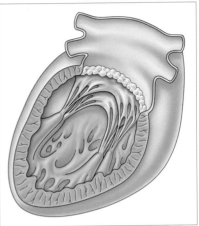

Figure 11.18 *Looking into the left ventricle and the left atrium. To show the normal mitral valve with its fibrous annulus (the ring), valve cusps, chordae tendinae, and the papillary muscles.*

Figure 11.19 *Age related change. Calcification of the annulus (ring) of the mitral valve.*

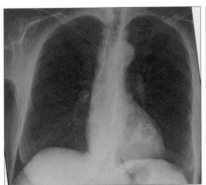

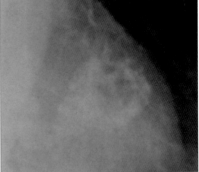

Figure 11.20 *Elderly patient. Female. Prominent age related calcification of the mitral valve ring. The doughnut shape, or reverse C shape, of this calcification (i.e. it adopts the shape of the annulus) is highly characteristic. This is a common incidental CXR finding in elderly people. It is very rarely of clinical significance.*

LEFT VENTRICULAR FAILURE (LVF)[6,9,10,11]

The following features may be present on a PA CXR.

1. Cardiac enlargement.

   Almost all patients with pulmonary opacities due to LVF have cardiomegaly. An occasional exception: a patient with an acute myocardial infarction may have pulmonary oedema and a normal CTR.

2. Changes in the calibre of the pulmonary vessels.

   When the pulmonary venous pressure is normal the upper lobe vessels are smaller in diameter than the lower lobe vessels on an erect CXR. As the venous pressure begins to rise these diameters are reversed and the upper lobe vessels enlarge and the lower lobe vessels constrict (Fig. 11.21). NB: this radiological appearance of upper lobe blood diversion is usually very, very, subtle, and often overdiagnosed.

3. Lung parenchymal and pleural changes.

   Various changes may occur as the pulmonary venous pressure rises even further (Table 11.2). The precise changes will differ between individuals. When a pleural effusion results from LVF it is commonly bilateral. Occasionally it will be unilateral; when this occurs it is usually on the right side. The mechanism for this right-sided selectivity is controversial...but may be related to the anatomical arrangement of lymphatics draining the lungs.

Table 11.2 LVF—signs on an erect CXR.	
Early	■ Enlarged heart
	■ Upper lobe vessels of wider diameter than lower lobe vessels
	■ Oedema: poorly defined (slightly blurred) margins of the hilar vessels
	■ Oedema: septal lines (Kerley B lines)
	■ Small pleural effusions—usually bilateral
Later	■ Interstitial shadowing (oedema) and/or
	■ Alveolar shadowing (florid oedema) and/or
	■ Pleural effusions of increasing size—usually bilateral

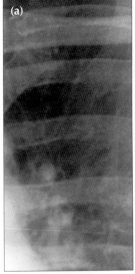
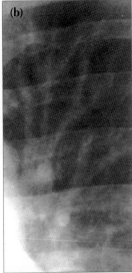

Figure 11.21 *Early LVF. Change in size of the upper lobe vessels. The pulmonary venous pressure was normal in (a). Subsequently (b), prior to developing florid pulmonary oedema. The upper lobe vessels are dilated in (b) as compared with (a). This example is provided to illustrate that changes in vessel size do occur. Nevertheless, it is emphasised that evaluation of vessel size in early pulmonary venous hypertension can be very, very difficult.*

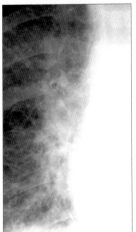

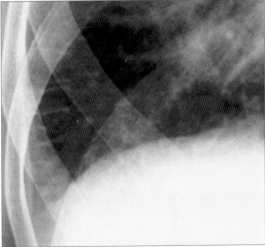

Figure 11.22 *Early LVF. Poorly defined margins of the hilar vessels due to perivascular oedema.*

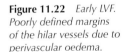

Figure 11.23 *Early LVF. Septal lines (Kerley B lines) caused by fluid in the interstitium. These short, straight lines reach the pleural surface and have this characteristic appearance.*

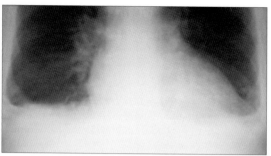

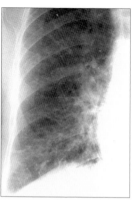

Figure 11.24 *Early LVF. Small pleural effusions. Slight blunting of the costophrenic angles. Effusions in LVF are usually bilateral.*

Figure 11.25 *Florid LVF. Extensive interstitial oedema. The fluid lies mainly in the interstitium of the lung.*

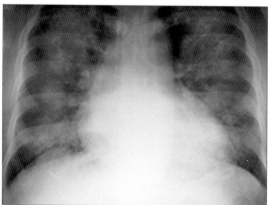

Figure 11.26 *Florid LVF. Extensive alveolar oedema. The alveolar air spaces have filled with fluid.*

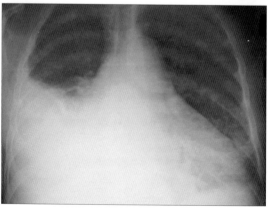

Figure 11.27 *Florid LVF. The main finding is a large pleural effusion. When pleural effusions occur they are usually bilateral. Unilateral effusions do occur and are most often situated on the right side. This predilection for the right side might be related to the differences in lymphatic drainage between the right and left lungs.*

CONGENITAL HEART DISEASE[2,11]

A detailed description of the numerous congenital cardiovascular conditions is beyond the scope of this book. In clinical practice most congenital cardiovascular abnormalities present in childhood (with heart failure or cyanosis) rather than in adults. Nevertheless, there is one condition where an adult's CXR can show abnormal features that may suggest the likely diagnosis.

Atrial septal defect (ASD)[2]

The defect between the low pressure atria can remain clinically silent until adulthood. Eventually, the patient may present with non-specific dyspnoea, a cardiac arrhythmia, and/or paradoxical arterial embolism. Normally, the left atrium is at a slightly higher pressure than the right atrium and so blood is shunted through an ASD from the left to the right side. This results in an increased blood flow through the lungs. If the shunt is very small—the CXR may appear entirely normal. The classical CXR features of a larger ASD are:

- Pulmonary plethora (prominent pulmonary vascular markings).

- Enlargement of the main pulmonary trunk and the pulmonary arteries.

- A small aortic knuckle. This is a constant feature[2]. The shadow of the ascending aorta on the right side of the mediastinum is absent because the aortic root is displaced by the dilated right atrium and right ventricle—i.e. causing leftward rotation of the heart and the great vessels.

- Eventually the pressure in the right side of the heart can become higher than in the left and the patient develops an Eisenmenger syndrome— i.e. pulmonary arterial hypertension, shunt reversal and cyanosis.

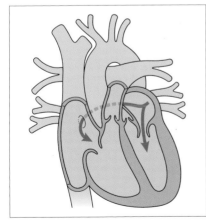

Figure 11.28 ASD. Pulmonary venous blood shunts across from the left atrium into the right atrium.

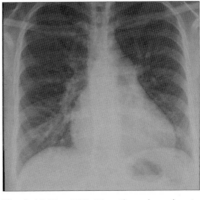

Figure 11.29 ASD. Note the enlarged main pulmonary artery, the plethora (overfilled) pulmonary vessels—arteries and veins—in the mid and distal thirds of the lung, and the small aortic knuckle.

PULMONARY ARTERIAL HYPERTENSION

■ Increased pressure in the pulmonary arteries causes the arteries to become enlarged (i.e. increased calibre), or hypertrophied...or both of these.

■ It is often difficult to distinguish between the various causes of pulmonary arterial hypertension (Table 11.3) from the CXR alone. Primary pulmonary hypertension is a diagnosis of exclusion. It is only accepted as the likely diagnosis after all the other causes for pulmonary arterial hypertension have been eliminated.

■ A common dilemma: when viewing a CXR—are these pulmonary arteries enlarged? **Rule of thumb**: The diameter at the mid point of a normal descending pulmonary artery should not measure more than 9 mm in women and 10 mm in men.

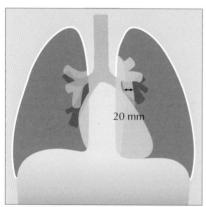

20 mm

Figure 11.30   *The diameter of the left descending pulmonary artery exceeds the normal 10 mm (male) or 9 mm (female). Pulmonary arterial hypertension.*

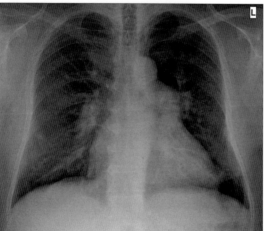

Figure 11.31   *The main pulmonary trunk and the proximal pulmonary arteries are dilated—but the pulmonary arteries in the mid and distal thirds of the lungs are conspicuously and disproportionately narrower. Pulmonary arterial hypertension.*

Table 11.3   Causes of pulmonary arterial hypertension[2,12].

■ Pulmonary venous hypertension (long standing)

■ Left-to-right shunt

■ Pulmonary embolism

■ Respiratory disease

■ High altitude

■ Drugs and poisons

■ Primary pulmonary arterial hypertension

REFERENCES

1. Felson B. Chest Roentgenology. Philadelphia, PA: WB Saunders, 1973.

2. Jefferson K, Rees S. Clinical Cardiac Radiology. 2nd ed. London: Butterworth, 1980.

3. Simon G. Principles of Chest X-ray Diagnosis. London: Butterworth, 1962.

4. Gammill SL, Krebs C, Meyers P et al. Cardiac measurements in systole and diastole. Radiology 1970; 94: 115–119.

5. Boxt LM, Reagan K, Katz J. Normal plain film examination of the heart and great arteries in the adult. J Thorac Imaging 1994; 9: 208–218.

6. Chen JT. The plain radiograph in the diagnosis of cardiovascular disease. Radiol Clin North Am 1983; 21: 609–621.

7. Carpentier AF, Pellerin M, Fuzellier JF et al. Extensive calcification of the mitral valve anulus: pathology and surgical management. J Thorac Cardiovasc Surg 1996; 111: 718–729.

8. Woodring JH, West JW. CT of aortic and mitral valve calcification. J Ky Med Assoc 1989; 87: 177–180.

9. Gluecker T, Capasso P, Schnyder P et al. Clinical and radiologic features of pulmonary edema. Radiographics 1999; 19: 1507–1531.

10. Fraser RG, Muller NL, Colman NC, Pare PD. Fraser and Pare's Diagnosis of Diseases of the Chest. 4th ed. Philadelphia, PA: WB Saunders, 1999.

11. Gross GW, Steiner RM. Radiographic manifestations of congenital heart disease in the adult patient. Radiol Clin North Am 1991; 29: 293–317.

12. Gaine S. Pulmonary hypertension. JAMA 2000; 284: 3160–3168.

12 PACEMAKER ASSESSMENT

The electrical stimulus which causes the heart to contract originates in the sinoatrial (SA) node in the right atrium. This incites the two atria to contract via a conduction pathway. The impulse also passes from the SA node to the atrioventricular (AV) node and thence along the bundle of His to the right and left ventricles (Fig. 12.1).

Various pathological conditions can affect these conduction pathways and cause dysrhythmias or heart block when this electrical system fails to conduct properly. Heart block can be managed by placing a permanent pacemaker within the heart. Some pacemakers have a lead which is positioned in the right ventricle. Others position a lead in the right atrium as well as in the right ventricle. In addition there are devices which resemble pacemakers which can treat some fast life-threatening dysrhythmias by means of pacing control or by defibrillation. These devices are known as implantable converter defibrillators (ICDs).

In an ideal world we would pace the left side of the heart, but the arterial pressure is high and this would cause haemostatic problems. Consequently, the low pressure right side of the heart is utilised.

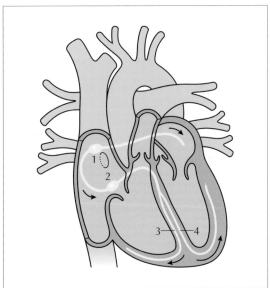

Figure 12.1 *Conducting system of the heart: 1 = SA node; 2 = AV node; 3 = right bundle branch; 4 = left bundle branch. The position of the foramen ovale is shown as a ring inferior to the SA node.*
Note the additional electrical pathway also originating in the SA node. This carries electrical impulses to the right and left atria.

PACEMAKER UNITS[1-4]

A permanent pacemaker has two components. The first is a power source. This is a pulse generator which contains semiconductor chips and a sealed lithium battery. It has a working life of approximately 10 years. The second component is a flexible lead (or leads). These are insulated wires which conduct the pulse to the metal electrodes positioned against the cardiac muscle.

The pacemaker lead is introduced via a cut down on a subclavian vein. The generator is placed in a chest wall pocket fashioned under the skin.

SINGLE CHAMBER : DUAL CHAMBER PACEMAKERS[1-4]

A single chamber pacemaker (i.e. one lead only) may be used to manage an atrial or a ventricular dysrhythmia. For atrial dysrhythmias—the electrode is positioned in the right atrial appendage. For a ventricular dysrhythmia—the electrode is placed against the myocardium at the apex of the right ventricle. Single chamber ventricular pacing is the most basic. It is activated when the ventricular rate falls too low, and only paces the ventricles. The activity of the atria is ignored. Nowadays these single lead systems are being inserted much less frequently.

A dual chamber pacemaker (i.e. two leads) attempts to synchronise the atrial and ventricular systems, since this is much more physiological. One electrode is positioned in the right atrium and the other electrode is placed at the apex of the right ventricle.

Some pacemakers have three electrodes: one in the right atrium, a second in the right ventricle, and a third lead is placed in the coronary sinus (Fig. 12.2). The coronary sinus lead paces the left ventricle. This system is referred to as biventricular pacing.

ICDs are used to manage specific ventricular dysrhythmias. These devices have a single lead and the majority of them have a radiographic appearance which is similar to that of a single chamber pacemaker.

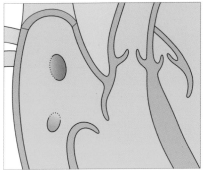

Figure 12.2 *The position of the coronary sinus opening (red) into the right atrium. The sinus is approximately 3 cm long and runs in the AV groove on the posterior border of the heart. The coronary sinus is the vessel which transmits most of the venous drainage of the myocardium. The site of the foramen ovale is shown in blue.*

POST-IMPLANTATION CXRS[1-7]

Why obtain a CXR? It is obtained in order to make sure that all is well. A clinically unsuspected complication from pacemaker insertion is infrequent. Nevertheless, complications do occur.

CXR practice varies between hospitals and clinics. Most physicians obtain a frontal CXR soon after insertion of the pacemaker. Others obtain lateral and frontal radiographs. If an atrial electrode is utilised then a lateral CXR is usually needed so as to ensure that the tip of the electrode (sited in the right atrial appendage) points towards the anterior wall of the thorax.

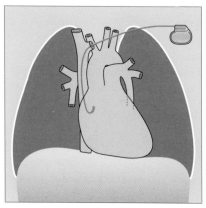

Figure 12.3 *Optimal electrode position. Atrial pacemaker. The tip is in the right atrial appendage.*

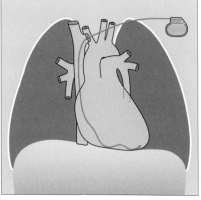

Figure 12.4 *Optimal electrode position. Single chamber pacemaker. The tip of the ventricular lead is situated at the apex of the right ventricle.*

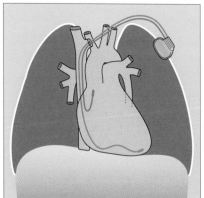

Figure 12.5 *Optimal electrode positions. Dual chamber pacemaker. Pacemakers tend to be introduced from the left side in right-handed patients.*

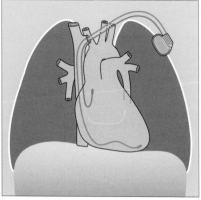

Figure 12.6 *Optimal biventricular electrode positions. The third lead has entered, and extends along, the coronary sinus.*

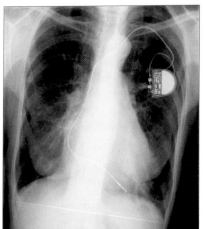

Figure 12.7 *Optimal electrode position. Single chamber pacemaker. The ventricular lead has its tip situated at the apex of the right ventricle. (Retouched.)*

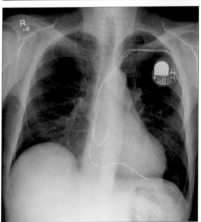

Figure 12.8 *Optimal electrode positions. Dual chamber pacemaker. The atrial lead has its tip in the right atrium; the ventricular lead has its tip at the apex of the right ventricle. (Retouched.)*

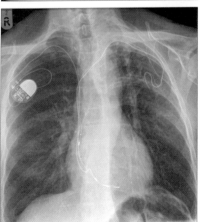

Figure 12.9 *Abandoned left subclavian lead. Pacemaker electrodes usually become adherent to the myocardium within a few weeks of implantation[7]. Some leads adhere to a vein or to the wall of the right atrium. When a pacemaker is being changed and the old lead is difficult to extract it is common practice to cut it short, cap it, and leave it to retract under the skin. (Retouched.)*

TWO CHECKLISTS

Following pacemaker insertion the CXR should be assessed using a checklist. We utilise a list for the frontal CXR and another for the lateral CXR.

PACEMAKER CHECKLIST—THE FRONTAL CXR

1. Electrode position:

    ❏ Atrial electrode in the right atrium (Fig. 12.3).

    ❏ Ventricular electrode in the apex of the right ventricle (Fig. 12.4).

    ❏ Biventricular pacing: the additional lead is in the coronary sinus (Fig. 12.6).

2. Leads/lead

    ❏ A direct course through the veins to the heart.

    ❏ Neither taut nor redundant—a lead is at risk of moving out of position if it is too tight or if it is overlong (Figs 12.10 and 12.11).

    ❏ No evidence of a fracture through a lead—always look at the at-risk pinch-off area between the first rib and the clavicle (Fig. 12.12).

3. Immediate post-placement complications. Check for:

    ❏ Myocardial penetration/perforation.

    – penetration…likely if electrode tip is within 3 mm of the epicardial fat

    – perforation…electrode tip is in the epicardial fat

    ❏ Pneumothorax.

    ❏ Pleural effusion.

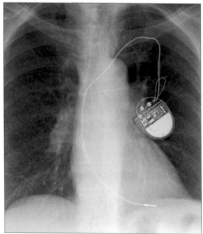

Figure 12.10 *A pacemaker lead can be too taut. Consequently, there is a risk of the tip becoming displaced. (Retouched.)*

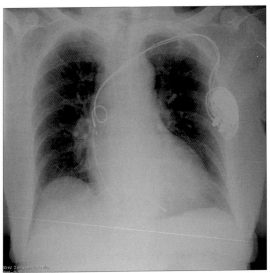

Figure 12.11 *Right atrial lead. Leads should curve smoothly through the cardiac chambers. Any kinks, coils or secondary loops may result in electrode displacement. This lead is coiled. (Retouched.)*

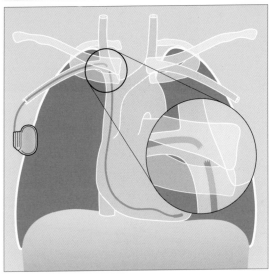

Figure 12.12 *Pacemaker lead fracture at the pinch-off area between the first rib and the clavicle[8]. Be careful: some pacemakers have a non-opaque connector and this joint lucency can be misdiagnosed as representing a lead fracture[2]. Pacemakers are usually introduced on the left side because most people are right-handed. In this illustration it can be presumed that the patient was left-handed or that access to the left subclavian vein was compromised.*

PACEMAKER CHECKLIST—THE LATERAL CXR

1. Ventricular lead:

   ❏ The tip should be directed anteriorly and inferiorly (Figs 12.13 and 12.14).

2. Atrial lead:

   ❏ The lead should have a smooth anterior curve as it is projected over the heart (Fig. 12.15).

   ❏ The electrode tip should be angled superiorly—i.e. positioned in the right atrial appendage (Figs 12.15 and 12.16).

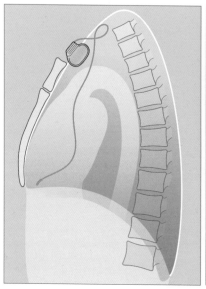

Figure 12.13 *Normal position of a ventricular lead.*

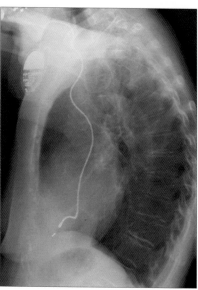

Figure 12.14 *Normal position of a ventricular lead. (Retouched.)*

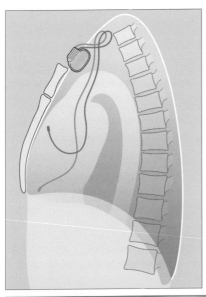

Figure 12.15 *Dual chamber pacemaker. Normal positions of the atrial and ventricular leads.*

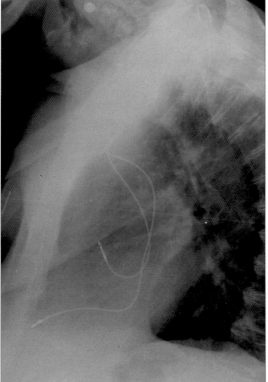

Figure 12.16 *Dual chamber pacemaker. Normal positions of the atrial and ventricular leads. (Retouched.)*

A RARE DISORDER—TWIDDLER'S SYNDROME[2,8]

Aetiology

Pacemaker in situ. Usually the patient has fiddled with the subcutaneous generator or with the lead. Fiddling/twiddling can cause the generator to become faulty, or the lead to fracture, or detachment of the electrode from the site of implantation. Sometimes the patient does not twiddle and the generator twists spontaneously because it is contained in an overlarge subcutaneous pocket.

Clinical features

The pacemaker fails to pace.

The CXR

Comparison with previous post-placement CXRs may alert the physician prior to an impending failure. The generator, or a lead, may have changed position/direction. The CXR appearance of the generator (i.e. its position) may suggest the reason why the tip of the electrode has moved or why a lead fracture, from too much twisting, has occurred.

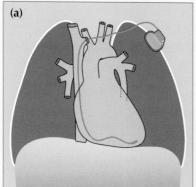 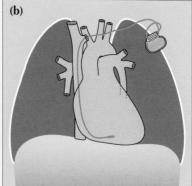

Figure 12.17 *A twiddler. (a) Post-implantation and the ventricular lead is in good position. (b) Some months later the position of the generator box has changed, loops have developed just proximal to the subclavian vein, and the tip of the electrode is no longer at the apex of the right ventricle. One or more of these findings should suggest twiddler's syndrome.*

A RARE DISORDER—SUBCLAVIAN CRUSH SYNDROME[9]

Aetiology

Mechanical friction applied to a pacemaker lead can cause damage to the wire. Most commonly this friction occurs against the clavicle or the first rib; it is then referred to as a subclavian crush.

Clinical features

The pacemaker fails to pace. Syncope or sudden death may occur.

The CXR

The wire may be thinned or fractured. On all CXRs—when a pacemaker is in situ and has been introduced via a subclavian vein puncture—the pacemaker lead should be evaluated for any damage including erosion. The most vulnerable site is where the lead crosses underneath the clavicle (Fig. 12.12).

REFERENCES

1. Bejvan SM, Ephron JH, Takasugi JE et al. Imaging of cardiac pacemakers. AJR 1997; 169: 1371–1379.

2. Burney K, Burchard F, Papouchado M et al. Cardiac pacing systems and implantable cardiac defibrillators (ICDs): a radiological perspective of equipment, anatomy and complications. Clin Radiol 2004; 59: 699–708.

3. Hertzberg BS, Chiles C, Ravin CE. Right atrial appendage pacing: radiographic considerations. AJR 1985; 145: 31–33.

4. Gregoratos G, Abrams J, Epstein AE et al. ACC/AHA/NASPE 2002 guideline update for implantation of cardiac pacemakers and anti-arrhythmia devices: summary article. A report of the American College of Cardiology/American Heart Association Task Force on Practice Guidelines. Circulation 2002; 106: 2145–2161.

5. Morishima I, Sone T, Tsuboi H et al. Follow up X-rays play a key role in detecting implantable cardioverter defibrillator lead fracture. Pacing Clin Electrophysiol 2003; 26: 911–913

6. Karthikeyan G. To Roentgen or not to Roentgen: Real dilemma or much ado about nothing? J Postgrad Med 2005; 51: 96.

7. Bohm A, Pinter A, Duray G et al. Complications due to abandoned non-infected pacemaker leads. Pacing Clin Electrophysiol 2001; 24: 1721–1724.

8. Weiss D, Lorber A. Pacemaker twiddler's syndrome. Int J Cardiol 1987; 15: 357–360.

9. Noble SL, Burri H, Sunthorn H. Complete section of pacemaker lead due to subclavian crush. Med J Aust 2005; 182: 643.

13 PATIENTS IN THE INTENSIVE THERAPY UNIT

In this chapter we concentrate on some of the pitfalls and difficulties that can occur when evaluating the bedside CXR in the intensive therapy unit (ITU).

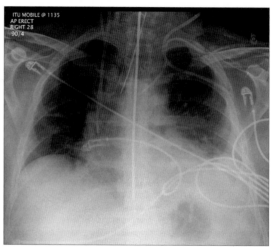

ITU MOBILE @ 1135
AP ERECT
RIGHT 28
90/4

Figure 13.1   *The CXR is essential for assesment of all lines, tubes and catheters. Careful analysis of the pulmonary and pleural appearances will assist clinical management.*

THE BEDSIDE CXR

Misleading appearances may result from the patient's position or be due to radiographic technique when a supine CXR is obtained.

POTENTIAL PITFALLS

■ The bedside AP projection magnifies the heart and the mediastinum (p. 5).

■ Slight patient rotation, angulation of the x-ray beam or variable x-ray tube to patient distances can produce deceptive features on the CXR.

   ❏ Rotation—normal aortic arch vessels can simulate an upper zone mass.

   ❏ Beam angulation—spurious left lower lobe consolidation[1].

   ❏ Differing x-ray tube to patient distances—alterations in mediastinal magnification on serial CXRs.

■ Exposures can vary. An underexposed CXR (everything too white) or an overexposed CXR (everything too black) can obliterate important abnormalities. Fortunately, problems resulting from under- or overexposure can be partially corrected using the windowing facility on digital images.

ASSESSING THE BEDSIDE CXR

A three-step sequence

1. Check the position of all lines, tubes and pacing leads.

2. Check the lungs and pleura. Check the mediastinum.

3. Apply the **three-film rule**: Always compare the present CXR with the immediately preceding one…and then with an even earlier CXR.

LINES AND TUBES

These must be correctly positioned (Table 13.1). False readings, inadequate drainage and iatrogenic injury do occur.

Table 13.1 Optimum positions.

Line, tube, wire	Purpose/function	Best position for the tip
Central venous pressure line	■ Monitoring right atrial pressure ■ Fluid infusion/nutrition ■ Drug administration	Superior vena cava or brachiocephalic vein
Swan–Ganz catheter (Pulmonary arterial catheter)	■ Monitoring pulmonary arterial pressure ■ To distinguish between cardiac and non-cardiac pulmonary oedema	Main or lobar pulmonary artery
Nasogastric tube	■ Gastric decompression/aspiration ■ Nutrition	At least 10 cm beyond the gastro-oesophageal junction
Nasoenteric tube	■ Nutrition	Beyond the gastric pylorus
Intercostal drain (thoracostomy tube)	■ Drainage of a pneumothorax/pleural effusion	In the pleural space
Endotracheal tube	■ Assisted ventilation	5–7 cm above the carina
Tracheostomy tube	■ Assisted ventilation	See p. 188.
Tunnelled venous catheter/Hickman line	■ Prolonged venous access ■ Nutrition ■ Chemotherapy administration	Junction of superior vena cava and right atrium
Oesophageal Doppler probe	■ Monitoring cardiac output via measurement of blood velocity in the descending aorta	Mid oesophagus

CENTRAL VENOUS PRESSURE (CVP) LINES

▪ Valves are present in the jugular and subclavian veins (Fig. 13.2). The tip of the central line must be distal to the valves otherwise central venous (i.e. right atrial) pressure readings will be inaccurate[2,3].

▪ **Rule of thumb:** On the CXR, the superior vena cava (SVC) commences at the level of the right first anterior intercostal space.

▪ A catheter tip situated in the right atrium or right ventricle may cause an arrhythmia.

▪ A curve at the tip of a CVP line suggests that the catheter is misplaced. Either it has entered a side vessel (Fig. 13.7), or it is jammed against the vessel wall, or it lies outside the vein.

VALVES[2]

▪ The last valve in the subclavian vein is 2 cm proximal to its junction with the internal jugular vein.

▪ The last valve in the internal jugular vein is approximately 2.5 cm above its junction with the subclavian vein.

▪ The brachiocephalic veins and the SVC do not contain valves.

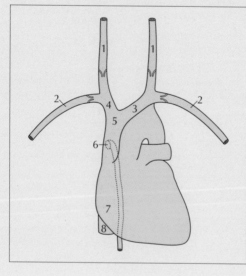

Fig. 13.2 *Vessels:*
1 = internal jugular vein;
2 = subclavian vein;
3 = left brachiocephalic vein; 4 = right brachiocephalic vein;
5 = SVC; 6 = orifice of the azygos vein;
7 = right atrium;
8 = inferior vena cava.

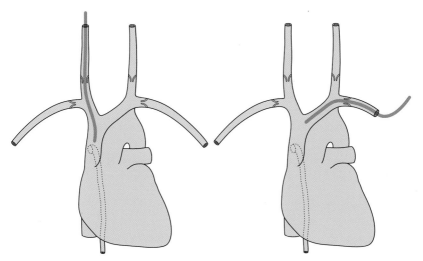

Figure 13.3 *The tip of the internal jugular line is correctly positioned in the SVC.*

Figure 13.4 *The tip of the left subclavian line is correctly positioned (i.e. well beyond the last valve in the vein).*

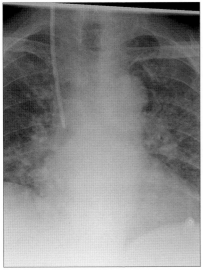

Figure 13.5 *Right internal jugular line in good position. (Retouched.)*

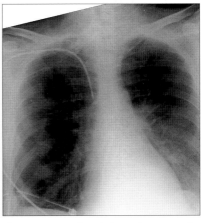

Figure 13.6 *Right subclavian line in good position with its tip in the SVC. The SVC commences at the level of the right first anterior intercostal space. (Retouched.)*

Faulty positions / complications

■ Line too high—inaccurate CVP measurements.

■ Line too low—risk of cardiac arrhythmia if in right atrium.

■ Vessel wall perforation resulting in:

❑ pneumothorax

❑ infusion of fluid into the mediastinum or the pleural space

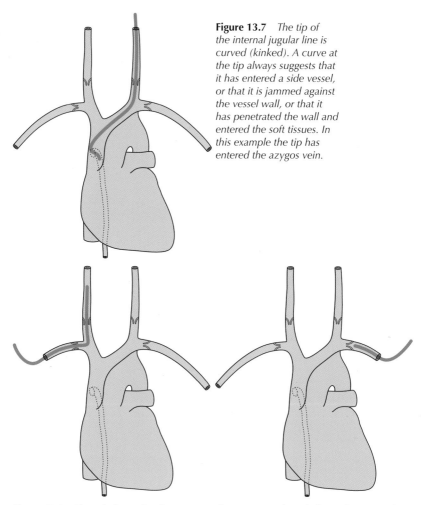

Figure 13.7 *The tip of the internal jugular line is curved (kinked). A curve at the tip always suggests that it has entered a side vessel, or that it is jammed against the vessel wall, or that it has penetrated the wall and entered the soft tissues. In this example the tip has entered the azygos vein.*

Figure 13.8 *The subclavian line has entered the internal jugular vein and the tip is directed towards the cranium.*

Figure 13.9 *The subclavian line is poorly positioned. Its tip lies proximal to a valve.*

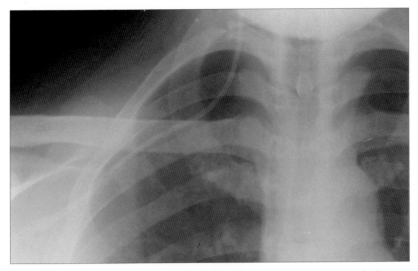

Figure 13.10 *The subclavian line has entered the internal jugular vein. (Retouched.)*

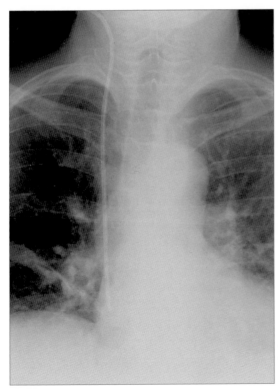

Figure 13.11 *The tip of the internal jugular line is situated in the right atrium. An unsatisfactory position; it may cause an arrhythmia. (Retouched.)*

SWAN–GANZ (SG) CATHETER

A SG catheter (pulmonary arterial line) measures the pulmonary capillary wedge pressure. This allows an assessment of the left atrial pressure and cardiac output. These pressure measurements have been regarded as crucial in complex ITU cases and help to distinguish between cardiac and non-cardiac pulmonary oedema. However, the usefulness of these catheters has been disputed and some studies suggest that pulmonary artery catheters do not improve patient outcome[4–7].

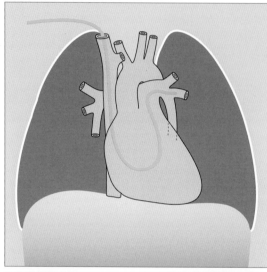

Figure 13.12 *The tip of the SG catheter is correctly positioned; i.e. the tip does not project more than 2 cm beyond the mediastinal outline.*

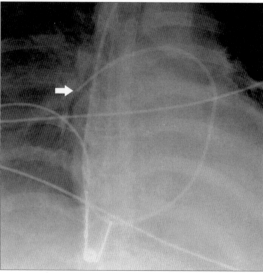

Figure 13.13 *SG catheter. Correct position. The tip (arrow) of the catheter overlies the border of the heart.*

- Optimum position. The SG tip should be situated between the main pulmonary artery and the interlobar arteries. Apply this rule: on the CXR the SG tip should extend no more than 2.0 cm beyond the mediastinal shadow.

- Faulty positions:

  ❏ Distal migration of the tip may cause pulmonary infarction.

  ❏ Proximal migration is common. If the tip is positioned in the right ventricle then there is a risk of an arrhythmia.

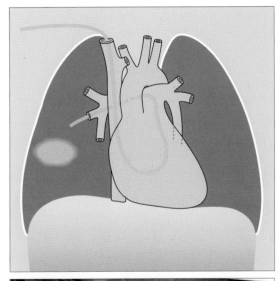

Figure 13.14 *SG catheter. The tip is situated well beyond the mediastinal shadow…in this example a pulmonary infarct has resulted.*

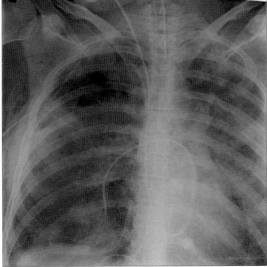

Figure 13.15 *SG catheter. Poor position. The tip of the catheter is well beyond the mediastinal shadow.*

NASOGASTRIC (NG) TUBE

- One or more side holes extend along the distal 5–10 cm of the tube (Fig. 13.16).

- The NG tip must be at least 10 cm beyond the oesophago-gastric junction… this will ensure that a side hole (Fig. 13.16) is not situated in the intra-abdominal portion of the oesophagus (Figs 13.17 and 13.18).

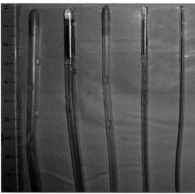

Figure 13.16 *A selection of large bore and small bore NG tubes. Note the positions of the side holes which extend along the distal 5–10 cm of the tubes.*

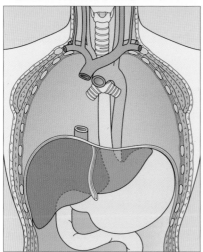

Figure 13.17 *Part of the oesophagus is normally situated just below the diaphragm. It is important that the tip of a NG tube is positioned 10 cm or more below the gastro-oesophageal junction—otherwise some of the side holes are likely to be within the oesophageal lumen.*

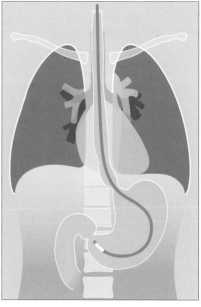

Figure 13.18 *The tip of the NG tube is in good position.*

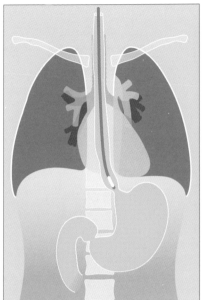

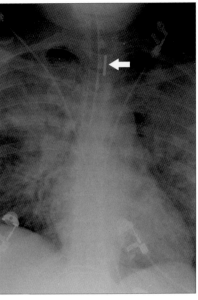

Figure 13.19 *Unsatisfactory position. The tip of the NG tube is positioned below the diaphragm— but it is still within the oesophagus.*

Figure 13.20 *The NG tube is curled on itself and its tip lies within the oesophagus at the level of the clavicles (arrow). The lung shadows represent extensive changes due to adult respiratory distress syndrome (ARDS).*

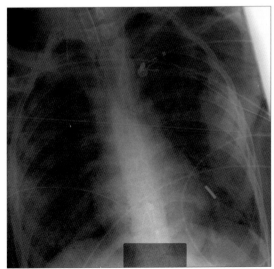

Figure 13.21 *The NG tube is identified by its dense tip. The tip has entered the trachea and lies within a left lower lobe bronchus.*

NASOENTERIC TUBE[8]

These feeding tubes are thin plastic catheters with a mercury/tungsten filled tip. The optimum position for the tip is distal to the pyloric sphincter.

Caution: because the tube is thin and flexible it can coil in the pharynx, oesophagus, or stomach. It may enter the trachea or the right main bronchus.

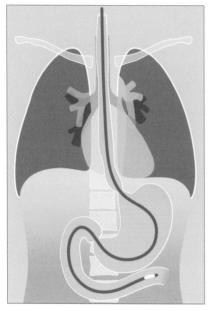

Figure 13.22 *The tip of the nasoenteric feeding tube is in good position; it lies distal to the gastric pylorus.*

PLEURAL DRAINAGE TUBES[3,8,9]

The various appearances and diagnostic problems associated with pneumothoraces and pleural effusions are addressed on pp. 82–106. Important aspects relating to pleural drainage are described on pp. 100–101.

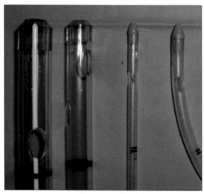

Figure 13.23 *A selection of intercostal and pleural drainage tubes. Note the number and position of the side holes. Most tubes have at least two side holes.*

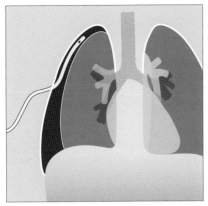

Figure 13.24 *Pneumothorax. Erect CXR. Pleural drainage tube in good position.*

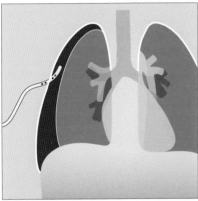

Figure 13.25 *Pneumothorax. Some of the side holes of the pleural drainage tube are outside the pleural space and are situated in the soft tissues of the chest wall.*

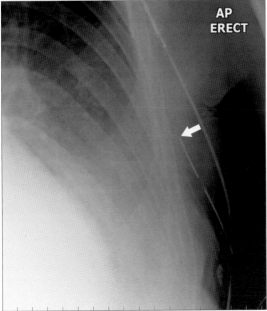

AP
ERECT

Figure 13.26 *The pleural drainage tube is not in the pleural space. Its side hole and tip (arrow) lie in the soft tissues of the chest wall.*

ENDOTRACHEAL TUBE (ETT)[3,8–14]

■ The ETT can move up or down[10,11]:

    ❏ Flex the neck and the tip can move 1.9 cm *downwards.*

    ❏ Extend the neck and it can move 1.9 cm *upwards.*

    ❏ Rotate the neck and it can move 0.7 cm *upwards.*

■ Ideally the tip should be situated midway between the carina and the vocal cords.

■ **Rule of thumb:** The tip of an ETT will be in a satisfactory position if it approximates to the level of the medial ends of the clavicles… i.e. approximately 5–7 cm above an adult's carina when the head is held in the neutral position.

Identify the carina

■ Its air shadow is visible on most CXRs.

■ If it is not visible—apply this **rule of thumb:** In 95% of people the carina is situated at the level of the T5–T7 thoracic vertebrae.

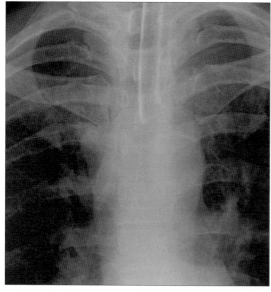

Figure 13.27 *ETT. Good position. Its tip lies 5–7 cm above the carina.*

Table 13.2 ETT problems.

ETT malposition 1	ETT malposition 2
Tip in the right main bronchus. May cause:	Tube in the oesophagus. CXR evidence:
■ Left lung collapse	■ ETT lateral to the tracheal air shadow
■ And/or: right upper lobe collapse	■ Oesophagus distended with air
■ Or: right lung over-distension and pneumothorax.	■ Stomach distended with air

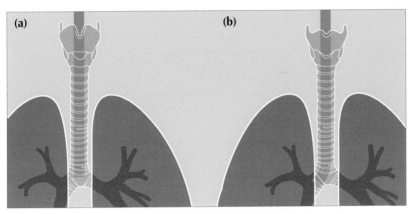

(a)   **(b)**

Figure 13.28 *ETTs. Faulty positions. (a) Tip at level of the carina—i.e. much too low. Flexing the neck from the neutral position can cause the tip of an ETT to descend 1.9 cm down the airway. (b) The tip of this ETT has entered the right main bronchus. Because of the obliquity of the angle of origin of the right main bronchus a much-too-low ETT will usually enter the right main bronchus rather than the left main bronchus.*

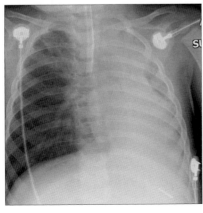

Figure 13.29 *ETT. Faulty position. The ETT has entered the right main bronchus. The left lung is no longer aerated. As a consequence, there is extensive collapse of the left lung.*

TRACHEOSTOMY TUBE

On a CXR the side walls of the tracheostomy tube should lie parallel to the outer margins of the trachea (Fig. 13.30).

Table 13.3 The CXR following introduction of a tracheostomy tube.

Normal	Abnormal
▪ Tracheostomy tube walls lie parallel to the long axis of the trachea.	▪ Widening of the mediastinum… a haematoma is developing.
▪ Tip lies several centimetres above the carina.	▪ Increasing mediastinal or subcutaneous air…a leak is occurring.
▪ The inflated cuff should not bulge the lateral walls of the trachea.	
▪ Initially, following the tracheostomy, a small amount of air in the mediastinum or subcutaneous tissues is to be expected and is unimportant.	

DOPPLER ULTRASOUND PROBE

An oesophageal probe is a minimally invasive instrument for monitoring cardiac output (via measurement of blood flow velocity in the descending aorta). Optimum probe position is at the level (approximately) of the mid oesophagus. Of course it is the clear ultrasound signal that confirms that probe position is good. Nevertheless, the doppler probe shadow (Fig. 13.31) should be familiar to those who evaluate ITU CXRs.

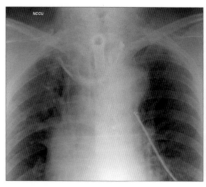

Figure 13.30 *Tracheostomy tube. Good position. Note that the walls of the tracheostomy tube parallel the walls of the trachea.*

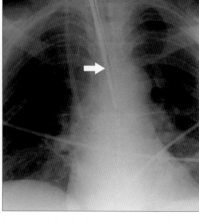

Figure 13.31 *Typical appearance of an oesophageal doppler ultrasound probe (arrow).*

THE LUNGS IN ITU

CONSOLIDATION, COLLAPSE, INFARCTION

The ITU patient is at risk of developing pneumonia, lobar collapse due to obstructive secretions, pleural effusion and pulmonary infarction. The relevant CXR appearances are described elsewhere:

- pneumonia—pp. 42–50
- lobar collapse—pp. 52–69
- pleural effusion—pp. 82–88
- pulmonary infarction—pp. 293–296

COMPLICATIONS OF MECHANICAL VENTILATION

Pneumothorax is common in ITU patients. It is usually consequent on mechanical ventilation. Sometimes it is a complication of subclavian artery line insertion. Detecting a pneumothorax on a supine CXR can be very challenging. The features to look for have been described earlier (pp. 97–106).

DIFFUSE LUNG PATHOLOGY[11,12,15–17]

- The CXR:
  - Frequently it is clinically—and radiologically—difficult to tell whether diffuse shadows are due to pneumonia, adult respiratory distress syndrome (ARDS), pulmonary oedema…or a combination of these. Table 13.4 provides some CXR features that can be helpful. But we must emphasise that assigning a specific pathological process to the shadows can be problematic. Indeed, extensive shadowing on a CXR often represents a combination of pneumonia, areas of lung collapse, pleural fluid, and ARDS.

- ARDS:
  - ARDS is a common cause for diffuse changes in the lungs. It results from an acute alveolar insult causing pulmonary inflammation and small vessel injury. The damaged endothelium leaks fluid and protein into the alveoli. There are numerous causes for ARDS including trauma, shock, systemic infection, head injury, multiple blood transfusions, severe pneumonia, smoke inhalation.
  - ARDS presents clinically as acute, severe, increasing respiratory distress. Onset of symptoms is usually within 24 hours of the original insult— invariably within three days.
  - The CXR shows diffuse consolidation in both lungs.
  - Sometimes the appearance of CXR changes is delayed…only becoming apparent 12 or more hours after the onset of symptoms.

Table 13.4 The CXR and diffuse lung shadows.

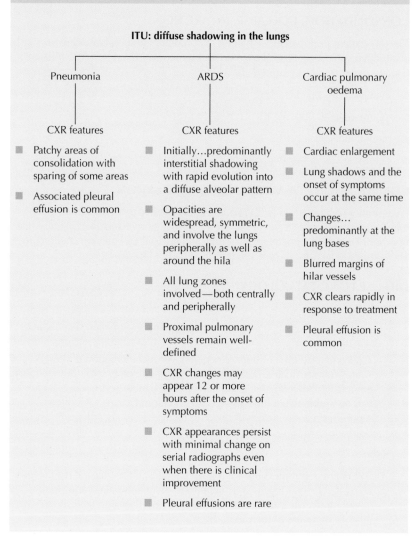

ITU: diffuse shadowing in the lungs

Pneumonia	ARDS	Cardiac pulmonary oedema
CXR features	CXR features	CXR features
■ Patchy areas of consolidation with sparing of some areas	■ Initially…predominantly interstitial shadowing with rapid evolution into a diffuse alveolar pattern	■ Cardiac enlargement
■ Associated pleural effusion is common	■ Opacities are widespread, symmetric, and involve the lungs peripherally as well as around the hila	■ Lung shadows and the onset of symptoms occur at the same time
	■ All lung zones involved—both centrally and peripherally	■ Changes… predominantly at the lung bases
	■ Proximal pulmonary vessels remain well-defined	■ Blurred margins of hilar vessels
	■ CXR changes may appear 12 or more hours after the onset of symptoms	■ CXR clears rapidly in response to treatment
	■ CXR appearances persist with minimal change on serial radiographs even when there is clinical improvement	■ Pleural effusion is common
	■ Pleural effusions are rare	

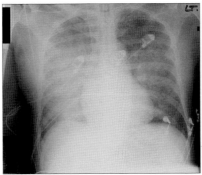

Figure 13.32 *ARDS. Typical pattern. Bilateral airspace (alveolar) shadowing.*

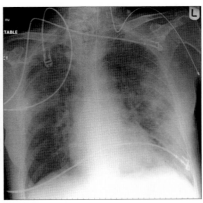

Figure 13.33 *ARDS. Typical pattern. Bilateral airspace (alveolar) shadowing.*

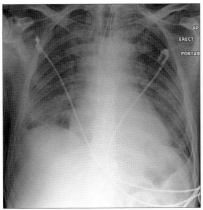

Figure 13.34 *Pulmonary oedema secondary to intracranial haemorrhage. Bilateral airspace (alveolar) shadowing.*

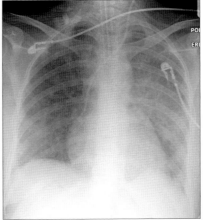

Figure 13.35 *Extensive pneumonia in both lungs. This appearance is indistinguishable from the diffuse alveolar shadowing that occurs in ARDS. The clinical history and examination together with the bacteriological findings indicated that the lung changes were due to infection—not to ARDS.*

FACTS AND FIGURES[18-24]

■ Analyse the CXR carefully. In one series of over a thousand consecutive ITU CXRs 35% had clinically unsuspected abnormalities[20].

■ An intravenous catheter or pacing wire may adopt a seemingly bizarre—but clearly intravenous—route as shown on the CXR. Several possibilities. It may have fortuitously entered a small but normal vein, e.g. the internal thoracic (i.e. mammary) vein. Alternatively, the patient may have a venous anomaly (e.g. a persistent left SVC). Thoracic venous anatomy—normal and anomalous—has been elegantly described by Godwin and Chen[2].

■ Pleural drainage tubes—position[21]:

❑ Conventional teaching: for pneumothorax drainage the tip is best placed antero-superiorly; for fluid drainage the tip is best positioned postero-inferiorly. However, several studies[22,23] suggest that the precise tube position in the pleural space is not that important.

❑ But be careful. Infected pleural fluid is a very different matter. If an empyema is to be drained then precise positioning of the tube is critical[21].

■ Pleural drainage tube enters a fissure:

❑ Occasionally this may lead to malfunction[24].

❑ However it has been shown that it is very common for a tube to be sited in a fissure[21]. In general this position does not adversely affect drainage.

REFERENCES

1. Zylak CJ, Littleton JT, Dinizch ML. Illusory consolidation of the left lower lobe: a pitfall of portable radiography. Radiology 1988; 167: 653–655.

2. Godwin JD, Chen JTT. Thoracic venous anatomy. AJR 1986; 147: 674–684.

3. Dunbar RD. Radiologic Appearance of compromised thoracic catheters, tubes, and wires. Radiol Clin North Am 1984; 22: 699–722.

4. Binanay C, Califf RM, Hasselblad V et al. Evaluation study of congestive heart failure and pulmonary artery catheterization effectiveness: the ESCAPE trial. JAMA 2005; 294: 1625–1633.

5. National Heart, Lung, and Blood Institute Acute Respiratory Distress Syndrome (ARDS) Clinical Trials Network. Pulmonary-artery versus central venous catheter to guide treatment of acute lung injury. N Engl J Med 2006; 354: 2213–2224.

6. Shure D. Pulmonary-artery catheters—peace at last? N Engl J Med 2006; 354: 2273.

7. Finfer S, DeLaney A. Pulmonary artery catheters. BMJ 2006; 333: 930–931.

8. Aronchick JM, Miller WT. Tubes and lines in the intensive care setting. Semin Roentgenol 1997; 32: 102–116.

9. Wechsler RJ, Steiner RM, Kinori I. Monitoring the monitors: the radiology of thoracic catheters, wires, and tubes. Semin Roentgenol 1988; 23: 61–84.

10. Conrardy P, Goodman L, Lainge F et al. Alteration of endotracheal tube position (flexion and extension of the neck). Crit Care Med 1976; 4: 8–12.

11. Goodman LR, Putman CE. Radiological evaluation of patients receiving assisted ventilation. JAMA 1981; 245: 858–860.

12. Sanders C. Chest radiography in the intensive care unit: pitfalls and potential. Current Imaging 1989; 1: 147–153.

13. Smith GM, Reed JC, Choplin RH. Radiographic detection of esophageal malpositioning of endotracheal tubes. AJR 1990; 154: 23–26.

14. Rollins RJ, Tocino I. Early radiographic signs of tracheal rupture. AJR 1987; 148: 695–698.

15. Greene R. Adult respiratory distress syndrome: acute alveolar damage. Radiology 1987; 163: 57–66.

16. Greene R, Jantsch H, Boggis C et al. Respiratory distress syndrome with new considerations. Radiol Clin North Am 1983; 21: 699–708.

17. Milne ENC, Pistolesi M, Miniati M et al. The radiologic distinction of cardiogenic and non-cardiogenic edema. AJR 1985; 144: 879–894.

18. Miller KS, Sahn SA. Chest tubes. Indications, technique, management and complications. Chest 1987; 91: 258–264.

19. Cameron EW, Mirvis SE, Shanmuganathan K et al. Computed tomography of malpositioned thoracostomy drains: a pictorial essay. Clin Radiol 1997; 52: 187–193.

20. Bekemeyer WB, Crapo RO, Calhoun S et al. Efficacy of chest radiography in a respiratory intensive care unit. Chest 1985; 88: 691–696.

21. Curtin JJ, Goodman LR, Quetteman EJ et al. Thoracostomy tubes after acute chest injury: relationship between location in a pleural fissure and function. AJR 1994; 163: 1339–1342.

22. Duponselle EFC. The level of the intercostal drain and other determining factors in the conservative approach to penetrating chest injuries. Afr J Med 1980; 26: 52–55.

23. Hegarty MM. A conservative approach to penetrating injuries of the chest: experience with 131 successive cases. Injury 1976; 8: 53–59.

24. Webb WR, La Berge JM. Radiographic recognition of chest tube malposition in the major fissure. Chest 1984; 85: 81–83.

14 PARTICULAR PAEDIATRIC POINTS

Children are not—medically—simply little adults.

Some pathological processes are shared by children and adults—the CXR patterns are often identical or similar. In this chapter we will concentrate on aspects of chest radiology that are different on a child's CXR.

NORMAL ANATOMY

THE THYMUS

■ The thymic shadow is visible at birth.

    ❑ Its size and shape varies widely between infants (Figs 14.1–14.4).

    ❑ When a child is ill the thymic shadow may decrease in size.

    ❑ The gland normally involutes between the ages of two and eight years.

    ❑ It is exceptional for the thymic shadow to be evident on the CXR after the age of eight years.

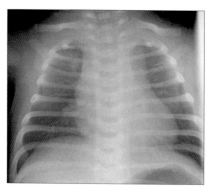

Figure 14.1 *33 weeks gestation. One day old. Mediastinum widened to the right and to the left by a normal thymus.*

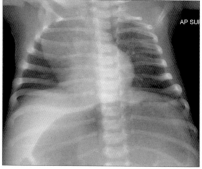

Figure 14.2 *Four weeks old. Lordotic AP projection. The rounded shadow projected over the right upper zone is a normal thymus.*

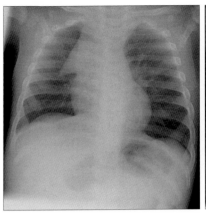

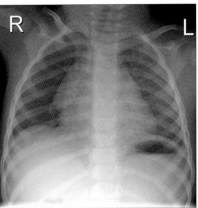

Figure 14.3 *Three months old. Cough. A triangular opacity overlies the right upper zone. Note that it has a sharp, well-defined, margin. This is a normal thymus.*

Figure 14.4 *Two years old. The right mid zone opacity blends with the border of the heart. Another normal thymic shadow. The thymic shadow usually disappears between the ages of two and eight years.*

THE HEART[1,2]

- **Two rules of thumb**: CXR evidence of cardiac enlargement.

  - On an infant's AP radiograph the normal cardiothoracic ratio (CTR) should not exceed 60%[1].

  - On a child's PA radiograph the normal CTR can be slightly above 50%, though by the second year it rarely exceeds 50%[1] (Fig. 14.5).

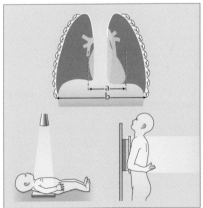

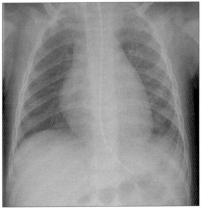

Figure 14.5 *An infant's CTR (a ÷ b) should not exceed 60% on an AP CXR. Over the age of 12 months, on a PA CXR, the CTR adopts the adult guideline—it should not exceed 50%.*

Figure 14.6 *Six months old. The initial impression is that the heart is enlarged. But...this is an AP CXR. The CTR does not exceed 60%. There is no reason to suggest cardiac enlargement.*

ABNORMAL CXRs—CHILD: ADULT

SIMILAR CXR PATTERNS

Several conditions that affect both children and adults show similar CXR features. For example: lobar collapse (pp. 52–66), pleural effusion (pp. 82–88), pneumothorax (pp. 96–104). See Figs 14.7–14.9.

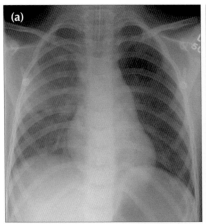

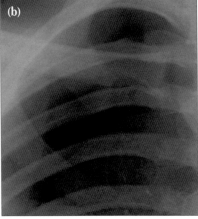

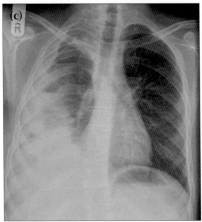

Figure 14.7   *(a) Right upper lobe pneumonia. (b) Pneumothorax. (c) Pleural effusion.*

Primary tuberculosis (PTB)

The CXR appearances are similar to those occurring in an adult with PTB. The possible CXR findings are described on pp. 134–136 but are worth repeating here:

- An opacity involving any segment of either lung.
- Enlarged hilar or mediastinal lymph nodes.
- Pleural effusion.
- Haematogenous spread producing miliary shadows (see Chapter 9, pp. 135–136).

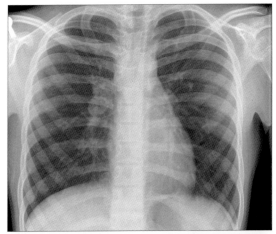

Figure 14.8 *Enlarged right hilum. A lumpy bumpy appearance. Consistent with lymph nodes. PTB.*

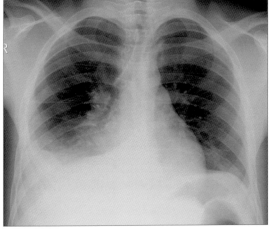

Figure 14.9 *Pleural effusion. PTB.*

CXR PATTERNS SPECIFIC TO CHILDREN

Bronchiolitis[3-5]

Infection occurring in children up to two years of age and caused by the respiratory syncytial virus. The inflammation mainly affects the bronchioles. These are narrowed by the inflammatory exudate and the narrowing causes air trapping (i.e. persistent distension) on expiration.

The CXR features of viral infection are not always recognised by those who have only episodic involvement with the CXRs of young children. Note:

- A pneumonic pattern does not occur.

- Bronchiolitis typically shows:

    ❏ Over-expansion (air trapping) of the lungs (Figs 14.10 and 14.11).

    ❏ Peribronchial cuffing (i.e. bronchial wall thickening) beyond the inner one third of the lung (Fig. 14.10).

    ❏ Small areas of linear collapse/peripheral atelectasis. These small shadows may change in position on subsequent CXRs[4].

- A small or poor inspiration in an infant (i.e. without bronchiolitis) often produces hazy peri-hilar shadows that can be misinterpreted as inflammatory change. In reality this appearance strongly suggests normality.

    Rule of thumb: If the CXR shows poor expansion of the lungs, i.e. they are not over-inflated…this suggests that the infant does not have bronchiolitis.

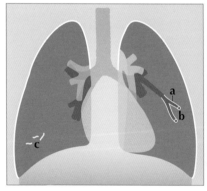 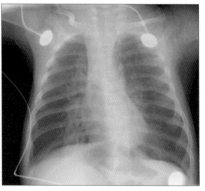

Figure 14.10 *Bronchiolitis. CXR features: (a) inflammation causes narrowing of the bronchioles and air trapping; (b) thickened bronchioles seen end-on will occasionally appear as small ring like densities (i.e. peribronchial cuffing); (c) small areas of linear collapse.*

Figure 14.11 *Three months old. Bronchiolitis. Note that the domes of the diaphragm are low due to the air trapping. Some streaky peri-hilar densities are also present; they represent inflammation of the bronchial walls and adjacent interstitium[5].*

Bacterial pneumonia[1,3,6,7]

Usually the CXR pattern will be identical to lobar pneumonia or broncho-pneumonia (p. 44) as they appear on an adult's CXR. Two additional specific features are worth noting:

- *Lymphadenopathy.* Obvious hilar lymph node enlargement is fairly common. This contrasts with adults in whom a simple pneumonia rarely causes a lymphadenopathy that is detectable on a CXR.

- *Round pneumonia (pseudotumour).* Sometimes pneumonic consolidation will appear as a rounded density simulating a lung mass. This rounded appearance does occur in adults—but it is much less common. It has been suggested that the round configuration is due to a gravitational effect in a child who sleeps in the supine position. Others offer a different explanation: an infant's system of collateral ventilation is relatively underdeveloped (i.e. few pores of Kohn and canals of Lambert). Inflammatory exudates accumulating in the alveoli cannot use these pathways to diffuse to adjacent alveoli as they would in an adult. Consequently, the exudate adopts the form of a sphere—the so-called round, or rounded, pneumonia. The importance of a round pneumonia appearance is that it can be misread as a primary or secondary tumour[3,6].

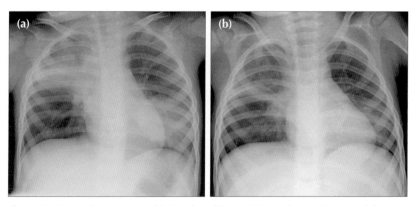

Figure 14.12 *Male. Two years old. Cough and fever. CXR (a) shows right upper lobe consolidation (pneumonia). A large round opacity in the left lower zone mimics a tumour. Following antibiotic treatment CXR (b) was obtained one week later. Both areas of shadowing have almost cleared. The spherical shadow represented a round pneumonia.*

SPECIFIC CLINICAL PROBLEMS

There are three common clinical scenarios in which the CXR may—or may not—play an important role: asthma; possible inhaled foreign body; and swallowed foreign body.

WHEEZING—IS IT ASTHMA?[7–9]

■ The most common CXR appearance in a child with asthma is an entirely normal radiograph.

■ The child with an established diagnosis of asthma does not require a routine CXR when an acute exacerbation occurs. However, if there is clinical deterioration then a CXR is indicated in order to exclude a complication (pneumothorax, pneumonia or lobar collapse).

■ Atypical CXR features should always raise the suspicion of another cause for wheezing, particularly foreign body inhalation. There is an important aphorism: beware the wheezing child too readily labelled as asthma who has a foreign body aspiration[5,8–10].

■ The lungs are over-distended when more than nine posterior ribs are visible above the domes of the diaphragm. **Rule of thumb:** Over-inflated lungs. Age two years and younger—likely viral infection. Older than two years—likely asthma (Table 14.1).

Table 14.1 Over-distended lungs. Bronchiolitis or asthma?

Pathology	CXR features	Note
Bronchiolitis	■ Over-distension of both lungs	The CXR appearances may be very similar in bronchiolitis and asthma. In a child under two years old bronchiolitis is the more likely diagnosis.
	■ +/– focal areas of linear collapse	
	■ +/– peribronchial cuffing *beyond the medial third of the lung* (Fig. 14.10)	
Asthma	■ Over-distension of both lungs	
	■ Peribronchial cuffing	

HAS A FOREIGN BODY BEEN INHALED?[7–14]

The most commonly inhaled foreign body is food, frequently a peanut[8–12]. A history of choking is usually obtained. Common clinical signs include coughing, stridor, wheezing and sternal retraction. Rapid recognition and treatment are essential. This is a medical emergency.

■ Radiography: if the child is able to cooperate then a frontal CXR should be obtained following a rapid forced expiration. Air trapping on the affected side is then more obvious (Fig. 14.13). Alternatively, fluoroscopy and observing the movement of the domes of the diaphragm relative to each other is an excellent method of detecting whether there is unilateral air trapping.

■ An inhaled foreign body may produce any one of three appearances[5,8,9,14]:

  ❏ Normal CXR. This is not necessarily reassuring. If a strong clinical suspicion persists (i.e. that a foreign body has been inhaled) then urgent referral for MRI or bronchoscopy is essential.

  ❏ Area of collapse or consolidation.

  ❏ Air trapping because the bronchial blockage has caused a ball valve effect. The affected lung appears blacker and larger than the opposite normal side (Fig. 14.13).

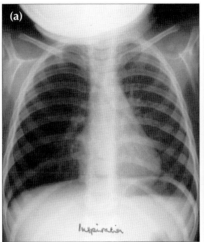
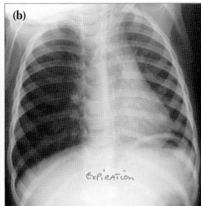

Figure 14.13 *Inhaled peanut has lodged in the right main bronchus. Inspiration CXR (a): the right lung is hypertransradiant (i.e. blacker) as compared with the left lung. Following a rapid expiration, CXR (b) shows the severe air trapping in the right lung with displacement of the mediastinum to the left side. These CXR findings indicate a medical emergency.*

IS THERE A FOREIGN OBJECT IN THE OESOPHAGUS?[15,16]

■ Occasionally, a coin will lodge in the oesophagus (Figs 14.14–14.16). Some of these patients may be asymptomatic. Erosion of the mucosa by a coin can cause an abscess or mediastinitis.

■ There is no danger to the child if the coin has passed into the stomach or the intestine. A radiograph of the abdomen (AXR) represents unjustified radiation exposure. Only a CXR is indicated.

■ Radiography: a single frontal CXR to include the neck.

■ If the CXR is normal, then the parents can be reassured that the coin has passed into the gut, will cause no harm and will be excreted within the next few days.

■ A caveat. Presently, coins minted in the UK are inert. In other countries this is not always the case. If a coin has a zinc core and a copper coating then gastric acid can dissolve the coating and the zinc can cause ulcers and anaemia. In countries where coins are potentially poisonous then an abdominal radiograph (if negative, to be followed by a CXR) would represent correct practice.

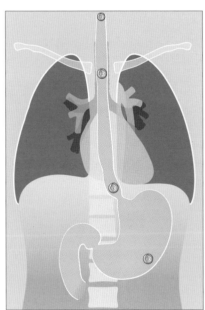

Figure 14.14 *Swallowed foreign bodies. A coin may impact in the oesophagus. Impaction usually occurs at one of three sites: in the cervical oesophagus, at the level of the arch of the aorta, or at the gastro-oesophageal junction. Once a coin passes into the stomach it invariably travels uneventfully through, and out of, the gastro-intestinal tract.*

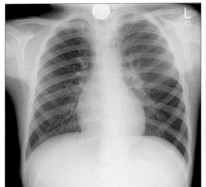

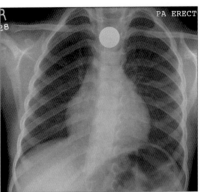

Figure 14.15   *Five years old. A coin has impacted in the cervical oesophagus. The neck must always be included on a child's CXR when a swallowed foreign body is a clinical possibility.*

Figure 14.16   *Four years old. A coin has impacted at the level of the aortic arch.*

AN INTERESTING CONDITION— CONGENITAL LOBAR EMPHYSEMA[5,7,17]

Aetiology / pathology

Most cases are thought to result from a bronchial obstruction affecting a lobe of the lung. Occasionally a structural occlusion (e.g. bronchial atresia) has been demonstrated. Usually one lobe alone is affected—invariably an upper lobe. Occasionally (less than 10%) two lobes are involved. Air enters the lobe via the canals of Lambert and pores of Kohn (collateral air drift) but cannot exit. Consequently the lobe gradually becomes very distended and it balloons to many times its normal size.

Clinical features

A few children present in the neonatal period. More commonly, symptoms occur between one and six months of age. Dyspnoea and cyanosis are the main features.

The CXR

■   Invariably an upper lobe (usually the left) is distended and hyperlucent. Adjacent lobes are compressed. Extreme distension will displace the mediastinum to the opposite side.

■   In the immediate neonatal period an affected lobe may appear opaque (i.e. dense) because the amniotic fluid in the lobe has not been cleared.

■   Occasionally, with congenital lobar emphysema, a hyperlucent lobe is found as an incidental finding on a CXR in an asymptomatic individual.

AN INTERESTING CONDITION—CYSTIC FIBROSIS[1,7,18,19]

Aetiology/pathology

Autosomal recessive. 1:1500 live births. An abnormality in chloride ion transport which results in viscid mucus production. Poor clearing of the mucus from the airway predisposes to chest infection, bronchiectasis, and other sequelae of chronic lung infection. Age of presentation in childhood is variable.

Clinical features

Recurrent pulmonary infections. Other organ involvement may suggest the diagnosis (e.g. involvement of pancreas, liver—biliary cirrhosis, paranasal sinuses).

The CXR

- Normal…if the disease is mild.
- Air trapping, hyperinflation.
- Peribronchial cuffing (see Fig. 14.10).
- Atelectasis, areas of infection, scarring.
- Bronchiectasis (see p. 322). Middle and upper lobes predominantly:
  - ❏ tubular (gloved finger appearance) and/or
  - ❏ cystic
- Prominent hila. Due to enlarged infected lymph nodes or to pulmonary arterial hypertension.

REFERENCES

1. Carty H, Shaw D, Brunelle F, Kendall B. Imaging Children. Edinburgh: Churchill Livingstone, 1994.

2. Jefferson K, Rees S. Clinical Cardiac Radiology. 2nd ed. London: Butterworths, 1980.

3. Branson RT, Griscom NT, Cleveland RH. Interpretation of chest radiographs in infants with cough and fever. Radiology 2005; 236: 22–29.

4. Griscom NT, Wohl MEB, Kirkpatrick JA. Lower respiratory infections: how infants differ from adults. Radiol Clin North Am 1978; 16: 367–387.

5. Rencken I, Patton WL, Brasch RC. Airway obstruction in pediatric patients. Radiol Clin North Am. 1998; 36: 175–187.

6. Rose RW, Ward BH. Spherical pneumonias in children simulating pulmonary and mediastinal masses. Radiology 1973; 106: 179–182.

7. Newman B, Oh KS. Abnormal pulmonary aeration in infants and children. Radiol Clin North Am 1988; 26: 323–339.

8. Lloyd-Thomas AR, Bush GH. All that wheezes is not asthma. Anaesthesia 1986; 41: 181–185.

9. Roback MG, Dreitlein DA. Chest radiograph in the evaluation of first time wheezing episodes: review of current clinical practice and efficacy. Pediatr Emerg Care. 1998; 14: 181–184.

10. Breysem L, Loyen S, Boets A et al. Pediatric emergencies: thoracic emergencies. Eur J Radiol 2002; 12: 2849–2865.

11. Baharloo F, Veyckemans F, Francis C et al. Tracheobronchial foreign bodies: presentation and management in children and adults. Chest 1999; 115: 1357–1362.

12. Metrangolo S, Monetti C, Meneghini L, et al. Eight years experience with foreign body aspiration in children: what is really important for a timely diagnosis? J Pediatr Surg 1999; 34: 1229–1231.

13. Silva AB, Muntz HR, Clary R. Utility of conventional radiography in the diagnosis and management of pediatric airway foreign bodies. Ann Otol Rhinol Laryngol 1998; 107: 834–838.

14. Svedstrom E, Puhakka H, Kero P. How accurate is chest radiography in the diagnosis of tracheobronchial foreign bodies in children? Pediatr Radiol 1989; 19: 520–522.

15. Macpherson RI, Hill JG, Othersen HB et al. Esophageal Foreign Bodies in Children: Diagnosis, Treatment, and Complications. AJR 1996; 166: 919–924.

16. Raby N, Berman L, de Lacey G. Accident and Emergency Radiology: A Survival Guide. 2nd ed. Philadelphia, PA: Elsevier Saunders, 2005.

17. Panicek DM, Heitzman ER, Randall PA et al. The Continuum of pulmonary developmental anomalies. Radiographics 1987; 7: 747–772.

18. Wood BP. Cystic fibrosis. Radiology 1997; 204: 1–10.

19. Robinson TE. Imaging of the chest in cystic fibrosis. Clin Chest Med 2007; 28: 405–421.

15 THE NEONATAL CXR

The newborn infant in respiratory distress is an emergency.

- **CXR essential (1). A fundamental principle**—as a rule the neonatologist cannot be absolutely certain of the cause of the distress without a CXR. The CXR will usually confirm the default diagnosis or reveal the true cause.

- **CXR essential (2).** Many of these infants will eventually have various lines and tubes inserted. Confirmation of correct positioning requires a CXR.

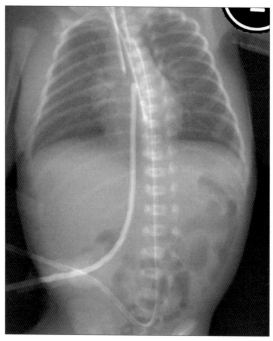

Figure 15.1 *Neonate. Can you list the abnormal findings on this chest and abdominal radiograph? Answer on p. 224.*

Respiratory distress in the newborn will occasionally be due to serious anatomical anomalies that usually require surgical intervention[1,2]. These include: oesophageal atresia/tracheo-oesophageal fistula; diaphragmatic hernia; cystic adenomatoid malformation of the lung; congenital lobar emphysema.

All of these are very rare conditions, but they must not be overlooked. If they are not recognised then morbidity and mortality will be high. These uncommon abnormalities will not be described here. Radiographic examples are illustrated on p. 213. In this chapter we will concentrate on the common day-in, day-out CXR problems encountered in the neonatal intensive care unit (NICU).

THE LUNGS

TERM INFANTS

Transient Tachypnoea of the Newborn (TTN)[1-5]

■ TTN occurs most commonly in pre-term infants following Caesarean section. All the same, TTN can occur in term infants.

■ Sometimes referred to as *wet lung*, because the fluid that filled the lungs prior to birth has not been cleared completely. Following delivery the infant breathes with some difficulty and requires oxygen.

■ The CXR shows indistinct pulmonary vessels bilaterally. There is lack of a sharp margin to the heart, mediastinum and diaphragm (Fig. 15.2). The lungs remain well inflated. Sometimes there is fluid in the horizontal fissure; occasionally some pleural fluid elsewhere.

■ The infant gradually improves and the CXR will be clear at 48 hours (Fig. 15.2).

Meconium Aspiration Syndrome[1,2]

■ Hypoxic stress *in utero* puts an infant at risk of discharging meconium into the amniotic fluid. When meconium is inhaled it irritates the respiratory tract and causes severe respiratory distress.

■ The CXR will show coarse reticular and nodular shadows representing scattered areas of collapse or consolidation. There may be associated areas of focal lung distension (i.e. emphysema).

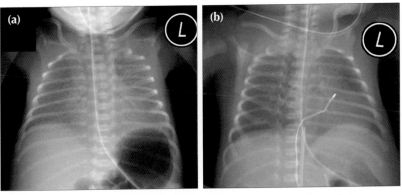

Figure 15.2 *Neonate. Slight respiratory distress. CXR (a) at age one day. Indistinct pulmonary vessels. Slightly indistinct margins of the heart and diaphragm. CXR (b) at age two days. The lungs are clear. Cardiac and diaphragm margins are sharp. The original CXR appearances were due to TTN (wet lung). Note that the umbilical vein catheter (UVC) is incorrectly positioned (see p. 216).*

PRE-TERM INFANTS

Respiratory distress syndrome/hyaline membrane disease (HMD)[1-5]

■ HMD is not simply due to surfactant deficiency. It represents an acute injury of immature lungs. One aspect of this immaturity is surfactant deficiency.

■ HMD affects mainly very pre-term infants. It can occur in term infants after Caesarean section and also when the mother is diabetic.

■ Symptoms develop soon after delivery because the infant simply cannot expand the lungs adequately.

■ Note: HMD and TTN are not always distinct and separate entities. They can overlap. All pre-term infants will have some degree of TTN.

■ **CXR appearances:**

These will be affected by the amount of lung distension produced by the assisted ventilation. The following are some useful generalisations.

1. **Early**

   The lungs show a homogeneous, bilateral, ground glass appearance (Fig. 15.3). Sometimes lung consolidation (i.e. airspace shadowing) also occurs.

2. **Within a few days**

   The lungs become consolidated as a result of a profuse exudation of fluid into the alveoli. They appear opaque. Frequently there are air bronchograms (see p. 227). A complete white out of both lungs may occur.

3. **Complications—early/short term**

   Severe HMD requires assisted respiration either with ventilation or with continuous positive airway pressure (CPAP). Complications may then result, either from lung pathology or from the treatment which is keeping the baby alive…or from both the pathological process and the treatment.

   Early complications include: pneumothorax, tension pneumothorax, pulmonary interstitial emphysema (PIE), and mediastinal emphysema[2,6]. These complications are usually short term, but some will be fatal if not recognised and treated (Figs 15.4 and 15.7).

4. **Complications—long term**

   Lung changes develop and persist in some infants (Fig. 15.8). The appearance is referred to as chronic lung disease (CLD) of prematurity… a synonym for the more traditional term of bronchopulmonary dysplasia.

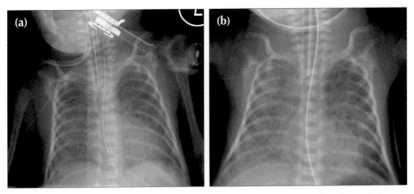

Figure 15.3 *Pre-term infant. Respiratory distress. CXR (a) at age one day. Ground glass appearance in both lungs. CXR (b) at age three days. Confluent airspace shadowing in both lungs. HMD. CXR (a) represents the typical early findings in HMD and CXR (b) shows the typical appearances that occur within a day or two.*

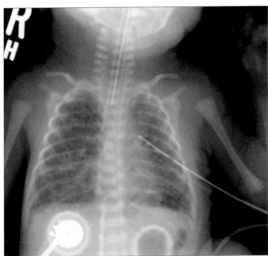

Figure 15.4 *Pre-term infant. Age five days. Respiratory distress. HMD and a complicating left pneumothorax has been treated with an intercostal drain. The bubbly appearance in both lungs represents air that has passed through ruptured alveolar walls and dissected through the interstitial tissues. This complication represents pulmonary interstitial emphysema (PIE).*

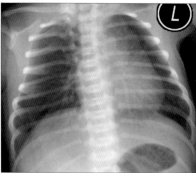

Figure 15.5 *Be careful. Neonate. Normal CXR. Two features could lead to erroneous diagnosis. (1) The infant is rotated to the left and the rotation distorts the mediastinal appearance. (2) A skin crease accounts for the line artefact overlying the right lung base. Vessels can be seen outside this line—i.e. it is not a pneumothorax.*

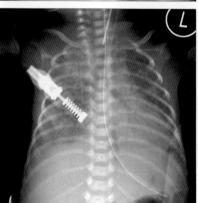

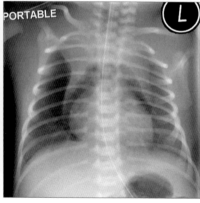

Figure 15.6 *Pre-term infant. HMD. An air bronchogram (see p. 227) is present in the consolidated left lung. Air bronchograms are often seen in lungs affected by HMD. There is no particular clinical connotation when an air bronchogram is present in HMD.*

Figure 15.7 *Pre-term infant. HMD. Pneumomediastinum. The air has arisen from an alveolar leak, dissected through the lung interstitium, and then entered the mediastinum. The normal thymus is outlined by the mediastinal air—a peculiar but characteristic appearance. It is often referred to as the angel wing sign.*

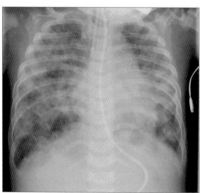

Figure 15.8 *Age five months. Previous HMD. The ring shadows and the coarse interstitial shadows are indicative of CLD of prematurity. Incidentally, the endotracheal tube (ETT) is too low; it is just above the carina.*

WATCH OUT FOR A PNEUMOTHORAX

A pneumothorax must be excluded on every single CXR. It is a common problem and it may produce a subtle change on the CXR.

■ **Easy to detect**

The typical CXR appearance is as described on p. 96. The features to look for are:

❏ The visible margin of the visceral pleural surface.

❏ A black area lateral to the visceral pleural surface.

❏ No vessels lateral to the visceral pleural surface.

■ **Much tougher**

Subtle features on the supine CXR (Fig. 15.9) may be overlooked. These are described on pp. 97–99. The air in the pleural space may show:

❏ A hyperlucent upper quadrant of the abdomen.

❏ The deep sulcus sign (see p. 97).

❏ A sharp black margin to the superior surface of the dome of the diaphragm (Fig. 15.10).

❏ A sharply defined cardiac border (Fig. 15.10).

■ **Really dangerous**

Tension pneumothorax. The CXR findings are described on pp. 100–102. Two cardinal features:

❏ The dome of the diaphragm on the affected side is almost always depressed or flattened (Fig. 15.11).

❏ The mediastinum and heart are usually—but not always—pushed to the opposite side (Fig. 15.11).

❏ **Potential pitfall:** With the baby lying supine the intrapleural air may collect anteriorly and a tension pneumothorax may compress and push the mediastinum in a posterior rather than in a lateral direction. Sometimes an anterior tension pneumothorax will only be revealed by a horizontal beam (i.e. a cross-table) CXR. Fig. 15.9 illustrates how an anterior tension pneumothorax can occur and be overlooked.

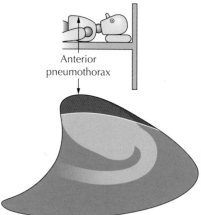

Figure 15.9 *In the NICU the CXR is obtained with the infant supine. Air in the pleural space will collect at the highest point, i.e. anteriorly, as shown on this lateral perspective of the thorax.*

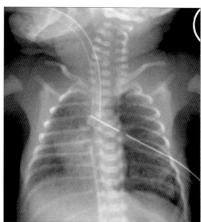

Figure 15.10 *Supine CXR. HMD. Extensive lung shadowing. Complicating pneumothorax… features to note: the sharp black line outlining the left heart border; the extreme clarity of the left dome of the diaphragm. Incidentally, the UVC tip is in the right atrium and the ETT is very low.*

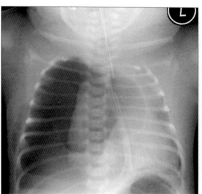

Figure 15.11 *Right-sided pneumothorax. It is under tension—the mediastinum is displaced to the left and the right dome of the diaphragm is low and flat. The right hemithorax is markedly hypertransradiant (i.e. very black).*

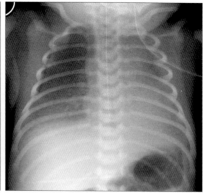

Figure 15.12 *Beware! Skin creases, clothing artefacts, or monitoring apparatus can mimic a visceral pleural line. In this infant a skin fold on the right simulates a pneumothorax.*

SOME RARE CONDITIONS CAUSING NEONATAL DISTRESS[1,2]

This chapter has concentrated on the everyday causes of neonatal distress. There are rare conditions that must not be overlooked. Four of these are illustrated below. The CXR is invaluable in suggesting the diagnosis.

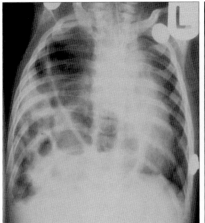

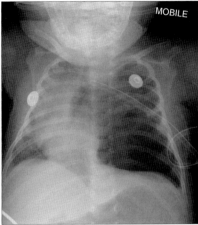

Figure 15.13 *Severe respiratory distress. The ring shadows at the right base represent multiple loops of bowel. Diaphragmatic hernia[1].*

Figure 15.14 *Be careful. The left lower zone lucency is not a pneumothorax, but is due to congenital cystic adenomatoid malformation of the lung (CCAM)[1].*

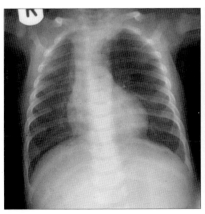

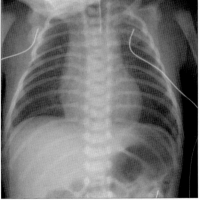

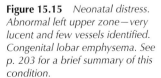

Figure 15.15 *Neonatal distress. Abnormal left upper zone—very lucent and few vessels identified. Congenital lobar emphysema. See p. 203 for a brief summary of this condition.*

Figure 15.16 *Neonatal distress. Grey skin appearance after delivery and intermittent grunting. The NG tube (illustrated) would not pass beyond the level of the T3 vertebra. Oesophageal atresia and a tracheo-oesophageal fistula.*

TUBES AND LINES[1,2,7–15]

Various tubes and lines are used to monitor, ventilate, hydrate and feed infants in the NICU (Table 15.1).

Table 15.1 The various tubes and lines.

Tube/line	Purpose
Umbilical vein catheter	■ Administration of fluids/drugs
	■ Transfusion
	■ Rarely—monitoring central venous pressure
Umbilical artery catheter	■ Measurement of blood gases/blood tests
	■ Monitoring arterial blood pressure
	■ Infusion of fluids
Central venous catheter	■ Administration of fluids/drugs
Endotracheal tube	■ Mechanical ventilation
Nasal prongs for continuous positive airway pressure	■ Assisted ventilation
Naso/orogastric tube	■ Gastric aspiration
	■ Enteral feeding
Jejunal feeding tube	■ Enteral feeding

UMBILICAL CATHETERS[1,7–9,11–14]

Basic post-natal anatomy

■ The single umbilical vein passes cephalad in the free margin of the falciform ligament just to the right of the mid line. The vein then divides into two branches (Fig. 15.17). One branch joins with the portal vein; the other continues as the ductus venosus (DV), terminating in the left (or middle) hepatic vein which joins the inferior vena cava. The length of the DV is approx. 2 cm in full-term infants; it is much shorter in tiny pre-term babies.

■ Each umbilical artery dips downwards into the pelvis to enter the internal iliac artery (Fig. 15.18).

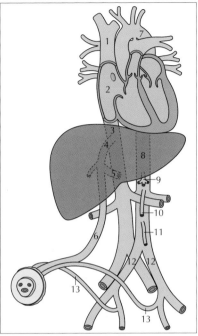

Figure 15.17 *Normal post-natal anatomy:*
1 = superior vena cava;
2 = right atrium;
3 = inferior vena cava;
4 = ductus venosus;
5 = branch vein joining the portal vein;
6 = umbilical vein;
7 = arch of the aorta;
8 = aorta;
9 = coeliac axis;
10 = superior mesenteric artery;
11 = inferior mesenteric artery;
12 = common iliac arteries;
13 = umbilical arteries.

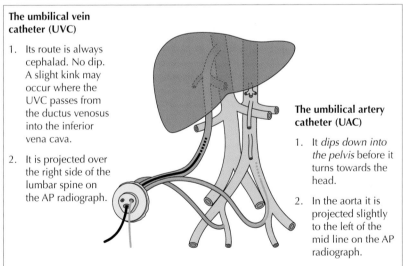

The umbilical vein catheter (UVC)

1. Its route is always cephalad. No dip. A slight kink may occur where the UVC passes from the ductus venosus into the inferior vena cava.

2. It is projected over the right side of the lumbar spine on the AP radiograph.

The umbilical artery catheter (UAC)

1. It *dips down into the pelvis* before it turns towards the head.

2. In the aorta it is projected slightly to the left of the mid line on the AP radiograph.

Figure 15.18 *Which catheter is which? To make an accurate assessment it is essential that the pelvis is included on the CXR/AXR. The question to ask: does the catheter take a dip into the pelvis? Yes = UAC. No = UVC.*

Umbilical Vein Catheter (UVC) [1,2,8,9,11,14]

■ Post-natal patency. The vein may be catheterised up to four days after birth. Eventually the vein closes, constricts, and forms the ligamentum teres extending from the umbilicus to the liver. The mesentery which surrounds the umbilical vein becomes the falciform ligament.

■ Catheter tip: optimum position (Figs 15.19a and 15.20).

  ❏ The requirement: the tip must be placed in a region of good blood flow and well away from branches that drain vital organs.

  ❏ There is no single correct position…a UVC tip position is acceptable so long as it is not in the liver nor in the heart. Sometimes it will be difficult to know whether the tip is just inside or just outside the liver because there are no anatomical landmarks that provide absolute certainty.

  ❏ An approach to adopt: a tip positioned in the inferior vena cava (approximately at the level of T8–T9 vertebrae) or at the porta hepatis (the opening on the visceral surface of the liver where the major arteries, ducts and portal vein enter and leave) is, in general, desirable.

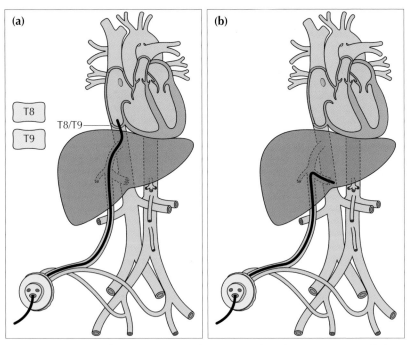

Figure 15.19 *UVC catheter tip. (a) In good position. In the inferior vena cava just below the right atrium. A tip positioned at the level of T8–T9 vertebrae is usually satisfactory. (b) The tip has entered the portal vein; thrombosis is a recognised complication.*

■ Wrong position...potential complications

   ❏ Tip...in the heart:

      – cardiac arrhythmia

      – valvular injury

      – pericardial perforation resulting in effusion/tamponade

   ❏ Tip...in a pulmonary artery:

      – pulmonary infarction

   ❏ Tip...in the portal venous system/DV (Figs 15.19b and 15.21):

      – portal vein thrombosis

      – hepatic necrosis

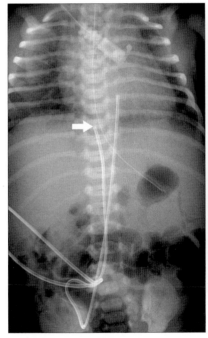

Figure 15.20 *UVC tip (arrow) in good position in the IVC.*

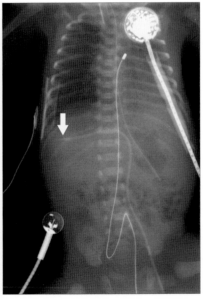

Figure 15.21 *UVC. Incorrect position. The tip (arrow) of the catheter has entered a portal vein and lies within the right lobe of the liver.*

Umbilical Artery Catheter (UAC)[1,2,7,9,11–13]

■ Post-natal patency. The paired umbilical arteries constrict and obliterate two to five days after birth. The obliterated arteries are covered with peritoneum and will persist as fibrous cords in the anterior abdominal wall outside the peritoneum—these are the medial umbilical ligaments.

■ Catheter tip: optimum position. Two choices (Fig. 15.22 and Table 15.2).

    ❏ The requirement is that the tip is situated in a region of rapid blood flow and well away from the origin of vessels supplying the vital organs.

    ❏ A high position ensures that the tip of the UAC is well above the origins of the coeliac axis (T12), the superior mesenteric artery (T12–L1), and the renal arteries (L1–L2).

    ❏ A low position ensures that the tip of the UAC is well below the origins of the same vessels and above the aortic bifurcation (L4–L5). All the same, the low position means that the tip can be close to the origin of the inferior mesenteric artery (which arises at the L3–L4 level).

    ❏ The UAC high position (Figs 15.22a and 15.23) is favoured in most NICUs.

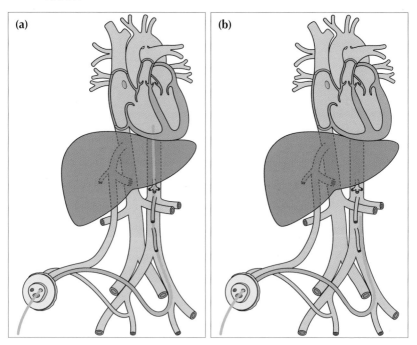

(a)   (b)

Figure 15.22 *UAC catheters in good positions. (a) High position. Tip in the aorta just above the level of the dome of the diaphragm. (b) Low position. Tip in the aorta at approximately the level of L3/L4 vertebrae.*

❏ Wrong position…potential complications.

– Tip…in the arch of the aorta—head vessels are at risk of thrombosis

– Tip…between T12 and L2—the major arterial branches of the aorta are at risk of thrombosis.

– Tip…into the buttock (via the gluteal artery)—ischaemia and muscle necrosis.

Table 15.2   UAC tip preferred position—two choices.

Position high (preferred by most units)	Position low
■ Thoracic	■ Lumbar
■ Above the diaphragm	■ Below the diaphragm and above the aortic bifurcation
■ Tip positioned between T7 and T10 vertebral bodies…level with (or just above) the dome of the diaphragm	■ Tip positioned between L3 and L4 vertebral bodies

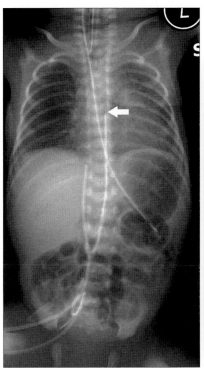

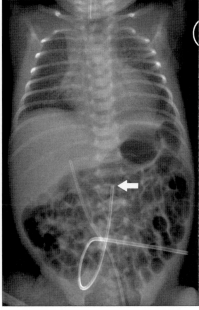

Figure 15.23   *UAC in good (high) position. The tip (arrow) lies above the dome of the diaphragm (at the level of the T7 vertebra). (Retouched.)*

Figure 15.24   *The tip (arrow) of the UAC is too low—it lies at the level of L2 vertebra, close to the origins of the renal arteries.*

CENTRAL VENOUS CATHETER—A LONG LINE

- If introduced via a subclavian, internal jugular or antecubital approach—the tip should lie in the superior vena cava just above the right atrium (Fig. 15.25).

- If a femoral approach is used—the tip should lie just below the right atrium outside the heart (guideline: at the level of T8–T9 vertebrae).

- If the position of the tip is uncertain then it can be checked by introducing contrast medium into the catheter, or by ultrasound examination. Many units carry out this check as a routine practice.

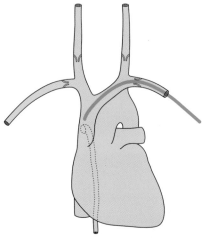

Figure 15.25 *Central line. Good position with the tip in the superior vena cava well beyond the last valve in the subclavian vein. The position of the last valve in each internal jugular vein is also shown. The dotted vessel is the azygos vein draining into the superior vena cava.*

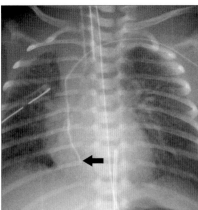

Figure 15.26 *Left ante-cubital long line. Unsatisfactory position. The tip (arrow) lies within the right atrium. Dysrhythmia is a recognised complication. (Retouched.)*

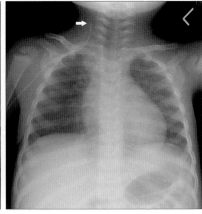

Figure 15.27 *Neonate. One day old. The lungs are clear, but the right ante-cubital long line has entered the internal jugular vein and its tip is directed towards the cranium. (Retouched.)*

ENDOTRACHEAL TUBE (ETT)[12]

- Optimum position of the tip is in the mid trachea…i.e. above the carina and below the vocal cords (Fig. 15.28).

- Malposition:

  ❑ Too low. The ETT may enter the right main bronchus (Figs 15.29 and 15.30).

  ❑ Too high. Rotation of the head from the neutral position can cause the ETT to move 1.0 cm upwards…and the ETT may pull out.

- **ETT rules of thumb:**

  ❑ If the clavicles are visible then the tip of the ETT should lie just below the medial ends of the clavicles.

  ❑ In some very small pre-term infants it can be difficult to identify the ends of the clavicles, but you can always see the carina. Make sure that the tip of the ETT is well above the carina.

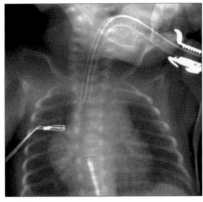

Figure 15.28 *ETT. Satisfactory position. Incidentally, note that the UVC tip is in the right atrium.*

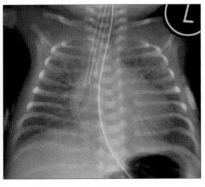

Figure 15.29 *HMD. The ETT has entered the right main bronchus. Lung collapse has not yet occurred. The ETT was pulled back to achieve a satisfactory position.*

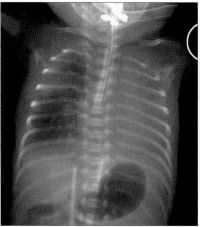

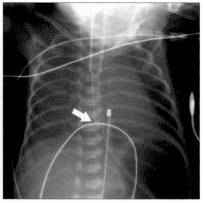

Figure 15.31 *ETT in the oesophagus. Note: (a) the tip (arrow) of the ETT is midline but well below the carina; (b) the distended and oxygen filled stomach. (Retouched.)*

Figure 15.30 *ETT in the right main bronchus. This has caused complete consolidation of the non-ventilated left lung. (Retouched.)*

FEEDING TUBES

Nasogastric (NG) tube[10,12]

■ Optimum position for the tip is within the stomach.

■ Wrong positions for the tip (Fig. 15.32):

❏ In the oesophagus. Common occurrence. Usually due to simple error in positioning. If re-positioning, in the neonate, fails to place the NG tip in the stomach then the possibility of oesophageal atresia must be considered.

❏ Into a bronchus.

❏ Elsewhere, outside the gastro-intestinal tract. Very rare occurrence. If it occurs then perforation of the pharynx, hypopharynx or cervical oesophagus must be considered. Any abnormal (i.e. non-anatomical) course of the NG tube in the thorax should always raise this possibility.

Jejunal feeding tube

Optimum position of the tip is in the fourth part of the duodenum (i.e. the tube has crossed the midline on the abdominal radiograph…from right to left).

Table 15.4 Checking the NG tube—three questions and three rules.

Question 1:	Is the tip in the stomach?
If not...	
Question 2:	Is it curled up in the oesophagus?
If not...	
Question 3:	Has it passed into the larynx and entered the trachea or a bronchus?
Rule 1:	If the tip cannot be positioned in the stomach—oesophageal atresia needs to be excluded.
Rule 2:	If the tube passes below the diaphragm but the tip is seen to be projected over the thorax (i.e. not over the abdomen) and away from the oesophagus—a diaphragmatic hernia needs to be excluded.
Rule 3:	Think perforation. Although perforation is very much rarer than incorrect positioning in the bronchus, its clinical importance means that perforation must be considered whenever there is any deviation of the NG tube from the normal anatomical course through the oesophagus.

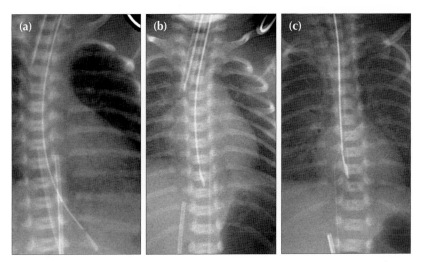

Figure 15.32 *NG tubes. (a) Normal position. (b) Tip in the oesophagus. (c) Tip in the oesophagus. Incidentally, note that the long line in (c), introduced via the femoral vein, has passed across an atrial septal defect into the left atrium.*

OTHER EQUIPMENT/MONITORING DEVICES

Assorted monitoring devices may produce shadows on the CXR (Fig. 15.33). These include:

- apnoea monitors
- pH monitor
- ECG leads
- transcutaneous blood gas sensors
- temperature probe

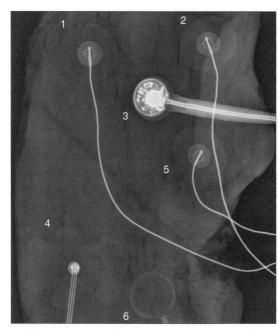

Figure 15.33 *Various external monitoring devices will produce shadows on the CXR. Their precise appearance will vary between different countries and between different units. Several of these devices were placed on a piece of steak—to simulate the chest wall soft tissues—and a radiograph obtained.*
1 = cardiac monitor;
2 = cardiac monitor;
3 = transcutaneous monitor (TCM) for blood gases;
4 = temperature probe;
5 = cardiac monitor;
6 = apnoea monitor.

Answer to Fig. 15.1 on p. 206:

The abnormal findings are...

1. Tip of the ETT unsatisfactory. At the origin of the right main bronchus.

2. Tip of NG tube unsatisfactory. In the lower oesophagus.

3. Tip of UVC unsatisfactory. In the right atrium.

4. Tip of the UAC unsatisfactory. Too high (at the level of T4 vertebra).

NB: some of the tubes and lines were retouched to make their positions clearer.

REFERENCES

1. Wood BP. The newborn chest. Radiol Clin North Am 1993; 31: 667–676.

2. Gibson AT, Steiner GM. Imaging the neonatal chest. Clin Radiol 1997; 52: 172–186.

3. Fraser J, Walls M, McGuire W. Respiratory complications of preterm birth. BMJ 2004; 329: 962–965.

4. Swischuk LE, John SD. Immature lung problems: can our nomenclature be more specific? AJR 1996; 166: 917–918.

5. Northway WH. Bronchopulmonary dysplasia: twenty five years later. Commentary. Pediatrics 1992; 89: 969–973.

6. Burt TB, Lester PD. Neonatal pneumopericardium. Radiology 1982; 142: 81–84.

7. Dyer C. Is inexperience a defence against negligence? BMJ 1986; 293: 497–498.

8. Kim JH, Lee YS, Kim SH et al. Does umbilical vein catheterization lead to portal venous thrombosis? Prospective US evaluation in 100 neonates. Radiology 2001; 219: 645–650.

9. Weber AL, DeLuca S, Shannon DC. Normal and abnormal position of the umbilical artery and venous catheter on the roentgenogram and review of complications. AJR 1974; 120: 361–367.

10. Grunebaum M, Horodniceanu C, Wilunsky E, et al. Iatrogenic transmural perforation of the oesophagus in the preterm infant. Clin Rad 1980; 31: 257–261.

11. Hogan MJ. Neonatal vascular catheters and their complications. Radiol Clin North Am 1999; 37: 1109–1125.

12. Cohen MD. Tubes, wires, and the neonate. Clin Radiol 1980; 31: 249–256.

13. Greenough A. Where should the umbilical catheter go? Lancet 1993; 341: 1186–1187.

14. Raval NC, Gonzalez E, Bhat AM et al. Umbilical venous catheters: evaluation of radiographs to determine position and associated complications of malpositioned umbilical venous catheters. Am J Perinatol 1995; 12: 201–204.

15. Das Narla L, Hom M, Lofland GK, et al. Evaluation of umbilical catheter and tube placement in premature infants. Radiographics 1991; 11: 849–863.

16 THE RADIOLOGIST'S TOOLBOX

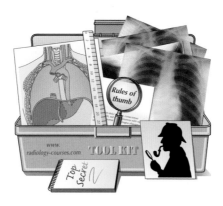

Some CXR appearances will be puzzling. Is the hilum enlarged or is it within the normal range? Where is that thoracic density? Is that shadow normal or abnormal?

Radiologists have a box of tricks—a toolbox—that helps them to sort out most of the puzzles. The box contains a mixed bag of rules, facts and figures. Here are some of the basic tools, a few power tools, and our assessment of 200 normal CXRs in patients aged 50 and older.

THE BASIC TOOLS

TOOL 1—A PREVIOUS CXR

Previous CXRs are the radiologist's—and your—best friend. You see a real or possible abnormality on the CXR. Was it there before? Has it got larger or smaller? Is it unchanged? A previous CXR will often highlight an important but subtle change. On the other hand it will frequently provide reassurance that all is well.

TOOL 2—THE SILHOUETTE SIGN[1,2,3]

An intrathoracic lesion touching a border of the heart, aorta, or diaphragm will obliterate part of that border on the radiograph. An intrathoracic lesion which is not anatomically contiguous with a border will not obliterate that border.

See pp. 45–50.

TOOL 3—AIR BRONCHOGRAM SIGN[3,4]

When the internal tubular outline of a bronchus is visible within a thoracic opacity...that is an air bronchogram.

- It is most commonly associated with a simple pneumonia. Sometimes it occurs with pulmonary oedema.

- It is usually very good news for the patient. An air bronchogram excludes a bronchial obstruction—i.e. the underlying pathological process is highly likely to be benign.

  - Like most things in life it is not 100% foolproof. Just occasionally—very occasionally—an air bronchogram will occur in an area affected by tumour. This very rare occurrence is most often associated with a bronchioloalveolar cell carcinoma or with lymphoma.

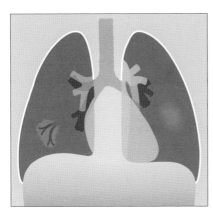

Figure 16.1 *The area of consolidation in the left lung does not show an air bronchogram because the bronchi are full of pus and debris. In the right lung some of the bronchi surrounded by lung consolidation happen to contain more air than debris; consequently an "air bronchogram" results.*

TOOL 4—HILA ASSESSMENT: RULE 1

The left hilum should be higher than the right. Occasionally the hila are at the same level...but the right hilum should never be higher than the left (see p. 240).

This toolbox rule is often overlooked by inexperienced observers. If the rule is broken then look carefully for evidence of lobar collapse.

TOOL 5—HILA ASSESSMENT: RULE 2

Most (unilateral) enlarged hila are both lumpy/bumpy and denser than the opposite normal side. Some normal hila will appear prominent—but are actually within the normal range. The three questions to ask yourself when a hilum appears equivocal are listed on p. 76.

TOOL 6—THE CARDIAC DENSITY RULE, FRONTAL CXR

The density (opacity) of the cardiac shadow should be equal on both sides of the spine. If there is any difference in density then look for evidence of pneumonia, or lower lobe collapse, or a lower lobe mass on the denser side.

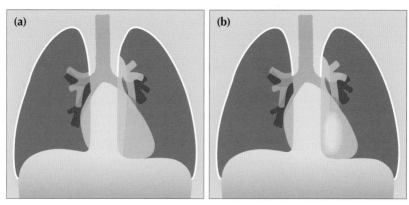

Figure 16.2 *(a) Normal CXR. Even density of the cardiac shadow on both sides of the spine. (b) Abnormal CXR. Increased density overlies the cardiac shadow on the left.*

TOOL 7—THE CARDIAC DENSITY RULE, LATERAL CXR

There should be no abrupt change in density across the cardiac shadow. Any abrupt change in density invariably indicates an abnormality in the overlying lung, on either the left or the right side.

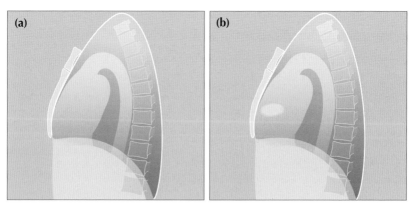

Figure 16.3 *(a) Normal lateral CXR. No abrupt change in density across the cardiac shadow. (b) Abnormal CXR. Focal area of density change.*

TOOL 8—PERIPHERAL OPACITIES

A peripheral opacity may be obvious, but is it really intrapulmonary? Could it be pleural, or alternatively, extrapleural?

Two rules to apply:

1. An intrapulmonary opacity abutting the pleura foms an acute angle at the interface. A pleural or extrapleural lesion forms an obtuse angle.

2. Many extrapleural lesions arise from a rib—e.g. tumour, infection, fracture. Always assess the ribs adjacent to, or overlying, any opacity.

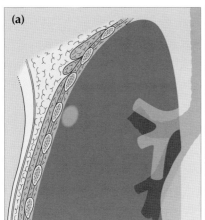

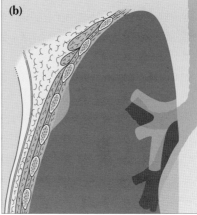

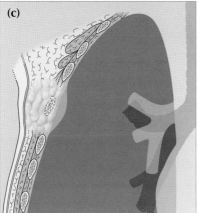

Figure 16.4 *(a) Intrapulmonary lesion. Acute angle between the opacity and the adjacent pleural surface. (b) The lesion is not intrapulmonary. It may arise from the pleura or originate outside the pleura. Obtuse angle between the lesion and the adjacent pleural surface. (c) The rib destruction indicates that the extrapleural lesion arises from bone.*

TOOL 9—RULES FOR LUNG APICES

Thickening of the apical pleura—sometimes referred to as an apical cap—occurs in 10% of middle-aged and elderly people (p. 238). Unfortunately, a flat superior sulcus carcinoma (e.g. a Pancoast tumour) can mimic an apical cap. The rules to apply are described in Fig. 16.5.

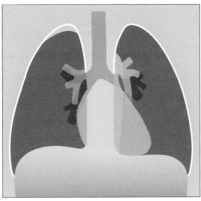

Fig. 16.5 *An apical pleural cap is present on the right. Apply these rules. (1) A benign apical pleural cap usually has a depth of less than 5 mm[5]. (2) If bilateral apical caps are present and one is deeper by 5 mm or more, then you need to rule out the possibility that the deeper one represents a superior sulcus tumour. (3) Always check that the ribs adjacent to a pleural cap are intact. (Superior sulcus: the groove in the lung created by the subclavian vessels. Pancoast tumour: the original description by the American radiologist Henry Pancoast, 1875–1939, included specific physical findings. The term is now used somewhat more loosely.)*

TOOL 10—THE DESCENDING PULMONARY ARTERIES

Always look for and identify the lower lobe pulmonary arteries…each will have a diameter similar to your little finger. If either is missing you must look for any other CXR features that suggest collapse of a lower lobe (see pp. 58–61). The right lower lobe pulmonary artery is identified just lateral to the cardiac border on approximately 94% of normal CXRs (p. 239). The left descending pulmonary artery will sometimes be more difficult to identify—it is visible in 62% of normal people (p. 239).

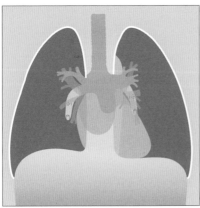

Figure 16.6 *Each main lower lobe pulmonary artery can be likened to a little finger pointing downwards. Sometimes—particularly on the left side—this arterial shadow comprises only the proximal phalanx of the finger.*

TOOL 11—A HELPFUL TRICK: THE DECUBITUS CXR

Problem 1:   A CXR may show extensive lower zone shadowing. The question arises: is this mainly pleural fluid or mainly lung consolidation?

Problem 2:   Sometimes a dome of the diaphragm appears high, and the configuration raises the possibility of a subpulmonary pleural effusion (p. 82).

The radiologist can sort out these problems by obtaining a lateral decubitus view. The patient lies with the abnormal side dependent and a cross-table CXR is obtained. Fluid that is free in the pleural space will layer out along the lateral chest wall.

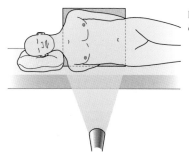

Figure 16.7   *Patient position for a (right) lateral decubitus CXR.*

TOOL 12—TWO TRICKS FOR RIBS

1. If a rib abnormality is suspected on clinical grounds (e.g. trauma) then before deciding that the ribs are normal:

   ❑ Rotate the image through 90° and assess the ribs in this second position.

   ❑ Then turn the original image through 180° (i.e. look at it upside down) and evaluate the ribs in this third position.

   Surprisingly, these moves can be helpful. Other distracting anatomy is discounted and the rib outlines stand out (p. 312).

2. If uncertain whether a thoracic density is in lung or in rib (e.g. an unimportant bone island), then:

   ❑ Obtain an AP CXR. If the lesion remains in the same position in relation to the rib as on the PA CXR—this confirms that it is a rib lesion.

   ❑ Alternatively, the density can be examined using fluoroscopy. If the lesion is in a rib then its position remains unchanged as the patient is turned slightly and breathes in and out.

THE POWER TOOLS

POWER TOOL 1 — RIGHT PARATRACHEAL STRIPE APPEARANCE[3]

The wall of the right side of the trachea can be visualised in approximately 60% of adult patients[3] (also see p. 242). The air within the trachea outlines its inside margin and the lung air outlines its outside margin. In 40% of normal adults the lung does not abut the outside wall and so this stripe (or line) will not be seen. When the stripe is visible it should measure no more than 2.5 mm in width (see p. 242). If the stripe is wider than 2.5 mm then suspect that there is adjacent lymph node enlargement.

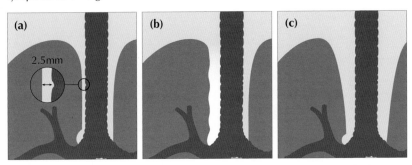

Figure 16.8 *(a) Normal right paratracheal stripe. (b) Thickened right paratracheal stripe—it exceeds the normal width of 2.5 mm. Lymphadenopathy should be suspected. Occasionally, widening of the stripe is due to haemorrhage. (c) Caution: superimposition of (age related) unfolded vessels arising from the arch of the aorta must not be mistaken for the paratracheal stripe.*

POWER TOOL 2 — PARAVERTEBRAL STRIPE DISPLACEMENT[6]

A left-sided vertical shadow is visualised on most normal frontal CXRs. This shadow is projected between the lateral margin of the descending thoracic aorta and the lateral margin of the thoracic vertebrae. It extends from the level of the arch of the aorta to the diaphragm. This is the left paravertebral stripe. It represents a deflection of the pleura posteriorly by the adjacent descending thoracic aorta (see Figs 8.7–8.9 on p. 113). A right paravertebral stripe is not visualised until middle age, when age related marginal osteophytes can cause pleural displacement. Two rules:

- Any focal bulge of the left paravertebral stripe…vertebral pathology requires exclusion.

- A visualised right paravertebral stripe is always abnormal…unless age related osteophyte formation is present.

NB: the most common pathological processes causing a bump or bulge of a paravertebral stripe are: haematoma following trauma, tumour, or infection arising in the vertebral column.

POWER TOOL 3—THE HILUM CONVERGENCE SIGN[3,6]

Sometimes referred to as the "hilus bifurcation sign". It allows an enlarged hilum due to enlarged pulmonary arteries to be distinguished from enlargement due to tumour. The sign is applied as follows:

- If vessels arise from or converge *directly* onto the hilar shadow—then the enlargement is vascular.

- If the vessels appear to arise or converge *medial* to the lateral aspect of the hilar shadow—then the enlargement is a mass.

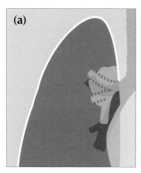
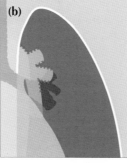

Figure 16.9 *Enlarged hila. Apply these rules. (a) If the vessels converge medial to the hilar shadow, then enlargement is due to a mass. (b) If the vessels converge and merge directly on to the hilar shadow, then enlargement is due to enlarged (or prominent) vessels. The vessel walls are outlined in red.*

POWER TOOL 4—THE HILUM OVERLAY SIGN[3,7]

This sign is often misunderstood and misrepresented. The original description carefully distinguished between cardiac enlargement and an anterior mediastinal mass, as follows:

- Hilum *lateral* to the lateral border of the "mass"—cardiac enlargement.

- Hilum *medial* to the lateral border of the "mass"—mediastinal mass present.

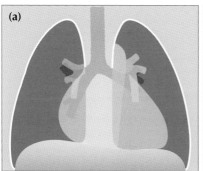
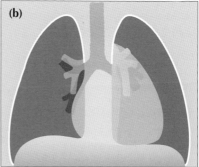

Figure 16.10 *Mediastinal enlargement. Apply these rules. (a) If the vessels at the hilum lie lateral to the enlargement—this indicates that the abnormality is due solely to cardiac enlargement. (b) If the vessels at the hilum lie medial to the lateral margin of the enlarged mediastinum then a true mediastinal mass is present.*

POWER TOOL 5—THE THORACO-ABDOMINAL SIGN[3]

This sign allows a lower mediastinal mass to be positioned accurately by analysing the frontal CXR. As follows:

■ A sharply marginated mediastinal mass projected over the diaphragm *on a CXR (or on an AXR)* will lie wholly or partly in the thorax...because it is outlined by the air in the lung.

■ Convergence of the lower lateral margin of the mass towards the spine indicates that the inferior aspect of the lesion is nearby. Consequently, the lesion is most likely to be entirely intrathoracic (Fig 16.11).

■ If the lower lateral margin of the lesion does not converge, and particularly if it diverges (Fig. 16.12), then a significant amount of the lesion lies within the abdomen (e.g. a paraspinal abscess).

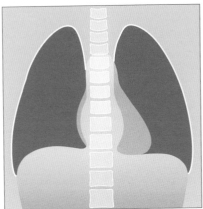 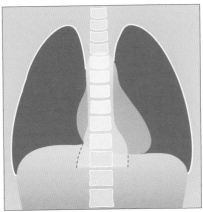

Figure 16.11   *The inferior margin of the mediastinal mass is converging towards the spine. This signifies that the mass is almost entirely intrathoracic. (Paraspinal abscess.)*

Figure 16.12   *The inferior margin of the mediastinal mass diverges away from the midline. This signifies that a large component of the mass lies within the abdomen. (Paraspinal abscess.)*

POWER TOOL 6—THE CERVICO-THORACIC SIGN[3,7]

This helps to decide whether a mass in the upper part of the mediastinum is situated anteriorly or posteriorly. The sign is based on a knowledge of normal anatomy and the application of the silhouette sign. Remember, the anterior aspect of a lung does not extend above the level of the clavicles. The sign applies to the frontal CXR as follows:

- If the lateral outline of the mass is visualised above the clavicle then the mass is situated posteriorly (Fig. 16.13a).

- If the lateral outline of the mass fades away as it reaches the lower border of the clavicle then the mass is situated anteriorly (Fig. 16.13b).

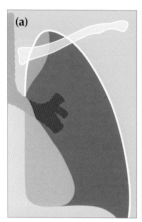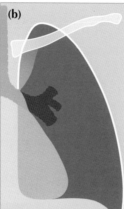

Figure 16.13 *The cervico-thoracic sign indicates that the mass in (a) lies posteriorly, and that the mass in (b) lies anteriorly…but may well extend into or originate from the soft tissues of the neck.*

POWER TOOL 7—THE SUBCARINAL ANGLE APPEARANCE

The carina is the site of the division of the trachea into the right and left main bronchi. The normal angle subtended at the carina[6] varies from 50° to 100°. If the angle is greater than 100° then the two main bronchi are being pushed apart (Fig. 16.14b). This pushing can be due to subcarinal tumour/lymph node enlargement or to an enlarged left atrium (e.g. mitral valve stenosis).

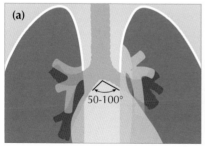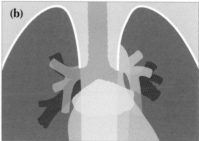

Figure 16.14 *(a) Normal carina. (b) The carina is splayed (its angle exceeds 100°). In this example a subcarinal mass/lymphadenopathy is present. Reminder: an enlarged left atrium in mitral valve disease will sometimes splay the carina.*

200 NORMAL CXRS: PATIENTS AGED 50 AND OVER

A tricky question: normal people vary…so what is normal?

There are some variations from the normal which occur so infrequently (or not at all) that finding a difference from the normal must be regarded as an abnormal finding.

Unfortunately, hard facts on the frequency of normal features are thin on the ground—apart from some data provided by Dr Ben Felson[3]. He painstakingly recorded statistical information from a large number of normal CXRs obtained on young men and women during World War II. His findings are used by radiologists as the benchmark in answer to the question—what is normal? Unfortunately, unlike Felson's fit young military recruits, most patients referred for a CXR are middle-aged or elderly.

We analysed an older group of patients, reviewing 200 digital or digitised PA CXRs of men and women aged 50 and over. This is how we tried to make sure that the CXRs were really normal:

■ All patients had been referred by primary care physicians for chest radiography during 2005. In each case the radiologist's report was normal. No further radiology had been obtained in the subsequent 12 months, or alternatively any subsequent examination (whether a CXR or thoracic CT) was also normal.

■ Two of us (GdeL, LB) reviewed each of the CXRs together (45% of cases); all three of us (GdeL, LB, SM) reviewed 55% of the cases together. At review we excluded any CXR with a cardio-thoracic ratio at or above 50%, and also any radiograph that did not appear to have been obtained during an adequate inspiration. The latter exclusion was based on a subjective impression.

THE PATIENTS

The 200 patients were living and working in or around the thriving and generally prosperous university town of Cambridge, in the south east of England. Gender: 47% were male, 53% were female. Age range: 50–91 years. Mean age (i.e. the average) = 64 years. Median age (i.e. the middle of the group) = 62 years. The mode (the age that occurred most often) = 61 years.

THE RESULTS

The following results are expressed mainly as percentages. On occasion we have provided numbers only.

1. DIAPHRAGM POSITION—ASSESSING INSPIRATORY EFFORT

Background: A technically adequate inspiration is important (p. 6). This assessment was carried out by relating the position of the diaphragm to the overlying anterior ribs. We wanted to determine whether an assessment as to an adequate inspiration is likely to be more accurate by looking at the position of the left or the right dome of the diaphragm.

Method/Results: Any CXR considered by us to be obtained during an inadequate inspiration had already been excluded from the study. This was based—as in everyday clinical practice—on an overall subjective impression. The levels of the domes of the diaphragm were recorded in relation to the nearest closely overlying costochondral junction (CCJ). If a CCJ was well below the dome, then the immediately superior CCJ was recorded. In two patients the costochondral junctions could not be assessed with precision—one because of developmental rib anomalies and the other because of extensive rib demineralisation. Thus, a total of 198 patients, all of whom—to us—showed an adequate inspiration, were assessed.

Table 16.1 198 patients. A good inspiration and the domes of the diaphragm

Height	4th CCJ	5th CCJ	6th CCJ	7th CCJ	8th CCJ
Right dome	0.5%	10%	67%	21%	1.5%
Left dome	0%	3%	50.5%	43%	3.5%

Comment: Our advice…evaluate for a good inspiration on a PA CXR by assessing the height of the left dome rather than the right dome. In the vast majority of patients a good inspiration has occurred when the left dome is at the level of the left 6th or 7th CCJ.

2. A WELL-DEFINED LEFT DOME OF THE DIAPHRAGM

Background: Loss of a clear silhouette of the left dome of the diaphragm is important in relation to detecting left lower lobe pathology (pp. 46–47).

Method/Results: We assessed how often the left dome was visualised from the costophrenic angle to the lateral margin of the vertebral column. The dome appeared sharp in 93% of cases. It was blurred (i.e. ill-defined) in 7%. When it was ill-defined then the loss of definition invariably affected only the medial 3–4 cm of the dome.

Comment: Left lower lobe consolidation or collapse frequently obliterates all or part of the outline of the left dome. The rules to apply: if you cannot see the whole of the left dome then you must check whether there is any added density above the diaphragm. Increased density often accompanies consolidation or tumour in a lower lobe.

3. APICAL PLEURAL CAP

Background: Thickening of the pleura over the lung apex is commonly referred to as an apical pleural cap (pp. 89 and 230). The shadow can be mimicked by malignant disease (e.g. a Pancoast tumour).

Results:

Table 16.2 200 patients. Apical pleural cap.

	%
Not present	90
Present on both sides	2.5
Present on right side only	6.5
Present on left side only	1

Comment: An apical pleural cap occurred in 10% of patients. When a cap is seen it is important to check for any features that might suggest that it could be a tumour. These features are described on p. 142.

4. BLURRED RIGHT HEART BORDER

Background: Blurring of the right heart border can be an important CXR finding as it may indicate middle lobe disease (p. 46).

Results: Blurring was present in 35 (17.5%) of the 200 patients.

Table 16.3 Cause of blurred right heart border (35 cases).

	No.
Heart not extending lateral to the vertebral margin	5
Impression: depressed sternum	1
Impression: adjacent cardiophrenic fat extending superiorly	8
Unexplained	21

Comment 1: A blurred, or ill-defined, right heart border was a relatively common appearance on normal CXRs in these patients. Several possible causes: a normal heart not extending to the right of the vertebral column; a depressed sternum; or fat extending upwards from the cardiophrenic angle. Blurring must not be regarded as pathognomic of middle lobe disease. Any further investigation must be tailored to the clinical presentation and clinical findings.

Comment 2: Our 17.5% figure is much higher than in Felson's series[3]. Most—or all—of Felson's cases were aged less than 25 years. The mean age in our cases was 64 years. Could some of our cases have had true middle lobe disease? That is possible, but we did not have any evidence to suggest that this was likely.

5. CARDIAC FAT PAD SHADOWS

Background: Collections of fat accumulate around the heart, particularly at the cardiophrenic angles. They can cause potentially misleading low density shadows, sometimes mimicking a mass lesion. Also, if not recognised, fat leads to inaccurate measurement of the transverse cardiac diameter.

Results: Fat was evident in 103 (51.5%) of cases. Of these 103 patients, fat cast a shadow only at the left cardiophrenic angle in 55%, at the right cardiophrenic angle in 6%, and at both angles in 39%.

Comment: A visible epicardial fat pad was very common in this group of patients. The most frequent pattern was fat on the left side only and producing a relatively small shadow. The next most common pattern was fat at both cardiophrenic angles and producing relatively small shadows. Occasionally a fat pad was exceptionally large.

6. VISIBLE PULMONARY VENOUS CONFLUENCE

Background: This is a convex opacity projected over the right side of the heart. Felson[3] attributed the appearance to a convergence of normal pulmonary veins draining into the left atrium. Others consider the shadow to be part of the normal left atrium. This shadow can be confused with a lung mass or a paravertebral soft tissue swelling (p. 151).

Results: The appearance occurred in 10% of our 200 cases. It was always on the right of the midline—never on the left side.

Comment: Being aware of this normal shadow will enable its significance to be properly attributed. See the example on p. 151.

7. MAIN LOWER LOBE PULMONARY ARTERIES

Background: The lower lobe pulmonary artery, on a PA CXR, can be likened to a little finger or to a finger's proximal phalanx (p. 71). The "little finger" appearance of the pulmonary artery is not seen when a lower lobe is collapsed. We evaluated how often the "little finger" appearance was seen.

Results: The "little finger" appearance was identified on both sides in 58.5% of patients, on the right side only in 35%, on the left side only in 3%, and was not identified on either side in 3.5%. Examples are shown on pp. 71–73.

Comment: If the right lower lobe pulmonary artery is not visible then pathology must be excluded (e.g. lower lobe collapse). However, the left lower lobe pulmonary artery is less frequently visible. If it is not identified, then check the position of the hilar vee (see below) before assuming abnormality.

8. HILAR HORIZONTAL VEES

Background: *The horizontal vee* is defined (p. 73) as follows: identify the lower lobe pulmonary artery and look for the site/point where the most superior *vertical or oblique* vessel (no matter if it is a vein or an artery) crosses close to the lower lobe pulmonary artery's lateral margin. The point of crossing forms a horizontal V shape.

The vee helps us to identify the hila precisely and with confidence. This is important when assessing whether there is any evidence of lower lobe collapse (pp. 56–61).

Results:

Table 16.4 The horizontal vees. 200 patients.

The vee identified	No.	%
On both sides	176	88
Right side only	18	9
Left side only	2	1
Neither identified	4	2

Comment: An absent vee on either side should raise a very strong suspicion—but not certainty—of lower lobe collapse.

9. LEVELS OF THE HILAR VEES WHEN BOTH ARE SEEN

Background: The position of the hilum is important for detecting lobar collapse because the hilum may move from its normal position when a lobe collapses. We assessed the positions of the hilar vees relative to each other.

Results: The left vee was higher than the right in 95% of cases. The vees were at the same level in 5%. The right vee was never higher than the left.

Comment: A cardinal rule…if the right vee is higher than the left then there is either volume loss in the left lower lobe or, alternatively, volume loss in the right upper lobe.

10. PROMINENT UNFOLDED OR TORTUOUS VESSELS

Background: Sometimes age related vessel unfolding (aorta or neck vessels), above and to the right or left of the aortic arch, can cause the inexperienced observer to be concerned that an apical mass is present.

Results: Prominent unfolding occurred in 5% of patients.

Comment: Potentially misleading vessel unfolding is a relatively uncommon occurrence on PA CXRs even in this age group. It is more likely to occur on AP CXRs where magnification and tube angulation distortions may occur.

11. HORIZONTAL FISSURE

Background: The absence of a visible horizontal fissure may lead to a concern as to normality. We assessed how frequently the horizontal fissure was visible.

Method / Results: The fissure was visualised in 134 of the 200 cases. On these 134 CXRs it appeared as a single line in 84% and as two lines in 16%. Frequently the second line was short—rarely longer than 2 cm. The reason why two lines are sometimes seen is explained on p. 55.

Comment: The horizontal fissure was not visible on 33% of normal CXRs. Its absence is not, on its own, of clinical significance.

12. AZYGOS VEIN SHADOW

Background: The azygos vein enters the superior vena cava to the right of the tracheal bifurcation (p. 176). Very small lymph nodes (not visible on the CXR) are also present at this site. Unless the patient is in right heart failure it is rare for the azygos vein to be enlarged. Consequently, enlargement of the azygos shadow is most commonly due to lymphadenopathy.

Results: The azygos vein was visible as a definite oval or rounded structure in 31% of patients. None of these visible azygos veins showed a transverse diameter in excess of 1.0 cm.

Comment: When a shadow is seen that appears to be a prominent azygos vein—measure its transverse diameter. The rule to apply: if this diameter exceeds 1.0 cm on a PA CXR: (a) presume that an abnormality is present; (b) determine whether the patient is in heart failure; and (c) check whether the clinical presentation might include the possibility of nodal enlargement.

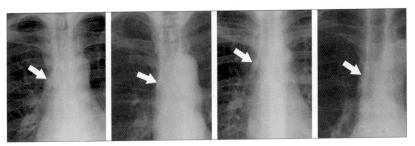

Figure 16.15 *Normal azygos vein (arrow) seen en face at its junction with the superior vena cava. Four examples. On a PA CXR the transverse diameter of the vein should not exceed 1.0 cm.*

13. THE RIGHT WALL OF THE TRACHEA

Background: Lymphadenopathy in the paratracheal region can be difficult to detect. The normal right paratracheal stripe can often be identified below the clavicle (see p. 112). The stripe represents both sides of the tracheal wall outlined by air. It is not seen in all patients, and it is rarely seen on the left side. Widening of the normal paratracheal stripe can be helpful in recognising early paratracheal lymph node enlargement. We assessed: (a) how frequently the normal right paratracheal stripe was seen; and (b) its width.

Results: Both sides of the right wall of the trachea were visible in 63% of patients. When both sides were visible (126 patients), in 98% of cases the wall thickness did not exceed 2 mm. In 2% of cases the wall thickness measured 2.5 mm. No cases exceeded 2.5 mm.

Comment: The rule to apply—when both sides of the right wall of the trachea are seen on a PA CXR then the wall thickness should not exceed 2.5 mm. If the wall thickness measures more than 2.5 mm then suspect that paratracheal lymphadenopathy is present.

14. STOMACH GAS POSITION

Background: A left-sided subpulmonary pleural effusion (p. 82) or subphrenic collection may be revealed by identifying inferior displacement of the gas shadow (or bubble) in the gastric fundus. We assessed the normal depth of separation between the gastric air and the diaphragm.

Method / Results: An unequivocal stomach gas bubble was visualised in 22% of cases. In these 44 patients the distance from the top of the stomach gas bubble to the immediately adjacent superior margin of the dome of the diaphragm was less than 7 mm in 98%. In one case the distance was 14 mm.

Comment: The distance between the left dome of the diaphragm and the superior surface of the gastric fundus is usually less than 7 mm. Very occasionally it can measure more than 7 mm. Thus, if a patient has a clinical presentation that might include the question of left-sided pleural fluid and the gastric air bubble is more than 7 mm below the dome then suspect a fluid collection. Applying this rule will lead to the occasional false positive diagnosis. No matter—an ultrasound examination will then rapidly confirm or refute.

15. UNILATERAL HYPERTRANSRADIANCY[8]

Background: Unilateral hypertransradiancy (blackening) can be a subtle but important sign of lung pathology. The causes of hypertransradiancy are described on p. 257.

Results: Hypertransradiancy was evident in 35% of patients. Of these CXRs (70 patients), 58% showed evidence of rotation. In 42% the cause was not apparent.

Comment: Detecting unilateral hypertransradiancy is subjective and depends on how meticulously you look for it. This will vary between observers. Some observers are very sensitive to a difference between the blackening of the two lungs. Be cautious about ascribing great significance to hypertransradiancy as an isolated finding. It is quite common. Frequently the cause is technical (p. 257). Work through our checklist (p. 258) to determine whether there is any other CXR evidence to suggest important pathology.

REFERENCES

1. Felson B, Felson H. Localization of intrathoracic lesions by means of the postero–anterior roentgenogram: the silhouette sign. Radiology 1950; 55: 363–374.

2. Glossary of terms for thoracic radiology: recommendations of the Nomenclature Committee of the Fleischner Society. AJR 1984; 143: 509–517.

3. Felson B. Chest Roentgenology. Philadelphia, PA: WB Saunders, 1973.

4. Reed JC. Chest Roentgenology: Plain Film Patterns and Differential Diagnosis. 5th ed. Philadelphia. PA: Mosby, 2003.

5. O'Connell RS, McLoud TC, Wilkins EW. Superior sulcus tumour: Radiographic diagnosis and work up. AJR 1983; 140: 25–30.

6. Fraser RG, Muller NL, Colman NC, Pare PD. Fraser and Pare's Diagnosis of Diseases of the Chest. 4th ed. Philadelphia, PA: WB Saunders, 1999.

7. Briggs G. Pocket Guide to Chest X-rays. 2004. Sydney, NSW: McGraw-Hill, 2004.

8. Joseph AE, de Lacey GJ, Bryant TH et al. The hypertransradiant hemithorax: the importance of lateral decentering and the explanation for its appearance due to rotation. Clin Radiol 1978; 29: 125–131.

Part B
Clinical Problems

17 THE CXR: ITS IMPACT ON CLINICAL DECISION MAKING

"Every diagnostic test causes additional cost if not additional risk. The cost and risk are justified if the test result is likely to change what is done for the patient. This includes a diagnostic test that does not alter therapy but provides important prognostic information to the patient, or to parents, or to the physician"[1].

In Part A the emphasis has been placed on the core knowledge—i.e. the basic principles that assist a physician to accurately and confidently assess a chest radiograph. In Part B we now turn to the practical use of a CXR in assisting with the individual patient's clinical management.

What impact does the CXR examination have on clinical management? This depends on whether or not the individual physician applies an informed evaluation of the CXR. This is not just shadow gazing. Informed evaluation requires the application of five important rules.

RULE 1 — CLINICAL DETAILS ARE PIVOTAL

Accurate interpretation of the CXR appearances always involves correlation with the findings obtained from the clinical history and physical examination. The CXR shadows should never be considered in isolation.

Example:

■ Age 20. Non-smoker in excellent health. CXR—a peripheral 2-cm diameter solitary pulmonary nodule. Likely diagnosis = hamartoma or carcinoid.

■ Age 75. Smoker with weight loss. CXR—a peripheral 2-cm diameter solitary pulmonary nodule. Likely diagnosis = bronchial carcinoma.

RULE 2 — ALWAYS ASK THE CXR A QUESTION

"What precise question do I want this CXR to answer?". The query will direct the analysis of the CXR to the specific clinical problem.

Example: this young man has acute chest pain. I think that a pneumothorax is likely. The question—is a pneumothorax, obvious or subtle, present? Formulating this query will lead to careful examination of the lung apex (p. 96).

RULE 3—RECOGNISE SOME IMPERFECTIONS

The CXR is a very useful but nevertheless imperfect test. It is good at providing information on some pathologies (e.g. is there pneumonia?) and poor with others (e.g. is there a pulmonary embolus?). Furthermore, a lung shadow merely represents a radiographic density. It does not provide the precise anatomical detail of CT nor the cellular diagnosis of histopathology.

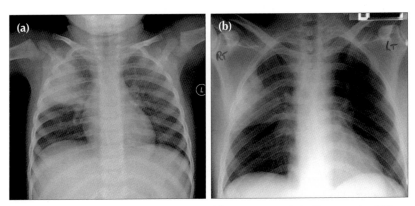

Figure 17.1 *Precise clinical details are crucial for accurate analysis. Compare the CXRs of patients (a) and (b). (a) presents with a cough, fever and green sputum. An acute illness. The lung opacity represents a lobar pneumonia. (b) presents with weight loss and haemoptysis. The CXR shows similar lung shadowing to (a). However, given the clinical history, a simple lobar pneumonia is unlikely. The illness is not acute. The eventual diagnosis...bronchioloalveolar cell carcinoma of the lung.*

RULE 4—A NORMAL CXR CAN BE VERY USEFUL[2]

It is tempting to think of the CXR as mainly a test for making diagnoses. In clinical practice a normal (i.e. negative) CXR is more common than an abnormal CXR. This does not mean that performing the CXR was a waste of time. In fact, a normal CXR can be extremely useful.

- It is very good at excluding some conditions with a high degree of confidence, e.g. pneumothorax.

- It can provide reassurance that a particularly serious condition is not present, or highly unlikely. In other words, a normal CXR may modify the pre-test probability of a particular disease so that the post-test probability (Rule 5) is so low that further investigation is unnecessary.

Example: haemoptysis—is it due to lung cancer? A normal CXR examination (in this instance, frontal and lateral projections) is very reassuring to both the physician and to the patient.

RULE 5—CARRY OUT PROBABILITY ASSESSMENTS[3–21]

"Diagnostic tests should be selected…in a way that allows them to influence the clinician's estimate of pre-test disease probability. This estimate is the major factor in determining whether to withhold treatment, order more tests, or treat without subjecting the patient to the risks of further testing"[4].

A probability assessment is valuable in enabling the physician to consider how useful a CXR will be in confirming or excluding a particular diagnosis.

PRE-TEST AND POST-TEST PROBABILITY

The physician will have in mind how likely it is that a particular diagnosis is present in the individual patient (i.e. the pre-test probability). The pre-test probability assessment will determine which diagnostic test the physician will then select. The likelihood that the disease is present is subsequently modified by the result of the test (i.e. a post-test probability is generated). These assessments help the physician to plan further management. This includes the option of deciding not to request any further tests. Thus:

■ It is a useful exercise for the physician requesting a CXR to note her pre- and post-test probability estimates of the disease being present both before and after a CXR. This is useful because probability assessments will:

a) Show that the physician has a clearly designed strategy for investigating the patient.

b) Assist in excluding unnecessary investigations.

■ Application of a pre-test probability assessment requires an understanding of the reliability of the CXR to diagnose or exclude the particular pathology in question (i.e. by knowing the positive and negative predictive values).

■ For those of us who do not like getting into statistics and numbers when making these probability assessments it is both practical and helpful to utilise a simple estimate of pre- and post-test probability as being either high, medium or low (see: Box A and Box B). For example: chest pain—rule out aortic dissection (Table 17.1).

BOX A		
Presence of disease X		
Estimate of pre-test probability	High	
	Medium	
	Low	

OR

BOX B		
No disease		
Estimate of pre-test probability	High	
	Medium	
	Low	

Table 17.1 Chest pain—rule out aortic dissection.

Stage 1

Pre-test probability

The physician has weighed the clinical evidence

Her view is that the probability of an aortic dissection (ie *the pre-test probability*) is either: High, Medium or Low

Stage 2

Establish a post-test probability

CXR requested and analysed

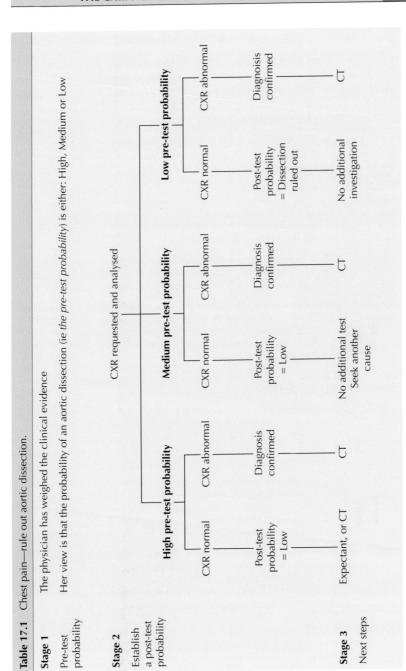

	High pre-test probability		**Medium pre-test probability**		**Low pre-test probability**	
	CXR normal	CXR abnormal	CXR normal	CXR abnormal	CXR normal	CXR abnormal
	Post-test probability = Low	Diagnosis confirmed	Post-test probability = Low	Diagnosis confirmed	Post-test probability = Dissection ruled out	Diagnoisis confirmed
Stage 3 Next steps	Expectant, or CT	CT	No additional test Seek another cause	CT	No additional investigation	CT

APPENDIX

Sometimes the terms used in discussions on the accuracy and selection of a diagnostic test (e.g. the CXR) can be confusing or poorly understood. This appendix provides some useful definitions and explanations.

DEFINITIONS AND EXPLANATIONS[3–26]

Bayes' Theorem	The predictive value of any particular test depends not only on the sensitivity and specificity of the test but also on the prevalence of the disease in the population being tested[8].
Clinical prediction rules	An assembly of symptoms and signs from a large number of patients with a specific disease. Points are assigned to the various symptoms and signs and the pre-test probability of disease is determined by adding up the points[4]. These rules (there are relatively few of them) permit a rough estimation of pre-test disease probability.
	NB: caution has been advised in too readily accepting an assumed consistency in pre-test probability estimates of some diseases, because there can be a large variation in pre-test estimations between clinicians[18].
Diagnostic accuracy	Accuracy measures how close to a true or accepted value a measurement lies. The accuracy (i.e. the performance) of a diagnostic test can be expressed in several different ways. These include: sensitivity and specificity; likelihood ratios; predictive values; the area under a receiver operator characteristic curve.
Gold standard	A method, procedure, or measurement that is widely accepted as being the best available[5].
Predictive value of a test	The probability that a person with a positive test is a true positive (i.e. does have the disease), or that a person with a negative test truly does not have the disease. The predictive value of a test is determined by the sensitivity and specificity of the test, and by the prevalence of the condition for which the test is used[5].
	■ **The negative predictive value** is the proportion of persons with a negative test who do not have the condition. In other words, given that a patient tests negative, what is the probability that she truly does not have the disease? This measure is critically dependent on the prevalence of the disease in the given population at a given time[4,6,9].
	■ **The positive predictive value** is the proportion of persons with a positive test who do have the condition. In other words, given that a patient tests positive, what is the probability that he truly has the disease? This measure is critically dependent on the prevalence of the disease in the given population[6,9].

Pre-test probability	The probability of disease (i.e. the target disorder) before performing a diagnostic test[5]. Statisticians commonly express pre-test probability[4,10] using numbers, i.e. a point on a continuum ranging from absent (0) to present (1). In practice, pre-test probability does not have to be expressed numerically. It can be described in terms of probability thresholds[11]. Thus the pre-test probability may usefully be expressed using the terms High, Medium and Low.
Post-test probability	The probability of disease (i.e. the target disorder) updated by the results of a diagnostic test[5].
Prevalence	The proportion of persons with a particular disease within a given population at a given time[5].
Sensitivity of a test	The probability of a positive test in those with the disease: i.e. the frequency of true positives. A sensitive test has few false negatives[6,7].
Specificity of a test	The probability of a negative test in those without the disease: i.e. the frequency of true negatives. A specific test has few false positives[6,7].
Test	Any method (laboratory; imaging; other) for obtaining additional information on a patient's health status.

AND

Likelihood Ratio	An index developed in order to indicate how reliably a diagnostic test detects a particular disease. Some statisticians prefer to use likelihood ratios[6] rather than positive and negative predictive values, because likelihood ratios are independent of disease prevalence[6]. Likelihood ratios have become incorporated into evidence-based medicine. The objective is to encourage physicians to make more accurate and cost-effective clinical management decisions[1,13,14,15].
Threshold Model	A clinical decision-making yardstick which utilises two thresholds[1,4,12]. Threshold 1 is a no-test threshold because the probability of a disease is so low that the value of not treating the patient is the same as that of performing the test. Threshold 2 is also a no-test threshold because the probability of the disease is so high that the value of performing the test is the same as that of administering treatment. If the probability of disease falls within either of these two thresholds (i.e. below Threshold 1 or above Threshold 2) then there is no point in carrying out the test. Thus the decision not to treat, to carry out the test, or to treat is determined by the pre-test disease probability and the two thresholds[1,4]. When the pre-test disease probability lies *between* the two thresholds then the test result could lead to a different (post-test) probability of disease that could alter the decision to treat, not to treat, or to instigate an additional test…thus, the test should be carried out.

REFERENCES

1. Moyer VA, Kennedy KA. Understanding and using diagnostic tests. Clin Perinatol 2003; 30: 189–204.

2. Gorry GA, Pauker SG, Schwartz WB. The diagnostic importance of the Normal Finding. New Engl J Med 1978; 298: 486–489.

3. Mishriki YY. When are liver tests warranted? Postgrad Med 2004; 116: 8.

4. Scherokman B. Selecting and Interpreting Diagnostic Tests. 1997. xnet.kp.org/permanentejournal/fall97pj/tests.html

5. The EBM Glossary, 2004. www.cebm.utoronto.ca/glossary

6. Attia J. Moving beyond sensitivity and specificity: using likelihood ratios to help interpret diagnostic tests. Aust Prescr 2003; 26: 111–113.

7. Fletcher RH, Fletcher SW, Wagner EH. Clinical Epidemiology: The Essentials. 3rd ed. Philadelphia, PA: Williams and Wilkins, 1996: 64–67.

8. Fleming J, Hersh J. Pulmonary Embolism: Diagnostic Evaluation. Am J Clin Med, 2004. www.aapsga.org/ajcm/2004/winter/article02.html

9. Guggenmoos-Holzmann I, van Houwelingen HC. The (in)validity of sensitivity and specificity. Stat Med 2000; 19: 1783–1792.

10. Kassirer JP. Our stubborn quest for diagnostic certainty: a cause of excessive testing. N Engl J Med 1989; 320: 1489–1491.

11. www.evidencebasedradiology.net

12. Pauker SG, Kassirer JP. The threshold approach to clinical decision making. N. Engl J Med 1980; 302: 1109–1117.

13. Sonis J. How to use and interpret interval likelihood ratios. Fam Med 1999; 31: 432–437.

14. Sackett DL, Haynes RB, Guyatt GH, Tugwell P. Clinical Epidemiology: A Basic Science for Clinical Medicine. 2nd ed. Philadelphia, PA: Lippincott, Williams & Wilkins, 1991.

15. Ebell MH. Evidence-Based Diagnosis: A Handbook of Clinical Prediction Rules. New York: Springer, 2001.

16. Wells PS, Anderson DR, Bormanis J et al. Value of assessment of pretest probability of deep vein thrombosis in clinical management. Lancet 1997; 350: 1795–1798.

17. University of Washington Department of Medicine. Advanced Physical Diagnosis, Learning and Teaching at the Bedside: Epidemiology Glossary, 2007. depts.washington.edu/physdx/eglossary.html

18. Phelps MA, Levitt MA. Pretest Probability Estimates: a pitfall to the clinical utility of evidence-based medicine? Acad Emerg Med 2004; 11: 692–694.

19. Altman DG, Bland JM. Statistics notes. Diagnostic tests (2): predictive values. BMJ 1994; 309: 102.

20. Altman DG, Bland JM. Diagnostic tests (1): sensitivity and specificity. BMJ 1994; 308: 1552.

21. Norcliffe PJ, Davies CWH. The validity of pre-test probability scoring to predict PE in routine practice. Thrombus 2006; 10: 1,3–5.

22. Fletcher RH. Interpretation of diagnostic tests. Indian J Pediatr 2000; 67: 49–53.

23. Camp BW. What the clinician really needs to know: questioning the clinical usefulness of sensitivity and specificity in studies of screening tests. J Dev Behav Pediatr 2006; 27: 226–230.

24. Coulthard MG. Quantifying how tests reduce diagnostic uncertainty. Arch Dis Child 2007; 92: 404–408.

25. Akobeng AK. Understanding diagnostic tests (1): sensitivity, specificity and predictive values. Acta Paediatr 2007; 96: 338–341.

26. Akobeng AK. Understanding diagnostic tests (2): likelihood ratios, pre- and post-test probabilities and their use in clinical practice. Acta Paediatr 2007; 96: 487–491.

18 ANALYSIS: ONE LUNG LOOKS BLACKER

One lung looks blacker: Unilateral hypertransradiancy of the thorax.

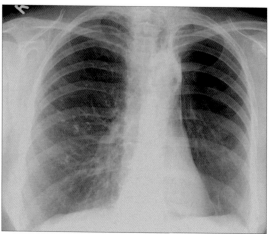

Figure 18.1 *Why does the left lung appear blacker than the right lung? Answer on p. 259.*

WHICH SIDE IS ABNORMAL?

Rule of thumb: In most instances the side that is blacker is the abnormal side.

Important rider: On occasion one side will appear blacker because the *opposite* side is abnormal (i.e. denser/more opaque) (Figs 18.2–18.5). A more dense hemithorax (e.g. on the right side) may result from:

- Any cause of right-sided hypertrophy or swelling of the chest wall soft tissues, such as:
    - ⨽ breast abscess
    - ⨽ chest wall haematoma
    - ⨽ right-handed sportsman with highly developed pectoral muscles (Fig. 18.2)
- Right-sided pleural fluid:
    - ⨽ particularly on a supine CXR
- Generalised right-sided pleural thickening.
- Right lung consolidation.

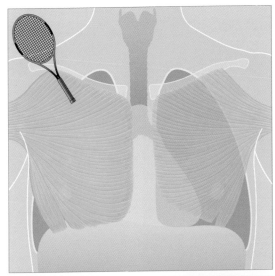

Figure 18.2   This patient's left side will appear blacker than the right on a CXR. This is because he is a right-handed tennis player whose right pectoral muscles are highly developed…they absorb more of the x-ray beam than does the less developed left side.

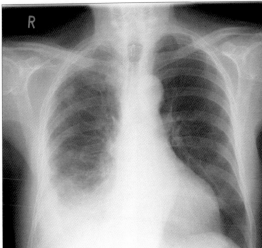

Figure 18.3   Right-sided malignant pleural effusion was treated with a pleurodesis. This additional pleural fluid and thickening absorbs more of the x-ray beam and so the normal left side looks blacker.

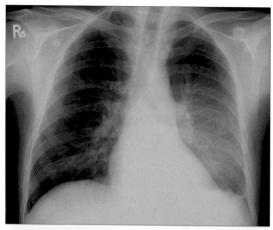

Figure 18.4 *Encysted (posterior) left pleural effusion causes increased absorption of the x-ray beam. Consequently the right lung looks blacker.*

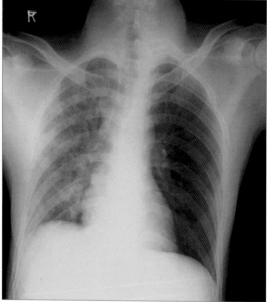

Figure 18.5 *Right-sided pneumonia. Consequently the left lung appears blacker.*

HYPERTRANSRADIANCY: HOW COMMON?

Unilateral hypertransradiancy is a common finding. In our analysis of 200 otherwise normal PA CXRs it occurred in 35% of patients (see Chapter 16, p. 243). The explanation was patient rotation in half of these cases. In 42% the cause was not obvious, though these are likely to have been due to other technical factors (Table 18.1).

HYPERTRANSRADIANCY: A HELPFUL CLASSIFICATION

Technical factors account for the vast majority of cases of unilateral hypertransradiancy. Nevertheless, there are occasions when the finding indicates underlying disease (Table 18.1) on the hypertransradiant, i.e. blacker, side. For this reason it is worth carrying out a simple step-by-step analysis whenever one lung appears blacker than the other (see p. 258).

Table 18.1   Unilateral Hypertransradiant Hemithorax.

	Cause
Technical	1. Unequal compression or positioning of the normal chest wall soft tissues against the cassette[1]
	2. Patient rotation[1,2]
	3. Incorrect centering of the x-ray beam to the grid = lateral decentering[2]
Chest wall abnormality	Asymmetric soft tissues[3,4]
	■ Mastectomy
	■ Absent or under-developed pectoral muscles (Poland Syndrome)
Skeletal abnormality	Scoliosis
Airways disease	1. Large pneumothorax
	2. Asymmetric emphysema
	3. Bronchial obstruction
	Adults: collapse of a lobe resulting in compensatory emphysema
	Children: inhaled foreign body[5]; congenital lobar emphysema[6]
	4. Previous bronchiolitis obliterans
	i.e. Swyer–James (= MacLeod's) syndrome[7,8]
Vascular disease	1. Pulmonary embolism[4,9]
	2. Extrinsic pulmonary artery obstruction secondary to:
	❏ tumour
	❏ lymph node enlargement
	3. Pulmonary artery hypoplasia or branch stenosis

HYPERTRANSRADIANCY: A STEP-BY-STEP ANALYSIS

If you have decided that the more opaque (denser) side is the normal side, adopt this step-by-step approach, concentrating on the side that is blacker.

STEP 1

Question: Is the medial end of each clavicle equidistant from the midline?

No—rotation is the likely explanation (Fig. 18.6).

The rule of rotation: The side with the medial end of the clavicle furthest from the midline will be blacker. If this rule is broken, suspect another cause[2].

STEP 2

Question: Are the soft tissues around the scapula and the axilla on the blacker side more penetrated (i.e. not quite so white as on the normal side)?

Yes—incorrect centering of the x-ray beam is the likely explanation (Fig. 18.7).

STEP 3

Question: Are the chest wall soft tissues asymmetric?

The clinical history and/or the physical examination is crucial: e.g. mastectomy; absent or hypoplastic pectoral muscles (Figs 18.8 and 18.9).

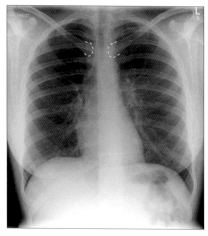

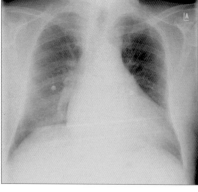

Figure 18.6 *The patient is rotated slightly to the right. The right side appears blacker. This obeys the rule of rotation[2].*

Figure 18.7 *The left side appears blacker. No rotation. Note that the scapula and soft tissues on the left side are less white (i.e. better penetrated) than those on the right. This indicates that the x-ray beam is decentred to the left—consequently the left-sided tissues (including the lung) appear blacker.*

STEP 4

Question: Is there a scoliosis?

■ This may result in alterations to the soft tissues in the path of the x-ray beam (Fig. 18.10). Also, a scoliosis may cause uneven compression of the anterior chest wall against the cassette.

■ NB: uneven compression of chest wall soft tissues against the cassette, even in the absence of a scoliosis, is a very common cause[1] of unilateral hypertransradiancy (Table 18.1).

STEP 5

NONE OF THE ABOVE? Now consider pulmonary or pleural pathology.

Question: Is there evidence of airways disease?

■ Large pneumothorax (Fig. 18.11).

■ Emphysema or an emphysematous bulla (Fig. 18.12).

■ Lobar collapse with compensatory hyperinflation. See p. 57.

■ Inhaled foreign body causing air trapping (children). See p. 201.

■ Congenital lobar emphysema (mainly children). See p. 203.

■ Swyer–James (= MacLeod's) syndrome (Fig. 18.13).

STEP 6

NONE OF THE ABOVE? Now consider vascular disease.

Question A: Are there any clinical features to suggest arterial disease?

■ Pulmonary embolism.

■ Pulmonary artery hypoplasia.

Question B: Is there any suggestion of a tumour at or adjacent to the hilum?

A tumour may cause secondary constrictive effects, including obstruction, to the adjacent pulmonary artery.

Answer to Fig. 18.1 on p. 254

Analysis: No evidence of rotation. Scapula density similar on the two sides. No scoliosis. The left hilum is elevated. Fibrotic shadowing in left upper zone. Fewer vessels in the left lung compared with a similar area in the right lung.

Conclusion: The left lung is blacker because there is major contraction (collapse and shrinkage) of the left upper lobe with consequent compensatory hyperinflation of the lower lobe.

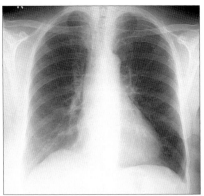

Figure 18.8 *The left side appears blacker. Left mastectomy.*

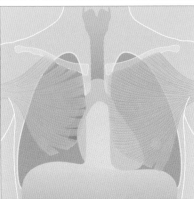

Figure 18.9 *Congenital under-development of the right pectoral muscles (Poland syndrome). The right lung will appear blacker on a CXR.*

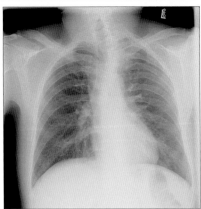

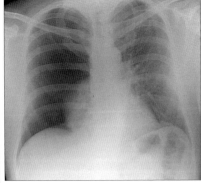

Figure 18.11 *The right side appears blacker. Large right pneumothorax with major collapse of the right lower lobe.*

Figure 18.10 *The right side appears blacker than the left. This is a consequence of the scoliosis which is presenting uneven thicknesses of soft tissue to the x-ray beam.*

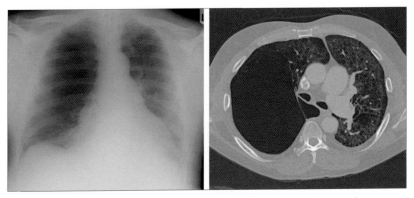

Figure 18.12 *The right side appears blacker. Airways disease…very large emphysematous bulla compressing the right lower lobe. CT section to illustrate.*

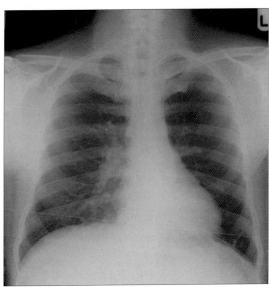

Figure 18.13 *The left side appears blacker. Airways disease. Note that there are fewer vessels in the left lung compared with a similar area in the right lung. There is a differential diagnosis for this appearance. In this patient the explanation proved to be the Swyer–James syndrome (also known as MacLeod's syndrome)…resulting from bronchiolitis obliterans in childhood[3,4,7,9].*

SPECIFIC CAUSES OF UNILATERAL HYPERTRANSRADIANCY

PNEUMOTHORAX

See Chapter 7, pp. 94–102.

EMPHYSEMA

See Chapter 22, pp. 285–286. Emphysematous changes are often asymmetric with one lung or one lobe predominantly affected.

BRONCHIAL OBSTRUCTION CAUSING LOBAR COLLAPSE

See Chapter 5, pp. 57–66. Major collapse of a lobe will result in compensatory emphysema (i.e. lobar over-expansion) in the unaffected lobe/lobes. The over-expansion of the lobe together with shunting of arterial blood to the opposite lung produces the unilateral hypertransradiancy. This effect is most commonly seen in adults with bronchial obstruction.

BRONCHIAL OBSTRUCTION DUE TO AN INHALED FOREIGN BODY[5]

See Chapter 14, p. 201. Occurs most commonly in young children. Though lobar collapse with compensatory emphysema in the unaffected lobe/lobes may occur it is more common for the foreign body to cause a ball valve obstruction and consequent air trapping. The affected lung appears blacker and larger than the opposite side.

CONGENITAL LOBAR EMPHYSEMA[6]

See Chapter 14, p. 203. There is developmental bronchial narrowing with progressive air trapping and over-expansion of the lobe or lung segment distal to the stricture. The majority of affected patients present within one month of birth. Presentation after six months is rare. The CXR shows an area of hypertransradiancy. Shift of the mediastinum to the opposite side and compression collapse of adjacent lung segments are commonly associated findings.

SWYER–JAMES SYNDROME[7,8]

Also known as MacLeod's syndrome. This results from viral bronchiolitis obliterans occurring in childhood which adversely affects normal development of the bronchial tree. Patients are thereafter usually asymptomatic. The CXR appearance of unilateral hypertransradiancy is often an incidental finding in adulthood. Characteristic findings on CT will confirm the diagnosis[8].

PULMONARY EMBOLISM

A massive pulmonary embolus producing a decrease in pulmonary blood flow may cause unilateral hypertransradiancy. A focal hypertransradiancy is often referred to as Westermark's sign[9]. It is a very rare finding. More often, any hypertransradiancy in a severely ill patient—even one who has sustained a pulmonary embolus—is due to a technical factor, e.g. patient rotation.

PULMONARY ARTERY HYPOPLASIA

Pathological hypertransradiancy, whether due to airways disease or vascular disease, is in large part the result of decreased pulmonary blood flow. Therefore a developmentally absent, under-developed or stenosed pulmonary artery can also cause one lung to appear blacker.

REFERENCES

1. Crass JR, Cohen AM, Wiesen E et al. Hyperlucent thorax from rotation: anatomic basis. Invest Radiol 1993; 28: 567–572.

2. Joseph AE, de Lacey GJ, Bryant TH et al. The hypertransradiant hemithorax: the importance of lateral decentering, and the explanation for its appearance due to rotation. Clin Radiol 1978; 29: 125–131.

3. Reed JC. Chest Radiology: Plain Film Patterns and Differential Diagnosis. 5th ed. Philadelphia, PA: Mosby, 2003.

4. Collins J, Stern EJ. Chest Radiology: The Essentials. Philadelphia, PA: Lippincott Williams and Wilkins, 1999.

5. Baharloo F, Veyckemans F, Francis C et al. Tracheobronchial foreign bodies: presentation and management in children and adults. Chest 1999; 115: 1357–1362.

6. Kennedy CD, Habibi P, Matthew DJ et al. Lobar emphysema: long-term imaging follow up. Radiology 1991; 180: 189–193.

7. Stokes D, Sigler A, Khouri NF, et al. Unilateral hyperlucent lung (Swyer–James syndrome) after severe mycoplasma pneumoniae infection. Am Rev Respir Dis 1978; 117: 145–152.

8. Moore AD, Godwin JD, Dietrich PA et al. Swyer–James syndrome: CT findings in eight patients. AJR 1992; 158: 1211–1215.

9. Worsley DF, Alavi A, Aronchick JM et al. Chest radiographic findings in patients with acute pulmonary embolism: observations from the PIOPED study. Radiology 1993; 189: 133–136.

A white out:	A frontal CXR shows homogeneous opacification of all or most of one hemithorax.

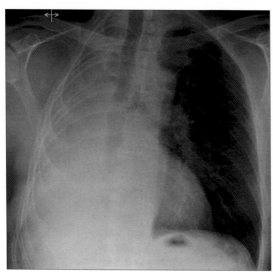

Figure 19.1 *Can you explain this white out? Answer on p. 266.*

When assessing a white out it is essential to be aware of the possible causes (Table 19.1).

Table 19.1 Causes of a white out.

Common	◼ Large pleural effusion...with minimal or moderate secondary compression collapse of the underlying lung.
	◼ Large pleural effusion...with major secondary compression collapse of the underlying lung.
	◼ Collapse of the entire lung. Minimal or no pleural fluid.
	◼ Previous pneumonectomy.
Uncommon	Extensive pneumonia involving the entire lung.
Extremely uncommon	Extensive tumour infiltration of the lung.
Extraordinarily rare	Congenital absence of a lung.

WHITE OUT—ANALYSING THE CXR[1-4]

■ The key to analysing a white out is determining whether the mediastinum is displaced. This requires assessment of the position of the heart and the position of the trachea.

  ❏ Mediastinum displaced to the opposite side = large effusion.

  ❏ Mediastinum displaced to the ipsilateral side = lung collapse.

■ An occasional dilemma: a white out but: (a) there is no displacement of the mediastinum and (b) the trachea is central.

  ❏ The most likely cause: a large pleural effusion associated with or causing major collapse of the lung. The net effect is no displacement.

  ❏ Much less common: an extensive lobar pneumonia affecting all the lobes of the lung. An air bronchogram (p. 227) may be visible.

  ❏ Very rarely: extensive tumour infiltration of the entire lung.

Table 19.2 White out.

CXR findings	Most likely cause
A ■ Mediastinum displaced to the opposite side. ■ Trachea central or deviated to the opposite side.	Large pleural effusion with minimal secondary compression collapse of the underlying lung.
B* ■ Mediastinum central. ■ No tracheal deviation.	Large effusion with major collapse of the underlying lung.
C ■ Mediastinum displaced to the ipsilateral side. ■ Trachea deviated to the same side.	Collapse of the entire lung. Minimal or no pleural fluid.
D Features as for C above, and: ■ Ribs missing/distorted.	Pneumonectomy. The clinical history is conclusive.

* Exceptionally...these findings may be due to an extensive pneumonia affecting all the lobes of a lung, or to extensive tumour infiltration of the entire lung.

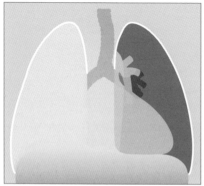

Figure 19.2 *White out. The mediastinum is displaced to the left and so is the trachea. Large right pleural effusion.*

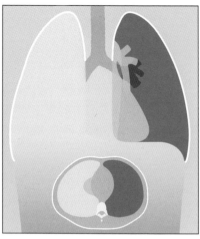

Figure 19.3 *White out. The mediastinum is central and so is the trachea. Large effusion with collapse of the underlying lung. The CT section shows the major compression collapse of the right lung caused by the large volume of fluid in the pleural space.*

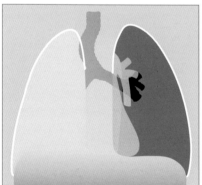

Figure 19.4 *White out. The mediastinum and trachea are displaced to the right side. Major collapse of the entire right lung.*

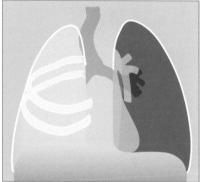

Figure 19.5 *White out. The mediastinum and the trachea are displaced to the right side. Several of the underlying ribs are abnormal. A previous right pneumonectomy accounts for the white out.*

Answer to Fig. 19.1 on p. 264

Analysis: Trachea and mediastinum are shifted to the right indicating a major loss of lung volume. But...always assess the bones. In this patient note the rib changes as well as the surgical clips.

Conclusion: A previous right pneumonectomy explains the white out.

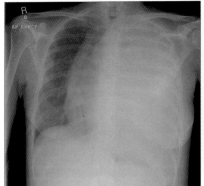

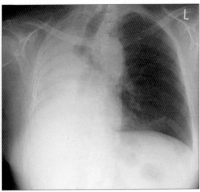

Figure 19.6 *White out. A large left pleural effusion is displacing the mediastinum to the right.*

Figure 19.7 *White out. The mediastinum and trachea are displaced to the right. Major collapse of the right lung.*

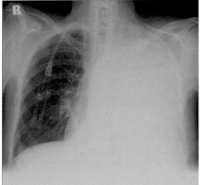

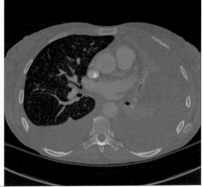

Figure 19.8 *White out. The mediastinum is not displaced and the trachea is midline. Large left pleural effusion with major compression collapse of the left lung. The CT section confirms the effusion and the collapsed left lung.*

REFERENCES

1. Ruskin JA, Gurney JW, Thorsen MK et al. Detection of pleural effusions on supine chest radiographs. AJR 1987; 148: 681–683.

2. Dee PM. The radiology of chest trauma. Radiol Clin North Am 1992; 30: 291–306.

3. Leung AN, Muller NL, Miller RR. CT in differential diagnosis of diffuse pleural disease. AJR 1990; 154: 487–492.

4. Kawashima A. Libshitz HI. Malignant pleural mesothelioma: CT manifestations in 50 cases. AJR 1990; 155: 965–969.

20 ANALYSIS: SOLITARY PULMONARY NODULE

> **Solitary pulmonary nodule (SPN):**
>
> *"to qualify as a nodule or cyst, a pulmonary lesion must present a reasonably sharp outline. Hence, a focal infiltrate with ill-defined borders is excluded.... I have set no upper limit of size for a pulmonary nodule, though I usually call the big ones a mass"[1].*
>
> *"a focal round or oval area of increased opacity in the lung that measures less than 3.0 cm in diameter"[2].*

A COMMON SCENARIO

An otherwise generally well patient has a CXR (e.g. for high blood pressure). A SPN is an unexpected finding.

Frequently, the clinical history will make a particular diagnosis highly likely. Examples: a man of 65 who has smoked two packs a day for 40 years—the default diagnosis will be a primary bronchial carcinoma. A history of carcinoma of the breast/kidney/colon some years previously will make a secondary deposit likely.

On the other hand there may be no clue from the history. In this case there are three steps:

1. Remind oneself of the causes of a SPN (Table 20.1).

2. Clinical assessment.

3. CXR analysis. This includes a search for CXR features which indicate a benign lesion and makes a CT examination unnecessary (Table 20.3).

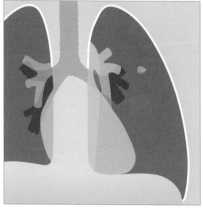

Figure 20.1 *A SPN is a common finding on adult CXRs. Approximately 60–70% are benign. Some 30–40% are malignant[2–4].*

CAUSES OF A SPN

A solitary pulmonary nodule is a very common finding on a CXR in adults. The vast majority are benign lesions (Table 20.1), usually old granulomas[2-4].

Table 20.1 Causes of a SPN.

Most common	Benign granuloma (previous infection)	
Less common	Bronchial carcinoma	Organising pneumonia
	Metastasis	Hamartoma
Much less common	Mucoid impaction	Rheumatoid nodule
	Abscess	Wegener's granuloma
	Infected bulla	Carcinoid
	Infarct	Sarcoid granuloma
	Haematoma	
Very rare	Arterio-venous malformation	Amyloid
		Hydatid cyst
	Intrapulmonary lipoma	

Table 20.2 Traps: simulated pulmonary nodules.

Overlap of normal pulmonary vessels	Encysted pleural fluid
Healing rib fracture	Electrocardiogram electrode pad
Rib density—benign	Nipple shadow
Rib density—malignant	Skin excrescence/mole
Cartilage calcification—first rib	Clothing artefact
Pleural plaque	

CLINICAL ASSESSMENT

CLINICAL DETAILS ARE CRUCIAL

- Is the clinical history helpful? Sometimes a recent low grade chest infection may result in a residual area of pneumonia. A history of asthma will raise the possibility of mucoid impaction. Perhaps there has been a recent injury to the chest, e.g. a haematoma.

- Is the clinical examination abnormal? Is there a mole or skin tag on the chest wall? A breast lump, an abdominal mass or an enlarged liver would raise the likelihood of malignancy.

STEP-BY-STEP CXR ANALYSIS

Step 1: Exclude any of the common traps (Table 20.2). A nodule may not be in the lung. A lateral CXR will confirm (or exclude) the lesion as intrapulmonary.

Step 2: Apply this rule: *"the best next step is comparison with a previous CXR"*. This will often remove the need for any further investigation.

■ If a CXR two or more years prior shows that the lesion has not changed in size...the SPN can be assumed to be benign, usually a benign granuloma. This is not a 100% guarantee[5,6]. Nevertheless, it is a highly reliable rule of thumb. Lack of growth implies a long doubling time (see opposite) which generally indicates a benign histology. This criterion has even greater power if earlier images (i.e. beyond two years) are also available for comparison.

■ If the previous CXR was clear...the SPN is an active lesion. It is highly likely to be malignant or inflammatory.

Step 3: No previous CXR available: look for benign features (Table 20.3).

Step 4: No previous CXR available: look for malignant features (Table 20.4).

Step 5: Is CT of the thorax necessary? Table 20.6 provides guidelines.

Table 20.3 SPN: benign characteristics.

CXR feature	Comment
Size	1. Almost all benign nodules are less than 3 cm in diameter.
	2. A nodule of less than 1 cm in diameter is very difficult to visualise[7]. Apply this maxim: *"this nodule is less than 1 cm in diameter but I can see it very well indeed. This means that it is almost certainly calcified and thus it will be benign."*
Shrinking	Rapid reduction in size in days or weeks on interval CXRs—the lesion is benign (often a resolving infection).
Calcification	Benign if central, shaggy, laminated, popcorn, or stippled.
Presence of Branching	Tubular branching leading up to the nodule suggests: ■ an arterio-venous malformation, or ■ a pulmonary venous varix, or ■ mucoid impaction within a bronchus
Stable	No change over two years is a strong feature suggesting a benign lesion[8]. Not an absolute guarantor[5,6] but indicates a high probability.

Table 20.4 SPN: malignant characteristics.

CXR feature	Comment
Size	Diameter of more than 3 cm is very suggestive of malignancy.
Margin	Ill-defined or spiculated border is a strong pointer towards malignancy.
Strands	Radiating strands at the margin—strong probability of a primary carcinoma...*but not an absolute certainty.*
Calcification position[9,10]	Eccentric calcification raises the suspicion of a scar carcinoma.

Table 20.5 SPN: unreliable characteristics...the indeterminate nodule.

CXR feature	Comment
Smooth margin	■ This is common with benign disease. Nevertheless, some primary carcinomas do have smooth margins. ■ A metastasis usually has a smooth margin.
Lobulated outline	May be present in benign as well as in malignant lesions.
The tail sign	Can occur in benign and malignant lesions[11] (Fig. 20.4).
Cavitation	Abscesses cavitate. Squamous cell carcinomas cavitate.
Doubling time/ rate of growth	■ Some granulomas grow slowly. ■ Some primary carcinomas grow very slowly...others grow very rapidly.

Doubling time—a summary[5,9–12]

The growth rate of a lesion is often expressed in terms of doubling time (i.e. the time in which a nodule doubles in volume[12]). It has been estimated that a nodule goes through some 30 doublings before it reaches 1 cm in diameter and becomes readily detectable on a CXR[13]. Bronchial carcinomas usually take 1–18 months to double in size.

Rule of thumb: A doubling time of less than one month, or alternatively more than 18 months, suggests benign disease. This maxim is a helpful guideline, but there are occasional exceptions.

Table 20.6 Is CT necessary?

CXR analysis	Feature	CT indicated?
Step 1	An artefact is confirmed (Table 20.2)	No
Step 2	Lesion unchanged over the previous two years	No (very occasionally, the clinical context—age, smoking history— will justify CT)
	Lesion has increased in size over the previous two years	Yes
Step 3	Classic benign features (Table 20.3)	No
Step 4	▪ Classic malignant features (Table 20.4)	Yes
	▪ Indeterminate features (Table 20.5)	Yes

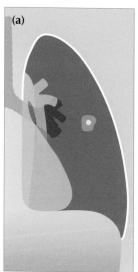
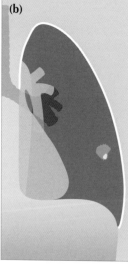

Figure 20.2 *(a) Central calcification in a SPN is usually a benign feature. (b) Eccentric calcification raises the suspicion of a carcinoma arising in an old scar.*

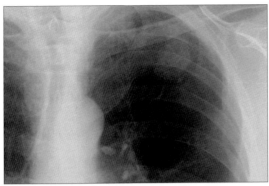

Figure 20.3 *SPN at the apex of the left lung. The margin is slightly irregular and ill-defined. These two features are suggestive of a primary bronchial carcinoma.*

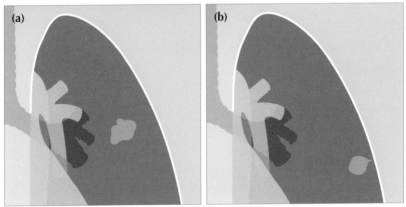

(a)   **(b)**

Figure 20.4 *SPNs. In (a) the margin is irregular. In (b) a tail sign is present. A "tail" is a strand-like or linear projection of tissue extending outwards from the margin of a nodule. Either (a) or (b) should raise the strong suspicion of malignancy.*

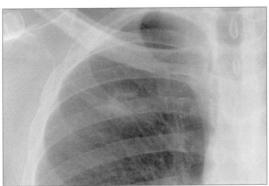

Figure 20.5 *The right upper zone nodule has a cavity within it. Some benign lesions do cavitate, e.g. abscess or rheumatoid nodule. All the same, in the appropriate clinical setting, cavitation should always suggest the probability of a squamous carcinoma. Subsequently confirmed squamous carcinoma of the bronchus.*

AN INTERESTING LESION—PULMONARY HAMARTOMA[2,10]

Pathology

Hamartomas are benign tumours found in various organs. All hamartomas contain cells of some of the tissues within the organ of origin. A pulmonary hamartoma invariably contains cartilage and bronchial epithelium; it often contains fat.

Clinical features

Usually an incidental, asymptomatic finding. Tuberous sclerosis is a rare association.

The CXR

■ 90% are situated peripherally in the lung. Very occasionally it is endobronchial.

■ Solitary.

■ Most are less than 3 cm in diameter. Exceptionally—may be as large as 10 cm.

■ Margins sharp and well-defined.

■ 10–20% contain calcification which may be stippled or popcorn shaped (Fig. 20.6)

■ Interval CXRs—slow growth does occur.

■ NB: fat within a SPN on CT is pathognomic of a hamartoma.

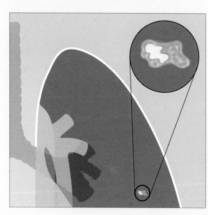

Figure 20.6 *Some hamartomas contain visible calcification. It is often stippled or popcorn shaped. This figure shows the appearance of popcorn calcification. Note the similarity to a popped kernel of corn[1].*

REFERENCES

1. Felson B. Chest Roentgenology. Philadelphia, PA: WB Saunders, 1973: 314–329.

2. Erasmus JJ, McAdams HP, Connolly JE. Solitary pulmonary nodules: Part I. Morphologic evaluation for differentiation of benign and malignant lesions. Radiographics 2000; 20: 43–58.

3. Gurney JW. Determining the likelihood of malignancy in solitary pulmonary nodules with Bayesian analysis. Radiology 1993; 186: 405–413.

4. Lillington GA, Caskey CI. Evaluation and management of solitary and multiple pulmonary nodules. Clin Chest Med 1993; 14: 111–119.

5. Sherrier RH, Chiles C, Johnson GA et al. Differentation of benign from malignant pulmonary nodules with digitized chest radiographs. Radiology 1987; 162: 645–649.

6. Yankelevitz DF, Henschke CJ. Does 2-year stability imply that pulmonary nodules are benign? AJR 1997; 168: 325–328.

7. Kundel HL. Predictive value and threshold detectability of lung tumours. Radiology 1981; 139: 25–29.

8. Good CA. Roentgenologic appraisal of solitary pulmonary nodules. Minn Med 1962; 45: 157–160.

9. Hansell DM, Armstrong P, Lynch DA, McAdams HP. Imaging of Diseases of the Chest. 4th ed. St Louis, MO: Mosby, 2005.

10. Collins J, Stern EJ. Chest Radiology: The Essentials. Philadelphia, PA: Lippincott Williams & Wilkins, 1999.

11. Webb WR. The pleural tail sign. Radiology 1978; 127: 309–313.

12. Reed JC. Chest Radiology: Plain Film Patterns and Differential Diagnoses. 5th Edition. Philadelphia, PA: Mosby, 2003.

13. Collins VP, Loeffler RK, Tivey H. Observations on growth rates of human tumors. Am J Roentgenol 1956; 76: 988–1000.

14. Erasmus JJ, McAdams HP, Connolly JE. Solitary pulmonary nodules: Part II. Evaluation of the indeterminate nodule. Radiographics 2000; 20: 59–66.

15. Dewan NA, Shehan CJ, Reeb SD et al. Likelihood of malignancy in a solitary pulmonary nodule: comparison of Bayesian analysis and FDG–PET scan. Chest 1997; 112: 416–422.

16. Woodring JH, Fried AM. Significance of wall thickness in solitary cavities of the lung: a follow-up study. AJR 1983; 140: 473–474.

21 ANALYSIS: MULTIPLE PULMONARY NODULES

Multiple pulmonary nodules:

"The term is generally accepted as indicating several or many separate and rounded lung densities varying in size up to 30 mm in diameter."

"miliary pattern (nodules)...a collection of tiny discrete pulmonary opacities that are generally uniform in size, widespread in distribution, and each of which is 2 mm or less in diameter."[1]

TWO SCENARIOS

Scenario 1:   A CXR shows multiple nodules. It is highly likely that the patient's clinical history will suggest the likely diagnosis. Examples:

■ A young intravenous drug addict...lung abscesses.

■ A history of renal carcinoma...metastases.

Scenario 2:   The clinical presentation does not provide an obvious clue to the likely diagnosis. We need to remind ourselves of:

1. The possible causes of multiple pulmonary nodules (Table 21.1).

2. Specific radiographic features that will suggest either: (a) the likely diagnosis; or (b) a snappy—but limited—differential diagnosis.

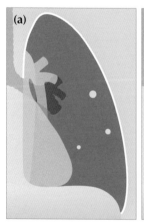 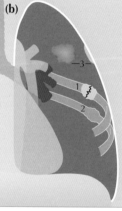

Figure 21.1   *(a) Multiple pulmonary nodules. The size of the nodules usually vary. Strictly speaking, a nodule has a maximum diameter of 30 mm. Above 30 mm an opacity is conventionally referred to as a mass. Some descriptive flexibility is accepted, particularly if most of the lesions are less than 30 mm in diameter. (b) Opacities outside the lung can simulate pulmonary nodules. These include healing rib fractures (1), old rib fractures (2), and pleural plaques (3).*

CAUSES OF MULTIPLE NODULES

A CXR showing clinically unexpected nodules is unusual. The default diagnosis is metastatic disease. In most instances the clinical history and examination will indicate whether an alternative diagnosis is likely.

Table 21.1   Causes of multiple pulmonary nodules[2-6].

Inflammatory / Infective	■ Granulomas
	■ Septic emboli/lung abscesses[7]
	■ Fungal pneumonia
	■ Tuberculosis
	❏ miliary
	❏ bronchopneumonia
	■ Chickenpox pneumonia
Neoplastic	■ Metastases[3-6,8]
	■ Bronchioloalveolar cell carcinoma
	■ Lymphoma
	■ Kaposi's sarcoma
	■ Mycosis fungoides
Autoimmune disease	■ Rheumatoid nodules
	■ Wegener's granulomatosis[9]
Vascular	■ Arteriovenous malformations
	■ Pulmonary infarcts
Other	■ Sarcoidosis
	■ Silicosis
	■ Langerhans cell histiocytosis (granulomatosis)

Table 21.2   Traps[10]: simulated pulmonary nodules.

■ Nipples	■ Pleural plaques (asbestos related)
■ Multiple cutaneous lesions	■ Bone islands in the ribs
■ Subcutaneous lesions	■ Healing rib fractures
❏ e.g. cysticercosis	■ Electrocardiogram electrode pads

NODULES—CXR FEATURES

Particular appearances will suggest a fairly limited differential diagnosis
(Table 21.3).

Table 21.3 Features and potential diagnoses.

Morphology	The possibilities
Calcified nodules	▩ Tuberculous granulomas
	▩ Histoplasmosis
	▩ Previous chickenpox pneumonia
	▩ Coccidioidomycosis
	▩ Metastases
	❏ osteogenic sarcoma, chondrosarcoma
	▩ Mitral stenosis with long standing elevated pulmonary venous pressure
	▩ Dust inhalation diseases. Silicosis
Miliary nodules	▩ Infection
"having the appearance of millet seeds"	❏ tuberculosis, histoplasmosis
	▩ Metastases
	❏ thyroid or breast carcinoma, melanoma, choriocarcinoma
	▩ Sarcoid
	▩ Silicosis
Cavitating nodules	▩ Abscesses
	❏ *Staphylococcus, Klebsiella, Streptococcus,* tuberculosis, fungal infection
	❏ hydatid disease
	▩ Metastases
	❏ squamous cell carcinomas, sarcomas
	▩ Areas of infarction
	▩ Rheumatoid nodules
	▩ Wegener's granulomatosis
	▩ Focal lung contusions
Beware	▩ Imposters—Not cavitation
	❏ multiple small bullae
	❏ cystic bronchiectasis

NODULES—A RULE OR TWO

Several useful rules of thumb can be applied (Table 21.4).

Table 21.4 Particular pathologies—CXR features.

Pathology	Features
Metastases	■ Margins are usually well-defined
	■ Occasionally ill-defined: choriocarcinoma
Abscesses	■ Ill-defined margins
	■ Edges may become harder and sharper when treated with antibiotics
Rheumatoid nodules	■ Can disappear spontaneuosly and later reappear
	■ Reappearance may be in different positions

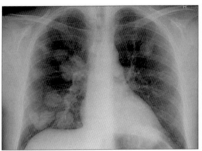

Figure 21.2 *Multiple nodules. Metastases from a renal cell carcinoma. The appearances are typical of metastases—rounded lesions with fairly well-defined margins.*

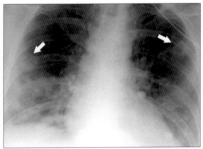

Figure 21.3 *Multiple nodules. Male. Age 38. Intravenous drug user. Endocarditis. Lung abscesses. Two of the nodules are cavitating (arrows).*

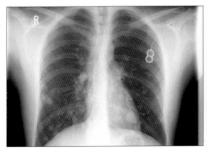
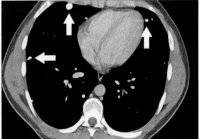

Figure 21.4 *Multiple small nodules. Some are much smaller than 10 mm but are readily visible. This suggests that they are calcified. Indeed, they do contain calcification as shown on the CT section (arrows). Secondary tumours from a primary osteogenic sarcoma.*

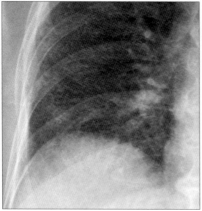

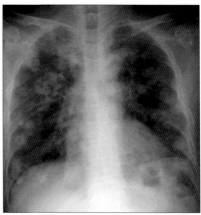

Figure 21.5 *Multiple miliary nodules. Tuberculosis. These very small densities (2 mm diameter) are visible because the lung interstitium has hundreds / thousands of exceptionally tiny lesions superimposed one in front of another.*

Figure 21.6 *Male. Cavitating nodules. Metastatic lesions from a primary tumour of the larynx. Metastases that cavitate are usually squamous cell lesions: in men, frequently a head and neck primary tumour; in women, often carcinoma of the cervix.*

INTERESTING NODULES—CHICKENPOX INFECTION[11]

Aetiology / pathology

Highly infectious viral infection (varicella). Spread by droplet infection / ruptured skin lesions / contact with herpes zoster.

Clinical features

Children are most commonly affected and it is then a relatively mild illness. Infected adults can be very ill. Characteristic rash appears centrally starting on the trunk and spreads centrifugally. In adults, chickenpox pneumonia may occur; it is a very rare complication in children. Pneumonia can be debilitating and occasionally fatal, particularly in immunocompromised individuals.

The CXR

■ Chickenpox pneumonia:

❏ Extensive, diffuse, ill-defined, air space shadowing.

❏ Subsequently: development of multiple calcified nodules in the lungs. Interestingly, an adult with chickenpox may subsequently develop calcified nodules whether or not pneumonia has complicated the illness.

■ The calcified nodules are characteristically:

❏ Scattered—mainly in the mid and lower zones.

❏ Small—less than 3 mm in diameter.

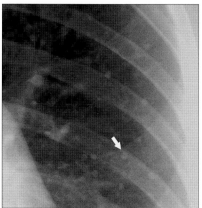

Figure 21.7 *Multiple small—very small—calcified nodules were present in the mid and upper zones of both lungs. One of the nodules is indicated by the arrow. Previous chickenpox pneumonia.*

REFERENCES

1. Glossary of terms for thoracic radiology: recommendations of the Nomenclature Committee of the Fleischner Society. AJR 1984; 143: 509–517.

2. Zitting AJ. Prevalence of Radiographic small lung opacities and pleural abnormalities in a representative adult population sample. Chest 1995; 107: 126–131.

3. Reed JC. Chest Radiology: Plain Film Patterns and Differential Diagnosis. 5th ed. Philadelphia, PA: Mosby, 2003: 259–286.

4. Collins SJ, Stern EJ. Chest Radiology: The Essentials. Philadelphia, PA: Lippincott Williams & Wilkins, 1999: 96–105.

5. Felson B. Chest Roentgenology. Philadelphia, PA: WB Saunders, 1973.

6. Fraser RG, Muller NL, Colman NC, Pare PD. Fraser and Pare's Diagnosis of Diseases of the Chest. 4th ed. Philadelphia, PA: WB Saunders, 1999.

7. Huang RM, Naidich DP, Lubat E et al. Septic pulmonary emboli: CT–radiographic correlation. AJR 1989; 153: 41–45.

8. Seo JB, Im JG, Goo JM et al. Atypical pulmonary metastases; spectrum of radiologic findings. Radiographics 2001; 21: 403–417.

9. Frazier AA, Rosado-de-Christenson ML, Galvin JR et al. Pulmonary angiitis and granulomatosis: radiologic–pathologic correlation. Radiographics 1998; 18: 687–710.

10. Gronner AT, Ominsky SH. Plain film radiography of the chest: findings that simulate pulmonary disease. AJR 1994; 163: 1343–1348.

11. Sargent EN, Carson MJ, Reilly ED. Roentgenographic manifestations of varicella pneumonia with post mortem correlation. AJR 1966; 98: 305–317.

22 SUSPECTED COPD

Chronic obstructive pulmonary disease (COPD): Disease characterised by the presence of airflow obstruction due to either chronic bronchitis or emphysema.

- **Chronic bronchitis is defined clinically:** A chronic productive cough on most days of the week for three months of the year in each of two successive years in a patient in whom other causes of chronic cough have been excluded.

- **Emphysema is defined anatomically:** Abnormal permanent enlargement of air spaces distal to the terminal bronchioles, accompanied by destruction of the alveolar walls but without obvious fibrosis.

Table 22.1 Avoid terminological confusions[1-3].

Term	Includes / represents	Notes
Obstructive pulmonary disorders	■ Asthma ■ Chronic bronchitis ■ Emphysema ■ Bronchiectasis ■ Cystic fibrosis	Diseases that are characterised by a reduction in expiratory airflow
COPD	■ Chronic bronchitis ■ Emphysema	■ The term COPD is limited to these two diseases ■ In some patients both diseases co-exist
Compensatory emphysema	Airspace dilatation (i.e. increased inflation) in response to loss of volume elsewhere in the lung	■ Very different to (COPD) emphysema ■ No destruction of alveolar walls ■ Example: compensatory emphysema of an upper lobe when there is total collapse of the lower lobe

CXR FINDINGS IN COPD

GENERAL

■ COPD is usually suspected clinically. The diagnosis is confirmed by spirometry demonstrating airflow obstruction that is not fully reversible. The CXR has a limited role in diagnosis but can be useful:

   ❏ To exclude other causes for the patient's symptoms.

   ❏ To assist in the management of a patient with known COPD whose clinical status shows an acute deterioration.

■ Even with extensive pathological changes (COPD) or severe clinical symptoms the CXR may appear normal—particularly if the dominant disease process is chronic bronchitis.

■ Caution (1): large volume lungs are not necessarily indicative of over-inflation[2]. They can occur in:

   ❏ healthy, well conditioned, young people

   ❏ tall people

   ❏ opera singers

   ❏ some athletes

■ Caution (2): be careful about making a diagnosis of COPD on the CXR alone without supporting clinical evidence.

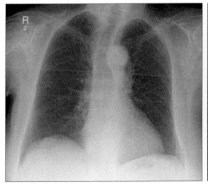 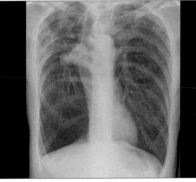

Figure 22.1 *Elderly female. Severe clinical and spirometry-confirmed COPD. The CXR is entirely normal. This is the most common CXR finding.*

Figure 22.2 *Elderly male. COPD. Abnormal CXR. The domes of the diaphragm are low and flat; large bullae in both upper zones; narrow, vertical heart. (Incidental and unrelated—the right hilum is pulled upwards and laterally by scarring from a previous infection involving the upper lobe.)*

CHRONIC BRONCHITIS

■ The diagnosis of chronic bronchitis is made clinically on the basis of well-defined and internationally accepted features. The CXR appearance may be normal or there may be abnormalities which are very subtle or non-specific (Table 22.2).

■ The principle role of the CXR is in helping to exclude diseases that can clinically mimic chronic bronchitis[2]. These include tuberculosis, carcinoma, bronchiectasis and lung abscess.

Table 22.2 CXR features in chronic bronchitis.

Symptoms	CXR
Mild to moderate	Normal
Severe	■ In most patients the CXR remains normal
	■ A few patients show non-specific findings:
	❏ Over-inflation—generalised
	❏ Thickened bronchial walls:
	– peribronchial cuffing (Fig. 22.3)
	– parallel tubular shadows
	❏ Areas of oligaemia (i.e. decrease in width of visible pulmonary vessels indicating reduced blood flow)
	❏ Saber sheath (UK: sabre sheath) trachea[4]

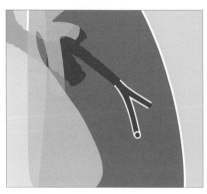

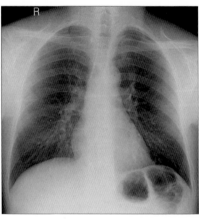

Figure 22.3 *The anatomical changes that explain peribronchial cuffing which is very occasionally seen in some patients with chronic bronchitis. The cuffing appearance is due to thickened bronchial walls seen en face on the CXR.*

Figure 22.4 *Chronic bronchitis. Normal CXR. This is the most common appearance.*

EMPHYSEMA

- The CXR is frequently normal. In some patients the CXR appearances are very abnormal.

- A low diaphragm does not of itself indicate emphysema. Over-inflation of the lungs due to emphysema should only be assumed when a dome of the diaphragm is both low and flat (Fig. 22.5).

Table 22.3 CXR features in emphysema.

Disease severity	CXR[2-9]
Mild to moderate	■ May appear normal
	■ Areas combining hyperlucency (blackness) and fewer vessel markings
Severe	■ A low, flat dome of the diaphragm is very suggestive
	❏ Flat: highest level of a dome is less than 1.5 cm above a line drawn between the costophrenic and the cardiophrenic sulci (Fig. 22.5)
	■ Vascular changes (see p. 286)
	■ Bullae
	■ Saber sheath trachea
	■ Other signs...are subjective and unreliable

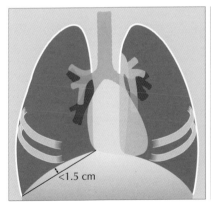
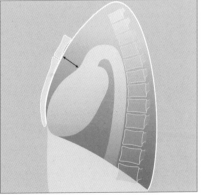

<1.5 cm

Figure 22.5 *Over-inflated lungs. Low domes of the diaphragm are not necessarily abnormal. It should only be assumed to indicate COPD if the domes are both low and flat. On a PA CXR a flat dome is one in which its highest point is less than 1.5 cm above a line connecting the costophrenic and cardiophrenic angles[2]. On a lateral CXR a flat dome is one in which the diaphragmatic peak is less than 1.5 cm above a line joining the sternophrenic and posterior costophrenic angles[2]. Note the enlarged retrosternal air space—on the lateral CXR—a regular finding in COPD when over-inflation is present.*

Vascular changes

Widespread emphysema may show the following abnormal appearances:

- A narrow, vertical, centrally situated heart. The explanation: over-inflation of the lungs causes the diaphragm to be low. Because the pericardium and the superior surface of the diaphragm are adherent, the heart is pulled inferiorly by the over-inflation. Consequently its transverse diameter appears narrow.

- The hilar vessels are prominent[10]. This is because there is less cardiac shadow overlap, or because the vessel margins at the hilum are sharply defined by the hypertransradiant over-distended adjacent air spaces, or because the pulmonary arteries are actually enlarged due to secondary pulmonary arterial hypertension.

- The vessels extending outwards into the lungs appear thinner or have a smaller diameter than is usual. This peripheral narrowing is in marked contrast to the very prominent hilar vessels. There may also be fewer vessels in affected areas (Fig. 22.6).

Bullae

- A bulla is a thin-walled air-filled structure measuring more than 1 cm in diameter. It represents a distended pulmonary lobule or group of lobules. Sometimes bullae are very large (5–20 cm in diameter) and are the result of groups of disrupted alveoli coalescing.

- Don't be surprised if a bulla disappears. This does happen—either spontaneously or following infection.

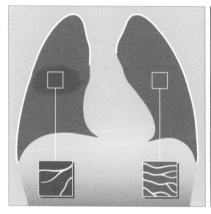

Figure 22.6 *Emphysematous area in the mid zone of the right lung. Compare the fewer and narrower vessels in the affected area with the appearance of the vessels at the same site in the normal left lung.*

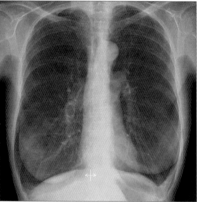

Figure 22.7 *COPD. Severe emphysema. Low, flat diaphragm. Large main pulmonary arteries resulting from pulmonary arterial hypertension.*

Saber sheath trachea (UK: sabre sheath trachea)

When a saber sheath appearance is present it is a reliable and sensitive sign of COPD. A saber sheath configuration is evident when the intrathoracic coronal diameter of the trachea is two-thirds of the saggital diameter or less, when measured 1 cm above the superior aspect of the aortic arch[4]. The precise mechanism causing this tracheal appearance remains speculative. This sign may appear in chronic bronchitis or emphysema (Figs 22.9 and 22.10).

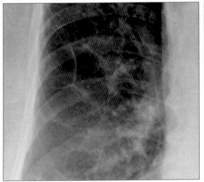
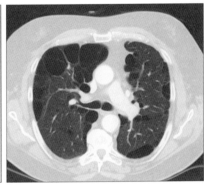

Figure 22.8 *Emphysematous bullae. Multiple ring-like shadows in all zones of both lungs. The CT confirms the presence of bullae.*

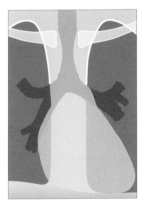
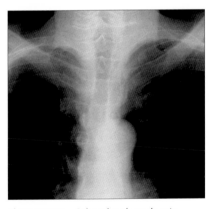

Figure 22.9 *Saber sheath trachea in COPD. The narrowing is limited to the intrathoracic part of the trachea. A saber sheath appearance exists when the coronal diameter of the trachea is two thirds of the sagittal diameter or less…measured 1 cm above the aortic arch[4]. Precise assessment requires a lateral as well as a PA CXR. Nevertheless, the tracheal narrowing is usually evident on the frontal CXR.*

Figure 22.10 *Saber sheath trachea in COPD.*

KNOWN COPD: INDICATIONS FOR A CXR

A CXR is only occasionally necessary during an acute exacerbation (Table 22.4).

Table 22.4 Indications for a CXR.

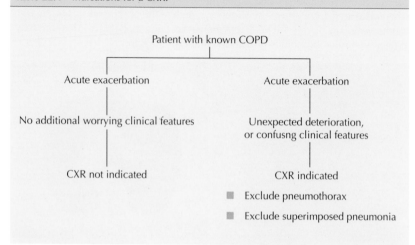

Patient with known COPD

Acute exacerbation	Acute exacerbation
No additional worrying clinical features	Unexpected deterioration, or confusng clinical features
CXR not indicated	CXR indicated

- Exclude pneumothorax
- Exclude superimposed pneumonia

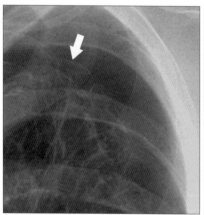

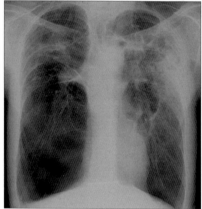

Figure 22.11 *COPD. Unexpected clinical deterioration. A pneumothorax is present. The visceral pleura (arrow) is visible.*

Figure 22.12 *COPD. Acute exacerbation with confusing clinical features. The CXR reveals an extensive pneumonia in the left mid zone. (NB: this is the same patient as shown in Fig. 22.2)*

FACTS AND FIGURES

■ The differential diagnosis in a patient with clinical symptoms suggesting COPD will include asthma, bronchiectasis, cystic fibrosis, left heart failure, interstitial lung disease, and upper airway obstruction.

■ Chronic bronchitis. The pathological changes: mucous gland enlargement, inflammation, and bronchial wall thickening. Airflow limitation results from the deformity of the bronchial walls and narrowing of the lumina.

■ Recognised causes of emphysema are: cigarette smoking, alpha 1-antitrypsin deficiency, intravenous drug abuse (cocaine, heroin, methadone), immune deficiency syndromes (including HIV infection).

■ Emphysema. Autopsy studies have shown that emphysema can involve as much as 30% of the lung tissue, and yet an individual may not have had any respiratory symptoms during life[5].

REFERENCES

1. American Thoracic Society. Standards for the diagnosis and care of patients with chronic obstructive pulmonary disease. Am J Respir Crit Care Med 1995; 152: 77–121.

2. Takasugi JE, Godwin JD. Radiology of chronic obstructive pulmonary disease. Radiol Clin North Am 1998; 36: 29–55.

3. Devereux G. ABC of chronic obstructive pulmonary disease. Definition, epidemiology, and risk factors. BMJ 2006; 332: 1142–1144.

4. Greene R. "Saber-sheath" trachea: relation to chronic obstructive pulmonary disease. AJR 1978; 130: 441–445.

5. Pratt PC. Role of conventional chest radiography in diagnosis and exclusion of emphysema. Am J Med 1987; 82: 998–1006.

6. Thurlbeck WM, Muller NL. Emphysema: definition, imaging and quantification. AJR 1994; 163: 1017–1025.

7. Collins J, Stern EJ. Chest Radiology: The Essentials. Philadelphia, PA: Lippincott Williams & Wilkins, 1999: 200–201.

8. Foster WL, Gimenez EI, Robidoux MA et al. The emphysemas: radiologic–pathologic correlations. Radiographics 1993; 13: 311–328.

9. Klein JS, Gamsu G, Webb WR et al. High-resolution CT diagnosis of emphysema in symptomatic patients with normal chest radiographs and isolated low diffusing capacity. Radiology 1992; 182: 817–821.

10. Simon G. Principles of Chest X-ray Diagnosis. 2nd ed. London: Butterworths, 1962.

Pulmonary embolism (PE):	Obstruction of a pulmonary artery by a thrombus.
Pulmonary infarction:	An area of tissue injury resulting from occlusion of a vessel—most commonly by an embolus. The injury may cause oedema and/or haemorrhage. It does not always result in necrosis of lung tissue.

BACKGROUND INFORMATION

■ The clinical diagnosis of a PE can be very difficult. The symptoms and signs are varied and diverse, and none are diagnostic[1-3]. The CXR has no role to play in making a definitive diagnosis of PE. However, it can be useful in:

❑ Excluding some other causes for the patient's symptoms.

❑ Supporting (i.e. lending weight to) the clinical suspicion of PE.

❑ Helping to decide which investigation should be performed next.

Continuing advances in multidetector CT scanning technology have established CT pulmonary angiography (CTPA) as the optimum imaging test for confirming or excluding a PE[4,5]. The present generation of CT machines are able to obtain very thin sections through the entire thorax in seconds. Establishing the precise accuracy of CTPA as a diagnostic test in suspected PE is difficult because meaningful research is constrained by the absence of a gold standard. Currently, the accepted view is that imaging carried out with high quality CTPA is very accurate.

■ What about D-dimer?

"D-dimer assays are commonly used as part of the screening assessment for patients with suspected venous thromboembolic disease (VTE). The assay results are best interpreted in conjunction with a formal clinical probability score. As D-dimer levels may be raised in many acute medical conditions, the clinical consensus is that the only useful D-dimer assay is a negative result as that has a high negative predictive value for VTE."[6]

■ The unreliability of clinical assessment in providing a definitive diagnosis of PE, together with the plethora of diagnostic tests[5-10], can lead to confusion and errors[11]. Pre-test probability assessments utilising clinical prediction rules (see Chapter 17) have helped to bring direction to the rational selection and use of the available diagnostic tests[2,7].

INVESTIGATION OF SUSPECTED ACUTE PE

This two-step approach is based on the British Thoracic Society 2003 Guidelines[2].

STEP 1

Clinical risk stratification—ask two clinical questions:

1. Is another diagnosis genuinely unlikely?

   The CXR and electrocardiogram findings may be helpful in suggesting other possible causes for the signs/symptoms.

2. Is there a major risk factor for PE?

   Examples: recent immobility, major surgery, lower limb trauma or surgery, pregnancy, post partum, major medical illness, previous proven venous thromboembolism.

If 1) and 2) answer NO	= low clinical probability of PE
If either 1) or 2) answer YES	= intermediate clinical probability
If both 1) and 2) answer YES	= high clinical probability

STEP 2

The clinical probability now determines the next investigation.

High clinical probability → proceed straight to CTPA
Intermediate or low clinical probability → perform a D-dimer test
D-dimer positive → proceed straight to CTPA
D-dimer negative: consider an alternative diagnosis and discharge

IS THERE A ROLE FOR ISOTOPE VQ SCANNING?[10,12]

"PE is often misdiagnosed—partly due to over-reliance on the ventilation perfusion (VQ) scan. It is important that clinicians continue to be aware of the limitations of the VQ Scan"[10].

■ Remember—the CTPA remains the optimum imaging investigation.

■ However, a VQ scan can be utilised if:

    1. The patient does not have known underlying cardio-respiratory disease.

    2. The CXR is normal.

    3. The VQ findings are interpreted in conjunction with the level of clinical probability (p. 291).

■ The next steps to be adopted are:

    ❑ Normal VQ—STOP.

    ❑ Any other result—proceed to CTPA.

THE ROLE OF THE CXR

The CXR has an important part to play in the diagnostic pathway outlined on p. 291—specifically in step 1.

THE MAJOR ROLE

To exclude conditions which can mimic the clinical features of PE. These include:

■ pneumothorax

■ rib fracture

■ left heart failure

■ pneumonia...but always be careful of making a diagnosis of pneumonia if lung consolidation is not associated with a fever and mucky sputum

A LESS IMPORTANT ROLE—BUT OCCASIONALLY USEFUL

An abnormal CXR (Table 23.1) may add strength to the clinical suspicion that a PE has occurred. This follows from the PISA-PED study which found that most patients with proven PE had an abnormality on the CXR[3,11]. Admittedly, most of these abnormalities are minor and non-specific (Table 23.1).

Table 23.1 CXR appearances in acute PE[3,11,12]

Acute PE without infarction
 	
(90% of affected patients)
	■ A completely normal CXR occurs in less than 20% of cases
	
	■ When abnormal the CXR findings (Fig. 23.1) are commonly minor and non-specific—including:
	
	  ❏ small areas of linear collapse
	
	  ❏ small areas of consolidation (i.e. alveolar shadowing)
	
	  ❏ small pleural effusion
	
	  ❏ slight elevation of a dome of the diaphragm
	
	  ❏ prominent main pulmonary artery
	
	■ Unilateral hypertransradiancy (if focal—the Westermark sign) does occur, but it is very rare

Acute PE with infarction
 	
(10% of affected patients)
	■ The CXR is invariably abnormal
	
	■ A spectrum of findings—including:
	
	  ❏ minor abnormalities such as small areas of linear collapse or a small pleural effusion
	
	  ❏ an area of consolidation (very similar to pneumonic consolidation; it represents haemorrhage/oedema)
	
	  ❏ a large effusion
	
	  ❏ consolidation and an effusion

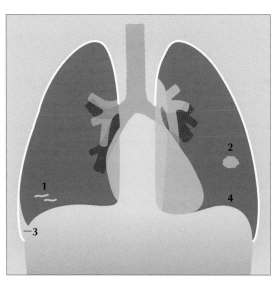

Figure 23.1 *The CXR is frequently abnormal in PE—but the changes are usually minor[12]. Some of these non-specific changes are illustrated: 1 = linear areas of collapse; 2 = small area of consolidation; 3 = small pleural effusion; 4 = elevated dome of the diaphragm.*

THE CXR AND TWO OVER-STATED SIGNS

Two CXR signs relating to acute PE are frequently emphasised. You may regard us as distrustful and cynical, but we prefer to see ourselves as streetwise when advising that you do not place too much weight on the presence or absence of either of these two signs.

THE WESTERMARK SIGN

■ This is a hyperlucent area of lung on the CXR due to reduced lung perfusion distal to an obstructed vessel. Be very careful. Placing too much reliance on an area of hyperlucency in these ill patients is usually unwise. Areas of local (or even whole lung) increased transradiancy (see pp. 254–263) can be produced by:

❑ patient rotation (Fig. 23.2)

❑ decentering of the x-ray beam (Fig. 23.3)

❑ differing amounts of chest wall compression against the cassette

❑ focal area of emphysema

❑ asymmetry of chest wall musculature

■ A hypertransradiant hemithorax is common in clinical practice. In our series, 35% of normal CXRs in people aged 50 years and older showed evidence of hypertransradiancy (see Chapter 16, p. 243).

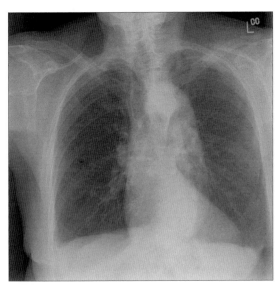

Figure 23.2 *Westermark sign? Be careful. Elderly female. Dyspnoeic. A PE is a clinical possibility. The right lung is hypertransradiant (blacker than the left lung). We need to be cautious and not too quick to call this the Westermark sign of PE. Two technical factors are causing the blackening on this CXR: (1) rotation to the right; (2) lateral decentering of the x-ray beam to the right side...this is evident from the increased definition of the scapula and soft tissues on the right side as compared to the left side.*

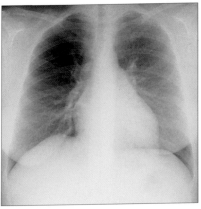

Figure 23.3   *Westermark sign? Be very careful. Middle-aged female. Intermediate clinical probability of a pulmonary embolus. The right lung is hypertransradiant (blacker) compared with the left lung. Two technical factors are contributing to this:*
(1) lateral decentering of the x-ray beam;
(2) asymmetric compression of the chest wall soft tissues on the right side. The VQ scan was entirely normal.

HAMPTON'S HUMP SIGN

This is the term given to what is often claimed to be the typical features of lung shadowing resulting from a pulmonary infarct. Hampton's hump is a wedge shaped density with its base against the pleural surface and a rounded medial margin directed towards the hilum. We have two reservations—particularly if only a frontal CXR is available:

■ A lobar pneumonia can produce an identical appearance.

■ On a frontal CXR a centrally situated density, seemingly well away from the pleura, will not show the features of Hampton's hump (Fig. 23.4). However, the density could still be based against the pleura, either peripherally in the lung or against a fissure. A lateral CXR may then reveal the characteristic features of Hampton's hump.

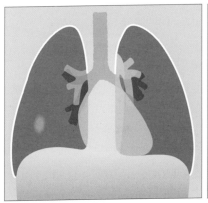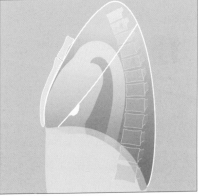

Figure 23.4   *Why no hump? The lung shadow produced by an infarct is situated centrally in the right lung. On the frontal view it has no distinguishing features, i.e. no Hampton's hump features. Only when a lateral CXR is obtained is it seen that the shadow is actually based against the pleura (the oblique fissure)—i.e. it fulfils a Hampton's hump criterion.*

FACTS AND FIGURES

The following are approximations[1-3]. Of patients with PE:

- 90% are tachypnoeic

- 70% are dyspnoeic

- 70% complain of chest pain

- 13% have haemoptysis

- < 20% of elderly patients have the classic combination of dyspnoea, chest pain, and haemoptysis

- 14% have a fever without any other identifiable cause for a pyrexia

- 70% have no clinical signs of a deep vein thrombosis

- 50% are shown to have lower limb thrombus on ultrasound examination of the lower limb veins

- 30–40% mortality if untreated

- 8% mortality if treated

Death results from acute pulmonary hypertension causing right heart failure and then circulatory collapse.

AN INTERESTING CONDITION—FAT EMBOLISM[13]

Aetiology / pathology

A complication following fracture of a long bone, extensive soft tissue injury, or severe burns. Fat globules can enter the venous system (thence to the lungs) or the arterial system. It probably occurs—in a mild form—more frequently than is diagnosed.

Clinical features

- Fat reaches the pulmonary arteries and causes dyspnoea, hypoxia, haemoptysis, chest pain. Fever and/or circulatory collapse can occur.

- Fat in the systemic arteries causes: confusion, coma, coagulopathy with skin petechiae, fat globules in the urine.

The CXR

The changes are mainly those of haemorrhagic pulmonary oedema, either an alveolar or interstitial pattern, as a result of a chemical pneumonitis. The alveolar densities are commonly peripheral and basal. The shadows usually appear 24–72 hours after the trauma and clear within 7–28 days.

REFERENCES

1. Robinson GV. Pulmonary embolism in hospital practice. BMJ 2006; 332: 156–160.

2. British Thoracic Society guidelines for the management of suspected acute pulmonary embolism. Thorax 2003; 58: 470–483.

3. Miniati M, Prediletto R, Formichi B et al. Accuracy of clinical assessment in the diagnosis of pulmonary embolism. Am J Respir Crit Care Med 1999; 159: 864–871.

4. Quiroz R, Schoepf UJ. CT pulmonary angiography for acute pulmonary embolism: cost-effectiveness analysis and review of the literature. Semin Roentgenol 2005; 40: 20–24.

5. Stein PD, Fowler SE, Goodman LR et al. Multidetector computed tomography for acute pulmonary embolism. New Engl J Med 2006; 354: 2317–2327.

6. Rose P. Very high D-dimers—what do they mean? Thrombus 2005; 9: 2.

7. Wells PS, Anderson DR, Bormanis J et al. Value of assessment of pretest probability of deep vein thrombosis in clinical management. Lancet 1997; 350: 1795–1798.

8. Tick LW, Ton E, van Voorthurzen T et al. Practical diagnostic management of patients with clinically suspected deep vein thrombosis by clinical probability test, compression ultrasonography, and D-dimer test. Am J Med 2002; 113: 630–635.

9. Daftary A, Gregory M, Daftary A et al. Chest radiograph as a triage tool in the imaging-based diagnosis of pulmonary embolism. AJR 2005; 185: 132–134.

10. Becket P, Biswas S. Clinicians' use of the VQ scan for diagnosis of pulmonary embolism. Thrombus 2005; 9: 8–9.

11. Miniati M, Pistolesi M, Marini C et al. Value of perfusion lung scan in the diagnosis of pulmonary embolism: results of the prospective investigative study of acute pulmonary embolism diagnosis (PISA-PED). Am J Respir Crit Care Med 1996; 154: 1387–1393.

12. Worsley DF, Alavi A, Aronchick JM et al. Chest radiographic findings in patients with acute pulmonary embolism: observations from the PIOPED study. Radiology 1993; 189: 133–136.

13. Feldman F, Ellis K, Green WM. The fat embolism syndrome. Radiology 1975; 114: 535–542.

24 SUSPECTED AORTIC DISSECTION

> **Aortic dissection:**
>
> - Occasionally the term dissecting aneurysm is used. This is inaccurate terminology. It is more correct to refer to the lesion as a dissecting haematoma.
>
> - Blood enters the aortic wall through a tear and dissects between the inner and middle layers (intima and media). The haematoma then tracks for a variable distance along the length of the aorta. Side branches supplying the major organs can be occluded.
>
> - Most dissections occur in the sixth or seventh decade.
>
> - 70–90% of patients are hypertensive or have a history of hypertension.
>
> - Mortality is high. Untreated, approximately 75% of patients with a dissection involving the ascending aorta will die within two weeks[1].
>
> - Aortic dissection is two to three times more common than a rupture of a thoracic or abdominal aortic aneurysm.

TWO DIAGNOSTIC PRIORITIES

1. To determine whether a patient with chest pain has an aortic dissection. The physician's working diagnosis is established primarily by the clinical features. Then, the CXR findings will often alter the physician's pre-test probability estimate (see Chapter 17, p. 249) of a dissection being present.

2. If the post-test probability of a dissection remains high or medium then it is essential that the precise type of dissection (if confirmed) is demonstrated, as this will determine further management. The type of dissection is established by CT, MRI or transoesophageal echocardiography.

CLASSIFICATIONS

Aortic dissections are classified anatomically. There are two main classifications: the DeBakey classification and the Stanford classification. We describe the Stanford classification as it is currently the one that is most commonly used.

DISSECTION: TYPES AND CLINICAL MANAGEMENT[1-10]

The Stanford Classification distinguishes between:

Type A Dissection: Any dissection involving the ascending aorta. These require surgical management.

Type B Dissection: Dissection limited to the aorta distal to the left subclavian artery. The ascending aorta is spared. These require medical management with antihypertensive medication.

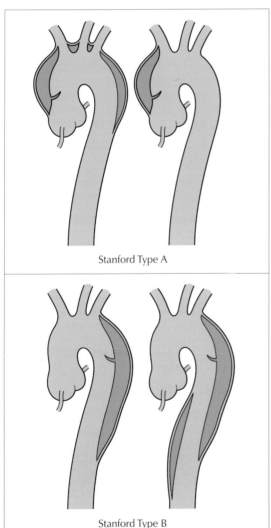

Stanford Type A

Stanford Type B

Figure 24.1 *Classification. Aortic dissection. Stanford Type A involves the ascending aorta. Stanford Type B spares the ascending aorta. Note: interventional radiology stenting has recently been introduced as an alternative strategy to conservative medical management.*

HOW CAN THE CXR HELP?

The CXR appearance can assist in influencing the physician's initial estimate of the likelihood of a dissection being present—i.e. it impacts on the post-test probability of aortic dissection (see Chapter 17, p. 249).

■ Approximately 12% of patients with an acute dissection will have a normal CXR[1].

■ In 88% of patients with an acute dissection[1], one or more of the following findings will be present: widened mediastinum; abnormal aortic knuckle; left pleural effusion; pericardial effusion.

Widened mediastinum[1,11–14]

■ Most importantly—whenever possible, compare present and previous CXRs. This is the most reliable way of confirming whether mediastinal widening is due to a dissection. Comparison may show that mediastinal widening is longstanding and likely to be due to simple age related unfolding of the aorta, or that mediastinal widening is new.

■ Widening of the mediastinum in a patient with a suspected aortic dissection has a high sensitivity (81–90%) but a low specificity.

■ The mediastinum enlarges to the right with a dissection of the ascending aorta and to the left with a dissection of the descending aorta.

■ The 8-cm rule[2]. This is a rough rule of thumb: on a portable AP CXR a widened mediastinum is one that exceeds a diameter of 8 cm at the level of the aortic arch.

■ The overall level of clinical suspicion is decisive. With a low level of clinical suspicion, comparison with previous CXRs will often provide sufficient reassurance that a dissection has not occurred. On the other hand, a high pre-test probability for dissection together with a widened mediastinum on the CXR will lead to a definitive cross-sectional investigation (as illustrated in Table 17.1).

Abnormal aortic knuckle…and calcification[11]

■ The aortic knuckle may be widened or show a bumpy or humped appearance.

■ **A useful rule of thumb**: If calcification within the aortic wall is displaced from the outer aortic margin by 1.0 cm or more…then the probability of a dissection is high. This rule becomes most useful if a lateral CXR shows absence of calcification in the anterior or posterior aortic wall (Fig. 24.2).

■ This calcium sign requires caution. Apparent displacement of intimal calcification from the outer margin of the ascending aortic wall on the frontal CXR can be misleading and spurious. The calcification may be in the descending aorta. In other words, calcification that appears displaced inwards from the lateral wall of the ascending aorta may actually be undisplaced and positioned on the posterior wall of a normal descending aorta (as illustrated in Fig. 24.3).

Left pleural effusion

An effusion is present in approximately 16% of patients with a dissection.

Pericardial effusion

A large globular shaped cardiac silhouette may be apparent. This is very bad news. It suggests that the dissection extends to the aortic root. These patients often die from a cardiac tamponade or coronary ischaemia.

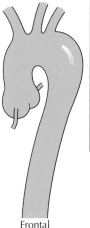
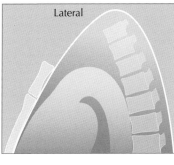

Frontal

Figure 24.2 *Intimal calcification. On the frontal projection the calcification appears to lie more than 1.0 cm from the outer margin of the aorta. The lateral projection does not show any intimal calcification either anteriorly or posteriorly. This appearance provides strong support for the diagnosis of dissection.*

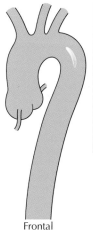
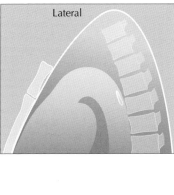

Frontal

Figure 24.3 *Intimal calcification. On the frontal projection the calcification appears to lie more than 1.0 cm from the outer margin of the aorta. However, the lateral projection shows that the calcification is situated posteriorly. This is not evidence of a dissection…the aortic arch is unfolded and the posterior calcification is (misleadingly) projected over the medial wall on the frontal view.*

NO CHEST PAIN—BUT THE CXR APPEARANCE IS WORRYING

It is common for CXRs in middle-aged or elderly people to show a widened mediastinum, because the aortic arch gradually unfolds as we get older. But is the widening in a particular patient due to simple aortic unfolding, to a Stanford Type A dissection…or to an aneurysm of the ascending aorta?

■ Usually, the widening will be due to age related aortic unfolding.

■ Analysis of the CXR appearance will often provide the necessary reassurance that it is unfolding only (Figs 24.4 and 24.5). If there is any persisting doubt then a lateral CXR will provide additional support.

■ Comparison with a previous CXR is mandatory if one is available.

■ A combination of the clinical history, clinical examination, and CXR analysis will almost always remove any worries.

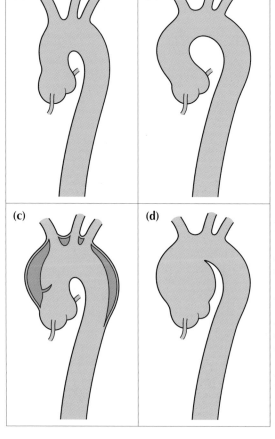

Figure 24.4 *A widened mediastinum at the level of the aortic arch may be vascular and due to either age related unfolding of the aorta (b), aortic dissection (c) or an aneurysm (d). A normal aorta—no unfolding—is shown in (a). Age related unfolding of the ascending and descending aorta from early middle age is a common CXR finding. Any unfolding will appear exaggerated, and often worrying, on an AP CXR because of the magnification effect.*

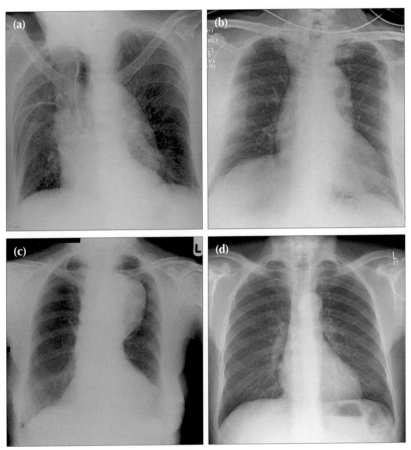

Figure 24.5 *Four patients, all middle-aged or elderly. Patient (a): age related aortic unfolding. Patient (b): the aortic shadow at the level of the ascending aorta and aortic arch is prominent in this patient who presented with tearing chest pain. Stanford Type A dissection. Patient (c): the aortic arch and the proximal descending aorta are very prominent and due to aneurysmal dilatation. Patient (d): a normal aortic outline—no unfolding. The amount of age related unfolding of the thoracic aorta shows a wide variation in middle-aged or elderly individuals—compare the CXRs of patient (a) and patient (d). Furthermore, in an elderly or frail patient, rotation (see patient a) is often present and will exaggerate any unfolding.*

CLINICAL SYNOPSIS: ACUTE CHEST PAIN[10,15]

■ In clinical practice the middle-aged or elderly patient presenting with acute chest pain is not only an emergency but frequently a diagnostic dilemma— is it a myocardial infarct or is it a dissection?

■ Wise advice has been provided by Schubert[10]:

> *"…acute myocardial infarction (AMI) and aortic dissection can present identically. For patients with chest pain, the most important first step in distinguishing AMI from aortic dissection is to consider both as diagnostic possibilities. After that, the strongest and most reliable indicators for aortic dissection are found in the history. Results of ECG and CXR investigations do not reliably discriminate between aortic dissection and AMI. A careful history focused on the quality of a patient's pain is the most useful tactic for distinguishing a dissection from AMI."*

■ Quality of pain:

  ❏ AMI. Gradual onset; heavy and crushing.

  ❏ Aortic dissection. Sudden onset; tearing and crushing.

GUIDELINES IN RELATION TO USEFULNESS OF THE CXR

■ The CXR will exclude some of the other causes of chest pain (e.g. pneumothorax, mediastinal emphysema).

■ A completely normal CXR makes the diagnosis of a dissection unlikely in a patient in whom clinical suspicion is low.

■ Any abnormal CXR feature in a patient with hypertension and an abrupt onset of chest or back pain warrants further definitive imaging (CT, MRI or transoesophageal echocardiography).

■ A reasonable clinical suspicion of dissection, even if the CXR is normal, should not delay further definitive imaging.

REFERENCES

1. Chen K, Varon J, Wenker OC et al. Acute thoracic aortic dissection: the basics. J Emerg Med 1997; 15: 859–867.

2. Nienaber CA, Eagle KA. Aortic dissection: new frontiers in diagnosis and management. Part 1: From etiology to diagnostic strategies. Circulation 2003; 108: 628–635.

3. Wiesenfarth J. Aortic dissection (monograph-on-line). Stanford, CA: Stanford University School of Medicine, 2001. www.emedicine.com/emerg

4. Hagan PG, Nienaber CA, Isselbacher EM et al. The International Registry of Acute Aortic Dissection (IRAD): new insights into an old disease. JAMA 2000; 283: 897–903.

5. Khan IA, Nair CK. Clinical, diagnostic, and management perspectives of aortic dissection. Chest 2002; 122: 311–328.

6. Erbel R, Zamorano J. The aorta. Aortic aneurysm, trauma, and dissection. Crit Care Clin 1996; 12: 733–766.

7. Rogers FB, Osler TM, Shackford SR et al. Aortic dissection after trauma: case report and review of the literature. J Trauma 1996; 41: 906–908.

8. Pretre R, Von Segesser LK. Aortic dissection. Lancet 1997; 349: 1461–1464.

9. Stultz DB, Gupta SC. Rapid assessment and treatment of aortic dissection. Emerg Med 2004; 36: 18–43.

10. Schubert H. Thoracic aortic dissection: distinguishing it from acute myocardial infarction. Can Fam Physician 2003; 49: 583–585.

11. Hansell DM, Armstrong P, Lynch DA, McAdams HP. Imaging of Diseases of the Chest. 4th ed. St Louis, MO: Mosby, 2005.

12. Cigarroa JE, Isselbacher EM, DeSanctis RW et al. Diagnostic imaging in the evaluation of suspected aortic dissection. Old standards and new directions. N Engl J Med 1993; 328: 35–43.

13. Jagannath AS, Sos TA, Lockhart SH et al. Aortic dissection: a statistical analysis of the usefulness of plain chest radiographic findings. AJR 1986; 147: 1123–1126.

14. Fisher ER, Stern EJ, Godwin JD. Acute aortic dissection: typical and atypical imaging features. Radiographics 1994; 14: 1263–1271.

15. Kelly BS. Evaluation of the elderly patient with acute chest pain. Clin Geriatr Med 2007; 23: 327–349.

25 SUSPECTED METASTATIC DISEASE

Metastasis...synonyms: secondary deposit; deposit

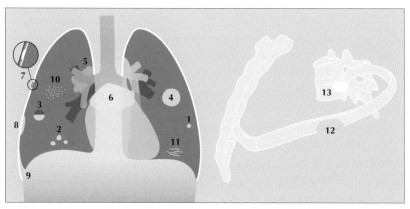

Figure 25.1 *Thoracic metastases: (1) and (2) solitary or multiple; (3) cavitating; (4) cannonball; (5) hilar lymphadenopathy; (6) subcarinal/mediastinal lymphadenopathy; (7) pleural; (8) subpleural; (9) pleural effusion secondary to pleural deposit(s); (10) miliary (resembling millet seeds); (11) lymphangitis carcinomatosa; (12) lytic; (13) sclerotic.*

This chapter concentrates on metastases arising from extrathoracic primary neoplasms (i.e. excluding bronchial carcinoma). Many patients with an extrathoracic primary tumour will undergo CXR examination in order to check for metastases. When this CXR examination is requested it is important to know: (a) which tumours are most likely to produce lung, hilar, mediastinal, lymphangitic, pleural or bone deposits; and (b) the various radiographic features of metastatic disease (Fig. 25.1).

SPREADING AND SEEDING

The precise mechanisms determining whether malignant cells enter the lymphatic or venous circulation and subsequently spread to and implant in the thorax are imperfectly understood[1-6]. Tumour affinity for a particular thoracic tissue (lung, pleura, bone, bronchial endothelium) varies between malignancies. How some malignancies reach and settle in the thorax is shown in Table 25.1. The various pathways give an inkling as to why some primary tumours metastasise to the thorax more commonly than do others.

Table 25.1 Tumour routes to the thorax[1,7–9].

Channel	Malignancy	Pathway
Lymphatic	Breast / stomach / pancreas / larynx/cervix	Draining lymphatics → lymph nodes → thoracic duct → vena cava → right atrium → pulmonary arteries → lungs
Venous (1)	Renal / thyroid / testicular / sarcomas / melanoma / head and neck	Draining veins → vena cava → right atrium → pulmonary arteries → lungs
Venous (2)	Colon / stomach / pancreas	Draining veins → portal vein → liver → hepatic veins → lungs
Venous (3)	Colon / stomach / pancreas	Batson's venous plexus (see below) → bones[7,8]
Dual venous (4)	Renal	(i) Renal vein → inferior vena cava → right atrium → pulmonary arteries → lungs (ii) Renal vein → Batson's venous plexus → bones[7,8]
Multiple	Breast[1,6,9]	▪ Draining veins → vena cava → right atrium → pulmonary arteries → lungs ▪ Lymphatics → thoracic duct → vena cava → right atrium → pulmonary arteries → lungs ▪ Intercostal veins and paravertebral venous plexus → vertebrae → other bones ▪ Direct invasion → chest wall ▪ Direct invasion → pleura

---

Batson's venous plexus

In 1940 Oscar V. Batson described the vertebral venous system[7,8]. The term Batson's venous plexus refers to the valveless plexiform vertebral veins that communicate freely with the superior and inferior vena cavae. This venous system, or plexus, is an important pathway for tumour spread to bone, and also to the brain and lungs.

SEARCHING FOR LUNG METASTASES[1,2,9,10]

GENERAL

■ **The basic rule:** Whenever possible compare the present CXR with any available previous CXR.

■ Deposits are commonly peripheral or subpleural. The lung bases are more frequently affected than are the upper lobes. The majority of deposits are round with fairly well-defined margins.

■ Lung deposits immediately adjacent to the pleura (ie subpleural) may not be round. They can appear plaque-like or stellate.

THE PRIMARY TUMOUR AND THE CXR

■ Malignancies that commonly metastasise to the lungs: sarcomas, renal cell carcinoma, choriocarcinoma, testicular cancer, some functioning thyroid carcinomas.

■ Lung metastases occur relatively infrequently with breast or colon cancer.

■ Lung metastases are often present at the time of the initial diagnosis of renal cell carcinoma, choriocarcinoma, Ewing's sarcoma, osteogenic sarcoma or Wilms' tumour.

■ Other CXR features are listed in Table 25.2.

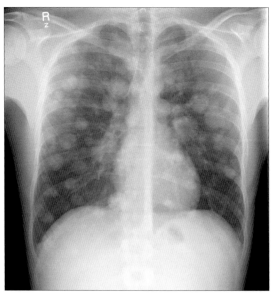

Figure 25.2 *Typical appearance and individual features of lung metastases: multiple lesions, variable size, well-defined margins. Testicular tumour.*

Table 25.2 Lung metastases[1–3,9–12].

CXR finding	Most common tumours	Other tumours
More than one deposit and: ❑ different sizes ❑ solid appearance	Kidney, head/neck, uterus, prostate, breast, colon	Choriocarcinoma, testicle, melanoma, thyroid, osteogenic sarcoma, Ewing's sarcoma, Wilms' tumour, rhabdomyosarcoma
Solitary lesion	Colon	Melanoma, sarcoma, breast, kidney, bladder, testicle
Cannonball (i.e. very large)	Colon, rectum, kidney, melanoma, sarcomas	
Cavitation[9]	Cervix in females, head and neck tumours in males, sarcomas	Colon
Miliary pattern	Thyroid, kidney	Osteogenic sarcoma, melanoma, choriocarcinoma
Calcified[9,13]	Osteogenic sarcomas	Chondrosarcoma, thyroid, colon, pancreas
Margins very ill-defined	Choriocarcinoma… occasionally[2]	

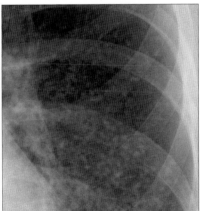

Figure 25.3 *Miliary metastases… multiple tiny secondary deposits. Thyroid carcinoma.*

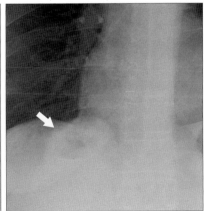

Figure 25.4 *Cavitating metastasis (arrow). Tough to detect because it lies below the horizon of the dome of the diaphragm. Remember…you only see what you look for.*

SEARCHING FOR HILAR AND MEDIASTINAL METASTASES

■ The appearances of hilar lymph node enlargement are described on pp. 76–77.

■ Extrathoracic tumours infrequently metastasise to mediastinal lymph nodes. If mediastinal lymphadenopathy is evident consider these tumours:

❑ bronchial carcinoma

❑ lymphoma

❑ kidney, testicle, head and neck

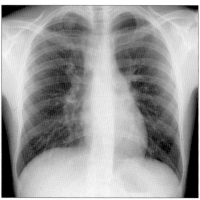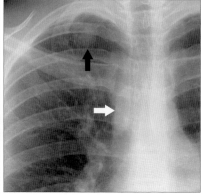

Figure 25.5 *Patient with weight loss. Paratracheal lymphadenopathy (white arrow). When enlarged mediastinal nodes are due to malignancy it is rare for the primary tumour to be extrathoracic. The most common primary tumour will be a bronchial carcinoma (black arrow).*

LYMPHANGITIS CARCINOMATOSA[1,2]

Tumour involvement of the lymphatics of the lung results from haematogenous spread. The CXR appearance is that of interstitial disease — i.e. reticular or reticulo-nodular shadowing. Initially, this may be indistinguishable from other interstitial processes such as pulmonary oedema. The most common primary is breast carcinoma.

■ Lymphangitic spread is usually bilateral, infrequently unilateral. Sometimes it is associated with a pleural effusion and/or enlarged hilar nodes.

■ Very occasionally a patient with a known primary carcinoma may develop dyspnoea due to lymphangitic deposits and the CXR may appear clear[1].

■ **Useful rule of thumb**: If an interstitial pattern is due to lymphangitis carcinomatosa then the patient will be short of breath.

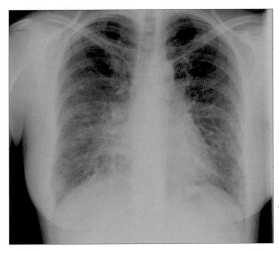

Figure 25.6 *Lymphangitis carcinomatosa. The reticular shadowing at the right base is fairly typical of the pattern of tumour involving the lymphatics. The primary tumour was a breast carcinoma.*

SEARCHING FOR PLEURAL METASTASES[14]

Some cancers have a predilection for the pleura.

- The CXR may show:
    - a pleural effusion, small or large
    - an isolated pleural mass
- The most common primary tumours:
    - any adenocarcinoma, including bronchus
    - breast carcinoma

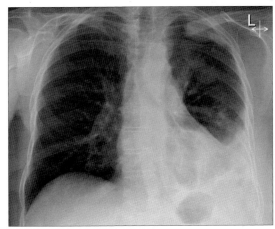

Figure 25.7 *Left pleural effusion. An effusion is the most common CXR finding in a patient who has metastatic disease involving the pleura. This patient had a previous carcinoma of the breast and a right mastectomy.*

SEARCHING FOR BONE METASTASES[3,8,9,15]

■ Some primary tumours have a propensity for metastasising to bone (Table 25.3). Other tumours rarely do so.

■ Bone metastases occur as a result of either: (a) tumour cells entering the venous system and being deposited in bone via arteries and capillaries; (b) retrograde venous flow (e.g. prostatic carcinoma); (c) dissemination via Batson's venous plexus; or (d) direct invasion of adjacent bone.

■ Bone deposits are usually either solely lytic (i.e. lucent) or solely sclerotic (i.e. dense)—see Table 25.3. Very occasionally a primary carcinoma may produce both lytic and sclerotic deposits in an individual patient.

■ A helpful trick. Any patient with bone or chest wall pain. When checking the ribs:

  ❑ Rotate the image so that the long axis of the CXR is parallel to the floor—assess the ribs again (Fig. 25.8).

  ❑ Then rotate the CXR through another 90° so that the CXR is upside down—assess the posterior aspects of the ribs again.

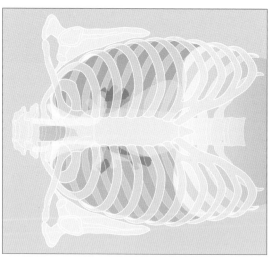

Figure 25.8 *Checking the ribs for metastases. Examining the ribs with the CXR aligned horizontally. This trick makes the ribs stand out. Note the destructive lesion in the posterior aspect of the left fifth rib. If you don't think that the lesion is shown particularly clearly— turn this page through 90° so that you are looking at the bones with the CXR upside down. Now what do you think?*

Table 25.3 Bone metastases[15].

Appearance	Most common primary	Less common primary
Sclerotic	■ Males—prostate ■ Females—breast	Pancreas, bladder, carcinoid, mucinous adenocarcinomas of the gastrointestinal tract Occasionally lymphoma
Lytic	■ Males—bronchus, kidney, thyroid ■ Females—breast, kidney, thyroid	Prostate, melanoma, neuroblastoma
Lytic…sometimes causing expansion of the affected bone	Renal, thyroid	

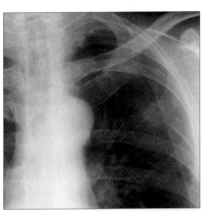

Figure 25.9 A destructive (lytic) metastasis in the posterior aspect of the left fifth rib.

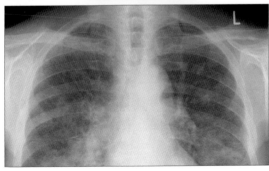

Figure 25.10 Sclerotic right sixth rib posteriorly. Metastasis from a prostatic carcinoma. Several other ribs showed a similar appearance.

AN UNEXPECTED RIB FRACTURE — IS IT PATHOLOGICAL?[15-17]

Most pathological fractures are due to a metastasis or to myeloma. Whenever a clinically unsuspected rib fracture is detected on a CXR:

1. Always link the fracture to the patient's present or past clinical history.

2. Look for other rib lesions.

3. Analyse the appearance carefully:

   ❏ Bone sclerosis. Two possibilities: a metastasis or callus around a healing simple fracture.

   ❏ Bone lucency — i.e. destruction. Consider metastasis or myeloma. Very rarely — lymphoma.

   ❏ Bone expansion. More commonly myeloma than a metastasis.

   ❏ Adjacent soft tissue extrapleural mass. More common with myeloma.

4. If carcinoma is considered to be a possibility then obtain an isotope bone scan. If the rib lesion is a secondary deposit then there will be multiple other deposits shown elsewhere in the skeleton.

5. If myeloma is likely then a myeloma haematological screen is necessary. If positive this should be followed by a radiographic skeletal survey. An isotope bone scan is often normal in myeloma because there is minimal or no bone turnover at the site of the lesion and consequently no increase in tracer uptake.

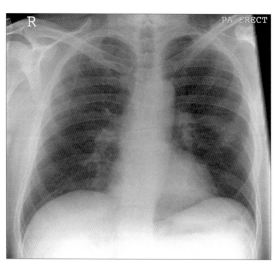

Figure 25.11 *Destructive lesion in the posterior aspect of the left seventh rib. The differential diagnosis is metastasis or myeloma. The prominent accompanying soft tissue shadow does favour myeloma. Myeloma was the diagnosis in this patient.*

REFERENCES

1. Coppage L, Shaw C, Curtis AM. Metastatic disease to the chest in patients with extrathoracic malignancy. J Thorac Imaging 1987; 2: 24–37.

2. Libshitz HI, North LB. Pulmonary metastases. Radiol Clin North Am 1982; 20: 437–451.

3. Collins J, Stern EJ. Chest Radiology: The Essentials. Philadelphia, PA: Lippincott Williams and Wilkins, 1999.

4. Janower ML, Blennerhassett JB. Lymphangitic spread of metastatic cancer to the lung. A radiologic–pathologic classification. Radiology 1971; 101: 267–273.

5. McCloud TC, Kalisher L, Stark P et al. Intrathoracic lymph node metastases from extrathoracic neoplasms. AJR 1978; 131: 403–407.

6. Viadana E, Bross ID, Pickren JW. Cascade spread of blood borne metastases in solid and non-solid cancers in humans. In; Weiss L, Gilbert HA (eds): Pulmonary Metastases. Boston MA: GK Hall, 1978: 143–167.

7. Batson OV. Function of vertebral veins and their role in spread of metastases. Ann Surg 1940; 112: 138–149.

8. Batson OV. The vertebral vein system. AJR 1957; 78: 195–212.

9. Seo JB, Im JG, Goo JM et al. Atypical pulmonary metastases: spectrum of radiologic findings. Radiographics 2001; 21: 403–417.

10. Crow J, Slavin G, Kreel L. Pulmonary metastasis: A pathologic and radiologic study. Cancer 1981; 47: 2595–2602.

11. Latour A, Shulman HS. Thoracic manifestations of renal cell carcinoma. Radiology 1976; 121: 43–48.

12. Libshitz HI, Baber CE, Hammond CB. The pulmonary metastases of choriocarcinoma. Obstet Gynecol 1977; 49: 412–416.

13. Maile CW, Rodan BA, Godwin JD et al. Calcification in pulmonary metastases. Br J Radiol 1982; 55: 108–113.

14. Raju RN, Kardinal CG. Pleural effusion in breast carcinoma: analysis of 122 cases. Cancer 1981; 48: 2524–2527.

15. Pagani JJ, Libshitz HI. Imaging bone metastases. Radiol Clin North Am 1982; 20: 545–560.

16. Grover SB, Dhar A. Imaging spectrum in sclerotic myelomas: an experience of three cases. Eur Radiol 2000; 10: 1828–1831.

17. Clayer MT. Lytic bone lesions in an Australian population: the results of 100 consecutive biopsies. ANZ J Surj 2006; 76: 732–735.

26 CHRONIC COUGH: WHAT TO LOOK FOR

Chronic cough:	Arbitrarily defined as a persistent cough lasting for more than eight weeks[1-3].

There are numerous causes for a chronic cough (Table 26.1). In adults the common causes can be identified[4]: cigarette smoking; medication with an angiotensin-converting enzyme (ACE) inhibitor; upper airway cough syndrome (UACS)…sometimes referred to as post-nasal drip syndrome (PNDS); asthma; gastro-oesophageal reflux disease (GORD); and non-asthmatic eosinophilic bronchitis (NAEB)[4].

Table 26.1 Causes of a chronic cough.

Pulmonary	■ Asthma
	■ NAEB*
	■ Infection—including tuberculosis
	■ Chronic bronchitis
	■ Post-viral cough[1]
	■ Pulmonary oedema secondary to left ventricular failure
	■ Bronchial carcinoma
	■ Bronchiectasis
	■ Interstitial lung disease
	■ Sarcoidosis
	■ Bacterial suppurative disease of the airways[5]
Extra-pulmonary	■ UACS; i.e. PNDS
	■ GORD
	■ Tracheal compression (usually a goitre)
	■ Subphrenic abscess
Drugs	■ Cigarette smoking
	■ ACE inhibitors[6]
Idiopathic[2,7]	■ Unexplained…a diagnosis by exclusion

*NAEB: Patients with a chronic cough, sputum eosinophilia, normal spirometry and normal peak expiratory flow variability. NAEB is responsive to inhaled corticosteroids[2].

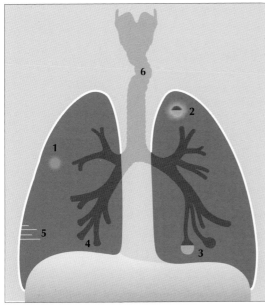

Figure 26.1 *Some causes for a chronic cough.*
1 = Bronchial carcinoma;
2 = Tuberculosis;
3 = Bronchiectasis—cystic changes;
4 = Bronchiectasis—tubular changes;
5 = Septal lines in pulmonary oedema;
6 = Tracheal compression by a goitre.

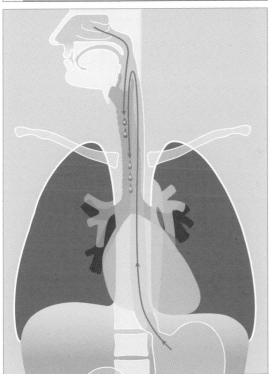

Figure 26.2 *Two common causes for a chronic cough.*
(a) UACS (synonym: PNDS).
(b) GORD.

INVESTIGATING A CHRONIC COUGH

A clinical approach...

A patient presents with a chronic cough and:

■ is a non-smoker

■ is not being treated with an ACE inhibitor

■ has no evidence of any other disorder

■ **has a normal CXR**

Then...

> "...an approach focused on detecting the presence of UACS, asthma, NAEB, or GORD, alone, or in combination, is likely to have a far higher yield than routinely searching for relatively uncommon or obscure diagnoses"[4].

CHRONIC COUGH — CXR FINDINGS

The CXR can be very helpful — whether abnormal or entirely normal.

CXR ABNORMAL — THE LIKELY DIAGNOSIS IS REVEALED

The CXR is obviously abnormal. As a consequence the physician's confidence as to the probable diagnosis will be high (Table 26.2).

Table 26.2 Abnormal CXR — likely diagnoses.

Appearance	Default diagnosis
Consolidation	■ Pneumonia — community acquired
	■ Tuberculosis or other chronic infection (Fig. 26.3)
Lobar collapse	■ Tumour (adults)
	■ Asthma (Fig. 26.4)
	■ Inhaled foreign body (children)
Ring shadows or tubular shadows	Bronchiectasis (Fig. 26.5)
Mass lesion	Tumour (Fig. 26.6)

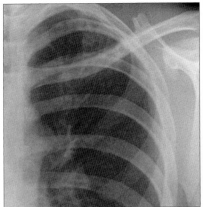

Figure 26.3 *Chronic cough. Ill-defined shadowing at the left apex raises the probability of post-primary tuberculosis. Subsequently, tuberculosis confirmed.*

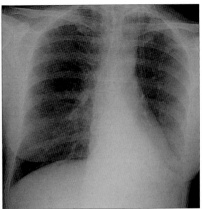

Figure 26.4 *Chronic cough. Asthmatic patient. A mucus plug has caused collapse of the left lower lobe. The collapse occurred some weeks previously. Note the collapsed lobe behind the heart gives the classic sail sign appearance.*

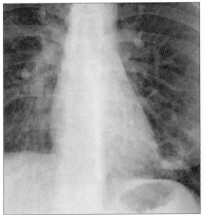

Figure 26.5 *Chronic cough. Tubular shadows in the right lower lobe; cystic changes in the left lower lobe. Bronchiectasis.*

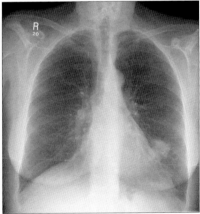

Figure 26.6 *Chronic cough. Lobulated mass in the left lower zone. Bronchial carcinoma.*

CXR ABNORMAL—A POSSIBLE DIAGNOSIS IS SUGGESTED

The CXR is abnormal but the abnormality is not in itself specific. Nevertheless, the CXR findings will suggest that a particular cause for the chronic cough now needs further consideration (Table 26.3).

Table 26.3 Abnormal CXR—possible diagnoses.

Appearance	Possible diagnosis
Large heart and interstitial or alveolar shadowing	Pulmonary oedema (Fig. 26.7)
Tracheal deviation in the neck	Goitre (Fig. 26.8)
Hiatus hernia	GORD (Fig. 26.9)

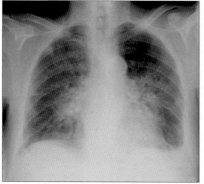

Figure 26.7 *Chronic cough. Small left pleural effusion and bilateral interstitial and alveolar shadows. Pulmonary oedema due to heart failure.*

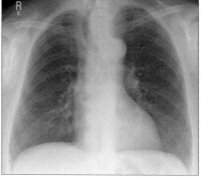

Figure 26.8 *Chronic cough. The trachea is compressed and deviated by a left-sided goitre.*

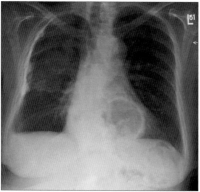

Figure 26.9 *Chronic cough. A hiatus hernia is shown as a gas shadow projected over the heart. This raises the possibility of GORD as the cause of the chronic cough. Note: in many instances, when a hiatus hernia is evident on a CXR it will have an air–fluid level within it.*

CXR NORMAL—REASSURANCE AND GUIDANCE

Reassurance: Middle-aged and elderly patients—both smokers and non-smokers—are concerned that the persistent cough signifies a cancer. Careful analysis of the CXR with particular attention to the hidden, tricky areas (Chapter 1, p. 13) enables the physician—with a high degree of confidence—to tell the patient that there is no evidence of a cancer.

Guidance: A normal CXR is an important negative finding. In an adult who is a non-smoker and is not being treated with an ACE inhibitor[6,7], a normal CXR allows the physician to concentrate further investigations on the remaining four most common possibilities (listed once more in Table 26.4).

Table 26.4 Reiteration: four common causes for a chronic cough[4].

- UACS (previously known as PNDS)
- Asthma
- GORD[9–11]
- NAEB[12]

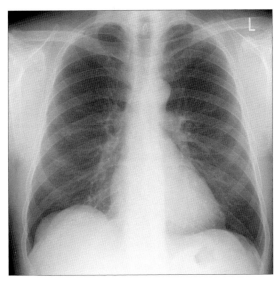

Figure 26.10 *Chronic cough. Normal CXR. This is a most useful finding. In an adult, it allows the physician to concentrate on a limited number of causes for a chronic cough (Table 26.4).*

AN INTERESTING CONDITION—BRONCHIECTASIS[13-15]

Aetiology / pathology

Bronchial obstruction causes severe inflammation which results in permanent damage to the bronchi and bronchioles.

Clinical features

Chronic cough. Usually with foul smelling sputum. Recurrent episodes of acute infection. Sometimes haemoptysis.

Recognised complications

Pneumonia, empyema, massive haemoptysis. Rarely: brain abscess, amyloid.

The CXR

■ Abnormal:

    ❑ tramline shadows—thickened bronchial walls

    ❑ ring shadows—dilated bronchi

    ❑ tubular shadows—fluid/pus filled bronchi

    ❑ focal scars

    ❑ volume loss—segmental or lobar

■ Normal...occasionally[13,14]

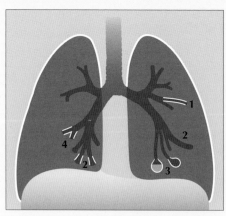

Figure 26.11 *In most cases of bronchiectasis the CXR will be abnormal. The abnormality may be subtle or gross, and may include any of the following: 1 & 4 = tramlines (thickened bronchial walls); 2 = tubular shadows (dilated & fluid filled bronchi); 3 = ring or cystic shadows (extreme bronchial dilatation). Slight or severe volume loss may also be present indicating fibrosis and shrinkage of the affected lung.*

REFERENCES

1. Morice AH. Epidemiology of cough. Pulm Pharmacol Ther 2002; 15: 253–259.

2. Haque RA, Usmani OS, Barns PJ. Chronic idiopathic cough: a discrete clinical entity? Chest 2005; 127: 1710–1713.

3. Pratter MR, Abouzgheib W. Make the cough go away. Chest 2006; 129: 1121–1122.

4. Pratter MR. Overview of common causes of chronic cough: ACCP evidence-based clinical practice guidelines. Chest 2006; 129: 59S–62S.

5. Schaefer OP, Irwin RS. Unsuspected bacterial suppurative disease of the airways presenting as chronic cough. Am J Med 2003; 114: 602–606.

6. Israili ZH, Hall WD. Cough and angioneurotic edema associated with angiotensin-converting enzyme inhibitor therapy. A review of the literature and pathophysiology. Ann Intern Med 1992; 117: 234–242.

7. Wood R. Bronchospasm and cough as adverse reactions to the ACE inhibitors captopril, enalapril and lisinopril. A controlled retrospective cohort study. Br J Clin Pharmacol 1995; 39: 265–270.

8. Pratter MR. Unexplained (idiopathic) cough: ACCP evidence-based clinical practice guidelines. Chest 2006; 129: 220S–221S.

9. Irwin RS. Chronic cough due to gastroesophageal reflux disease. ACCP evidence-based clinical practice guidelines. Chest 2006; 129: 80S–94S.

10. Sifrim D, Dupont L, Blondeau K et al. Weakly acidic reflux in patients with chronic unexplained cough during 24 hour pressure, pH, and impedance monitoring. Gut 2005; 54: 449–454.

11. Chang AB, Lasserson TJ, Kiljander TO et al. Systematic review and meta-analysis of randomised controlled trials of gastro-oesophageal reflux interventions for chronic cough associated with gastro-oesophageal reflux. BMJ 2006; 332: 11–17.

12. Brightling CE, Ward R, Goh KL et al. Eosinophilic bronchitis is an important cause of chronic cough. Am J Respir Crit Care Med 1999; 160: 406–410.

13. Gudbjerg CE. Roentgenologic diagnosis of bronchiectasis. An analysis of 112 cases. Acta Radiol 1955; 43: 210–226.

14. Fraser RG, Muller NL, Colman NC, Pare PD. Fraser and Pare's Diagnosis of Diseases of the Chest. 4th ed. Philadelphia, PA: WB Saunders, 1999.

15. Morrissey BM. Pathogenesis of bronchiectasis. Clin Chest Med 2007; 28: 289–296.

27 CHEST PAIN: WHAT TO LOOK FOR

CHEST PAIN — POSSIBLE CAUSES

There are numerous causes for a pain in the chest[1-10]. They can be sub-divided into non-cardiac causes (common and uncommon), and cardiac or aortic causes. These sub-divisions are shown in Tables 27.1–27.3.

Table 27.1 Non-cardiac chest pain: the most common causes.

Occurrence	Origin	Includes	Notes
Very common	Musculo-skeletal	■ Costochondritis (Tietze's syndrome)	Costochondritis is probably the most common cause of chest pain
		■ Degenerative change— shoulder or thoracic spine	
		■ Rib fracture	
		■ Muscle tear…often an intercostal muscle. Torn as a result of injury/ over-exertion/coughing.	
		■ Cervical spondylosis	
		■ Injury to the chest	
	Gastro-intestinal	■ Gastro-oesophageal reflux disease (GORD)	Any of these can mimic the pain of myocardial infarction
		■ Oesophageal spasm… or any excessive uncoordinated contraction of the oesophagus	
		■ Tear of oesophageal mucosa	
Common	Pulmonary	■ Acute bronchitis	
		■ Pneumonia	
		■ Pleural effusion	
		■ Pneumothorax	
		■ Asthma	
Common in healthy young people	Benign chest wall pain		Cause unknown

Table 27.2 Non-cardiac chest pain: the uncommon causes.

Occurrence	Origin	Includes	Notes
Uncommon	Viral infection of intercostal muscles	◼ Bornholm disease	Headache, fever, sore throat and systemic features will be present.
	Pulmonary embolism		
	Pneumo-mediastinum		
Very uncommon	Gastro-intestinal	◼ Gall bladder disease ◼ Peptic ulcer disease ◼ Pancreatitis	
	Miscellaneous	◼ Herpes zoster ◼ Psychological...this diagnosis is usually made by exclusion. It includes anxiety, panic attack	

Table 27.3 Cardiac or aortic chest pain.

Occurrence	Includes	Notes
Fairly common	◼ Angina pectoris ◼ Myocardial infarction	
Uncommon	◼ Aortic dissection ◼ Pericarditis ◼ Myocarditis ◼ Arrhythmia ◼ Mitral valve prolapse	
Often overlooked	◼ Cocaine usage	Causes cardiac blood vessels to constrict.

Stash

CHEST PAIN—THE ROLE OF THE CXR

The CXR is just one of several diagnostic tools. When a CXR is requested it will:

Sometimes...provide the precise diagnosis (Figs 27.1–27.3).

Occasionally...suggest a possible diagnosis (Fig. 27.4).

Often...exclude several causes for the pain.

CXR ABNORMAL—DIAGNOSIS REVEALED

- Pneumothorax.
- Pneumonia.
- Rib fracture.
- Perforated peptic ulcer.

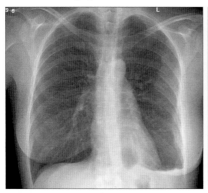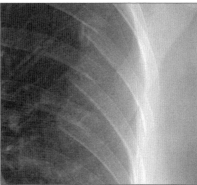

Figure 27.1   *Female, 35 years. Drunk and disorderly. Complaining of chest pain. Multiple posterior rib fractures. Note also the shallow left pneumothorax.*

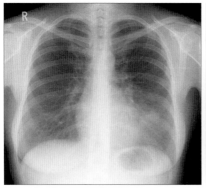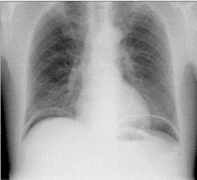

Figure 27.2   *Female, 38 years. Chest pain. Silhouette sign...pneumonia in the lingual segments of the left upper lobe.*

Figure 27.3   *Male, 54 years. Chest pain, but difficult to localise. Free air under the domes of the diaphragm. Perforated duodenal ulcer.*

CXR ABNORMAL—A POSSIBLE DIAGNOSIS IS SUGGESTED

■ Ischaemic heart disease. Left heart failure…subtle pulmonary oedema.

■ GORD…a fixed hiatus hernia.

■ Musculo-skeletal…clear evidence of degenerative change in the thoracic spine.

■ Acute asthma or ruptured oesophagus…mediastinal emphysema.

■ Smoking marijuana or cocaine…mediastinal emphysema.

■ Aortic dissection…a widened mediastinum (see Chapter 24).

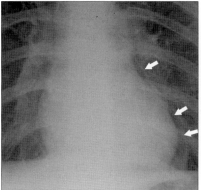 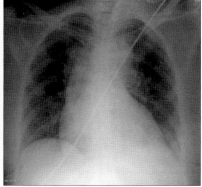

Figure 27.4 *Young male. Recent vomiting episode. Now complains of chest pain. Air is present in the mediastinum (arrows). Oesophageal rupture. Boerhaave's syndrome.*

Figure 27.5 *Male. Acute tearing chest pain. The mediastinum is widened at the level of the aortic arch. Aortic dissection (Stanford Type A).*

CXR NORMAL—DIAGNOSTIC SIGNIFICANCE

"A normal finding, when assessed quantitatively, can sometimes be extremely valuable in differential diagnosis…only when a normal test result occurs with equal or nearly equal frequency among all the diseases being considered will a negative finding contribute little or nothing to the diagnostic process."[11]

A normal CXR will exclude some very common causes of chest pain:

■ Pneumothorax.

■ Pneumonia.

■ Pleural effusion.

FACTS AND FIGURES

- Costochondritis (Tietze's syndrome):
    - ❏ Probably the most common cause of chest pain.
    - ❏ Invariably accompanied by tenderness at the site of pain.
- Pneumothorax and/or pneumomediastinum are recognised complications when smoking cocaine[12]; or marijuana. The mechanism appears to be use of the valsalva manoeuvre to obtain a high input of the drug into the alveoli. Reflex coughing may raise the intra-alveolar pressure even higher and cause alveolar rupture.
- 10–30% of patients with chest pain who undergo cardiac catheterisation are found to have normal coronary arteries[9].
- 40% of patients with non-cardiac chest pain have an abnormal degree of acid reflux[9].
- Cough-induced rib fractures. In patients with a chronic cough, 78% of fractures are in women. The lateral aspects of the middle ribs are most commonly affected and the sixth rib is particularly vulnerable[10].

AN INTERESTING CONDITION— DIFFUSE OESOPHAGEAL SPASM[7,9,13–15]

Aetiology/pathology

Excessive, uncoordinated, contractions of the smooth muscle of the oesophagus.

Clinical features

Chest pain is common.

The CXR

No abnormal findings.

A barium swallow examination will often show the characteristic features (Fig. 27.6).

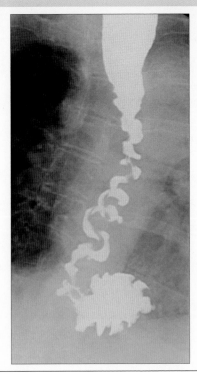

Figure 27.6 *Female. Age 65. Recurrent episodes of chest pain. Diffuse oesophageal spasm demonstrated on a barium swallow examination. This is the so-called nutcracker oesophagus.*

REFERENCES

1. Spalding L, Reay E, Kelly C. Cause and outcome of atypical chest pain in patients admitted to hospital. J R Soc Med 2003; 96: 122–125.

2. Just RJ, Castell DO. Chest pain of undetermined origin. Gastrointest Endosc Clin N Am 1994; 4: 731–746.

3. Crea F, Gaspardone A. New look to an old syndrome: Angina pectoris. Circulation 1997; 96: 3766–3773.

4. Minocha A. Noncardiac chest pain. Where does it start? Postgrad Med 1996; 100: 107–114.

5. Fam AG. Approach to musculoskeletal chest wall pain. Prim Care 1988; 15: 767–782.

6. Wise CM. Chest wall syndromes. Curr Opin Rheumatol 1994; 6: 197–202.

7. Hong SN, Rhee PL, Kim JH et al. Does this patient have oesophageal motility abnormality or pathological acid reflux? Dig Liver Dis 2005; 37: 475–484.

8. Chun AA, McGee SR. Bedside diagnosis of coronary artery disease: a systematic review. Am J Med 2004; 117: 334–343.

9. Paterson WG. Canadian Association of Gastroenterology Practice Guidelines: management of non-cardiac chest pain. Can J Gastroenterol 1998; 12: 401–407.

10. Hanak V, Hartman TE, Ryu JH. Cough induced rib fractures. Mayo Clin Proc 2005; 80: 879–882.

11. Gorry GA, Pauker SG, Schwartz WB. The diagnostic importance of the normal finding. N Engl J Med 1978; 298: 486–489.

12. Eurman DW, Potash HI, Eyler WR et al. Chest pain and dyspnea related to "crack" cocaine smoking: value of chest radiography. Radiology 1989; 172: 459–462.

13. Richter JE. Oesophageal motility disorders. Lancet 2001; 358: 823–828.

14. Adler DG, Romero Y. Primary esophageal motility disorders. Mayo Clin Proc 2001; 76: 195–200.

15. Tutuian R, Castell DO. Review article: oesophageal spasm—diagnosis and management. Aliment Pharmacol Ther 2006; 23: 1393–1402.

28 DYSPNOEA: WHAT TO LOOK FOR

Dyspnoea:	Difficult, laboured or uncomfortable breathing...the sense of not getting enough air. A symptom, not a sign.
Acute dyspnoea:	Dyspnoea arising over the preceding 24–48 hours[1].
Chronic dyspnoea:	Dyspnoea lasting more than one month[2].

Golden Rule 1:	The usefulness of the CXR findings — positive or negative — depends on the input derived from the clinical history and the physical examination.
Golden Rule 2:	Always tailor your inspection of the CXR to the individual patient...asking the CXR a specific question.
Golden Rule 3:	You only see what you look for — you only look for what you know.

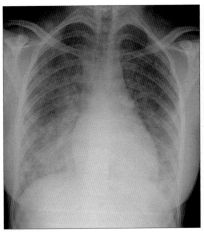

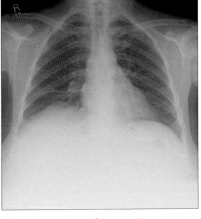

Figure 28.1 *Chronic dyspnoea. Extensive alveolar shadowing. Wide differential diagnosis. Apply Golden Rule 1—clinical details are crucial. Known renal failure with fluid retention. CXR conclusion—alveolar pulmonary oedema.*

Figure 28.2 *Acute dyspnoea. Lungs clear. Both domes of the diaphragm are high. Apply Golden Rule 1—clinical details are crucial. Abdomen is distended with a succussion splash when shaken. CXR conclusion—ascites displacing the diaphragm upwards.*

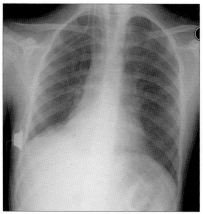

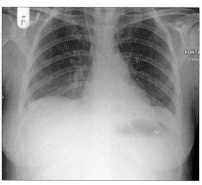

Figure 28.3 *Chronic dyspnoea. Shadowing in the right lower zone. Apply Golden Rule 3—you only look for what you know. CXR conclusion—collapse of the right lower lobe.*

Figure 28.4 *Acute dyspnoea. Left dome of the diaphragm appears to be high. Apply Golden Rule 3—you only look for what you know. Note the inferior displacement of the stomach air bubble. CXR conclusion—large subpulmonary effusion, not an elevated dome of the diaphragm (See p. 82).*

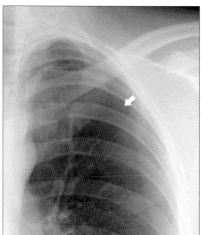

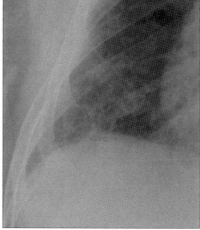

Figure 28.5 *Acute dyspnoea. No obvious CXR abnormality. Apply Golden Rule 1—clinical details are crucial. History of left sided pleuritic pain. Apply Golden Rule 2—ask the CXR a specific question…and Golden Rule 3—you only look for what you know. CXR conclusion—careful inspection of the left apex reveals a shallow pneumothorax. The arrow indicates the visceral pleura.*

Figure 28.6 *Chronic dyspnoea. Apply Golden Rule 3—you only look for what you know. Fine interstitial lines and nodules in the right lower zone. The same appearance was evident in the left lower zone. CXR conclusion—interstitial fibrosis. Subsequently confirmed.*

DYSPNOEA — POSSIBLE CAUSES

The clinical history and examination will predict the precise diagnosis in 70–80% of patients presenting with dyspnoea[1,3–6]. In many instances the CXR findings—normal or abnormal—will confirm or support the pre-test clinical diagnosis (see Chapter 17). On the other hand, the pre-test clinical diagnosis may be uncertain. The physician will know whether the dyspnoea is acute or chronic, and based on this and the clinical findings she needs to compose the question that she wishes the CXR to answer.

Examples:

■ Acute dyspnoea: is there a subtle pneumothorax? A hidden pneumonia? Left lower lobe collapse?

■ Chronic dyspnoea: are there any features to suggest bronchiectasis? Any evidence of elevated pulmonary venous pressure? Is there any subtle shadowing that would suggest interstitial fibrosis?

Table 28.1 Acute dyspnoea: pulmonary and cardiac causes.

Pulmonary disease	■ Acute exacerbation of chronic obstructive pulmonary disease (COPD)	■ Lung or lobar collapse
	■ Asthma exacerbation	■ Non-cardiac pulmonary oedema
	■ Bronchitis	■ Pleural effusion
	■ Epiglottitis	■ Pneumonia
	■ Foreign body aspiration… especially in children	■ Pneumothorax
		■ Pulmonary embolus
Cardiac disease	■ Acute myocardial infarct	■ Pulmonary oedema
	■ Cardiomyopathy	■ Septal defects
	■ Pericarditis	■ Unstable angina

Table 28.2 Acute dyspnoea: other causes.

■ Acute blood loss	■ Psychogenic:
■ Metabolic acidosis	❑ anxiety
■ Drugs:	❑ post-traumatic stress disorder
❑ cocaine or crack cocaine… may cause an acute coronary syndrome or a spontaneous pneumothorax or a pneumomediastinum	❑ panic attack

Table 28.3 Chronic dyspnoea: pulmonary and cardiac causes.

Pulmonary disease	■ COPD
	■ Bronchiectasis
	■ Parenchymal lung disease
	❏ interstitial lung disease (p. 40)
	❏ malignant infiltration
	■ Pleural effusion
	■ Pulmonary arterial hypertension
Cardiac disease	■ Coronary arterial disease
	■ Left heart failure
	■ Valvular disease
	■ Arrhythmia
	■ Cardiomyopathy

Table 28.4 Chronic dyspnoea: other causes.

Anaemia	
Neuromuscular...	Weakness of respiratory muscles
Thyroid disease...	Hyperthyroidism
Deconditioning...	Poor physical condition

CXR EVALUATION

It is important that the CXR is analysed in a systematic manner in order not to overlook subtle evidence of disease (see p. 10). If you think that the CXR is normal, then take a few more seconds to re-examine or exclude:

1. The tricky hidden areas (p. 13).

2. Lobar collapse (pp. 52–69).

3. Pneumothorax (pp. 94–99).

4. Borders of the heart and domes of the diaphragm (pp. 45–48).

DYSPNOEA—CXR IMPACT ON DIAGNOSIS

Sometimes the CXR will provide the precise diagnosis, sometimes it will suggest a possible diagnosis…and a normal CXR will often exclude several diagnoses.

CXR ABNORMAL—DIAGNOSIS CONFIRMED OR DISCLOSED

Examples:

■ pneumothorax

■ pneumonia

■ malignant disease causing lung or lobar collapse

■ pleural effusion

■ pulmonary oedema

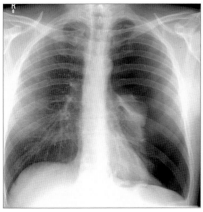

Figure 28.7   *Acute dyspnoea. Large left pneumothorax.*

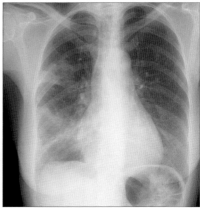

Figure 28.8   *Acute dyspnoea. Cough and fever. Scattered areas of consolidation in the right upper and lower lobes. Pneumonia.*

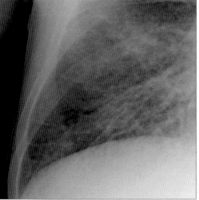

Figure 28.9   *Acute dyspnoea. Extensive interstitial shadows with septal lines at the right base. Pulmonary oedema.*

CXR ABNORMAL—A POSSIBLE DIAGNOSIS IS SUGGESTED

A CXR finding may not be definitive—in terms of diagnosis—but will assist by directing the physician towards a likely possibility.

Examples:

- Enlarged heart and vessel margins slightly blurred
    - left heart failure[6]

- Low—and flat—diaphragm
    - COPD
    - asthma

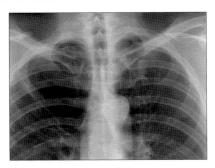

Figure 28.10 *Chronic dyspnoea. Large bulla in the right upper zone. COPD suggested as a cause for the dyspnoea.*

- Lung "shadows"
    - interstitial disease[7] (e.g. interstitial fibrosis)
    - bronchiectasis

- Enlarged hilum or hila
    - enlarged pulmonary arteries
        - pulmonary arterial hypertension
        - pulmonary thrombo-embolic disease

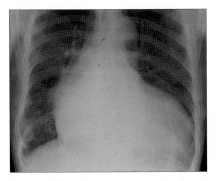

Figure 28.11 *Chronic dyspnoea. The heart is enlarged. Cardiac disease suggested as a cause for the dyspnoea.*

- Plethoric lungs
    - left-to-right cardiac shunt

- Fixed hiatus hernia
    - gastro-oesophageal reflux disease (GORD) and aspiration as a possible cause of chronic dyspnoea

- Abnormally high dome or domes of the diaphragm
    - phrenic nerve paralysis
    - displacement upwards by an intra-abdominal mass or ascites

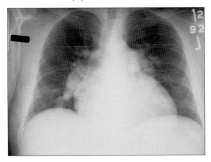

Figure 28.12 *Chronic dyspnoea. The proximal pulmonary arteries are large and the arteries in the mid zones of both lungs are disproportionately smaller. Pulmonary arterial hypertension suggested as the cause for the dyspnoea (see pp. 162–163).*

CXR NORMAL...BUT HELPFUL[8]

■ A negative (i.e. normal) CXR can be very valuable in excluding several causes for the dyspnoea.

　❑ A normal CXR excludes:

　　– pneumothorax

　　– pneumonia

　　– pleural effusion

　❑ A normal cardiothoracic ratio excludes acute left heart failure— unless the patient has suffered an acute myocardial infarct.

■ An important reminder. A normal CXR does not exclude:

　❑ Pulmonary thromboembolic disease...in many patients pulmonary embolism will be the default diagnosis and this must be excluded or confirmed by utilising other tests (pp. 291–292).

　❑ Asthma.

　❑ Acute bronchitis.

　❑ Acute infection superimposed on COPD.

　❑ Bronchiectasis...though most CXRs will be abnormal[9].

　❑ *Pneumocystis carinii* infection...early (p. 139).

　❑ Interstitial fibrosis...though most CXRs will be abnormal[10].

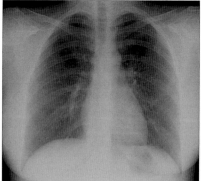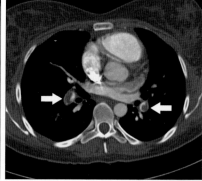

Figure 28.13 *Female. Age 24. Acute dyspnoea. Normal CXR. The CT pulmonary angiogram reveals large thrombi in the pulmonary arteries (arrows). Acute pulmonary embolism.*

FACTS AND FIGURES

■ Two thirds of patients presenting with dyspnoea have a cardiac or pulmonary cause.

■ One third of patients presenting with dyspnoea have more than one causative factor[5].

■ Acute myocardial infarction but no chest pain...dyspnoea is a common presenting symptom. Particularly in:

❑ women

❑ patients with diabetes mellitus

❑ patients age 70 and older

REFERENCES

1. Boyars MC, Karnath BM, Mercado AC. Acute dyspnea: a sign of underlying disease. Hosp Physician 2004; 7: 23–27.

2. American Thoracic Society. Dyspnea. Mechanisms, assessment, and management: a consensus statement. Am J Respir Crit Care Med 1999; 159: 321–340.

3. Mulrow CD, Lucey CR, Farnett LE. Discriminating causes of dyspnea through clinical examination. J Gen Intern Med 1993; 8: 383–392.

4. Schmitt BP, Kushner MS, Weiner SL. The diagnostic usefulness of the history of the patient with dyspnea. J Gen Intern Med 1986; 1: 386–393.

5. Michelson E, Hollrah S. Evaluation of the patient with shortness of breath: an evidence based approach. Emerg Med Clin North Am 1999; 17: 221–237.

6. Wang CS, Fitzgerald JM, Schulzer M et al. Does this dyspneic patient in the emergency department have congestive heart failure? JAMA 2005; 294: 1944–1956.

7. American Thoracic Society. Idiopathic pulmonary fibrosis: diagnosis and treatment. International consensus statement. American Thoracic Society (ATS) and the European Respiratory Society (ERS). Am J Respir Crit Care Med 2000; 161: 646–664.

8. Gorry GA, Pauker SG, Schwartz WB. The diagnostic importance of the normal finding. N Engl J Med 1978; 298: 486–489.

9. Gudbjerg CE. Roentgenologic diagnosis of bronchiectasis. An analysis of 112 cases. Acta Radiol 1955; 43: 210–226.

10. Johnston ID, Prescott RJ, Chalmers JC et al. British Thoracic Society study of cryptogenic fibrosing alveolitis: current presentation and initial management. Thorax 1997; 52: 38–44.

29 ASTHMATIC ATTACK: WHAT TO LOOK FOR

Acute asthma:	A disorder characterised by paroxysmal narrowing of the bronchi. The bronchoconstriction causes wheezing, shortness of breath and a tight feeling in the chest.

CXR FINDINGS IN ACUTE ASTHMA

In 95% of patients the CXR is normal. In a few patients the lungs demonstrate hyperinflation—i.e. generalised hyperlucency (increased blackening) with the domes of the diaphragm unusually low.

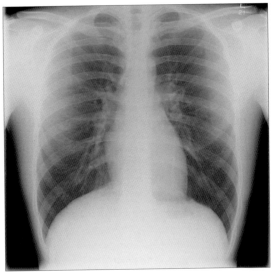

Figure 29.1 *Acute asthma. Normal CXR. This is the most common finding in a patient with an acute asthmatic episode.*

IS A CXR NECESSARY?[1–4]

- Very rarely. A CXR is not necessary in the vast majority of patients presenting with an acute episode.

- Caution…this is providing that the clinical diagnosis of asthma is unequivocal[5,6]. In small children an inhaled foreign body can cause wheezing.

WHEN IS A CXR USEFUL?

In four circumstances. When:

1. The diagnosis of asthma is equivocal.
   - ❏ A CXR may reveal another cause for the dyspnoea (e.g. foreign body inhalation, see p. 201).
2. Pleuritic pain occurs.
   - ❏ Pneumothorax and/or pneumomediastinum are recognised complications.
3. There is a pyrexia.
   - ❏ Pneumonia can induce or increase symptoms.
4. Unexpected and unexplained clinical deterioration develops.
   - ❏ Mucus plugging may cause a lobe to collapse.

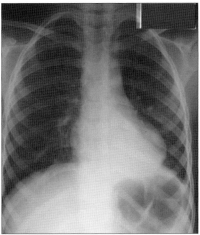

Figure 29.2 *Acute asthma. Unexplained clinical deterioration. Collapse of the left lower lobe due to a mucus plug in the bronchus.*

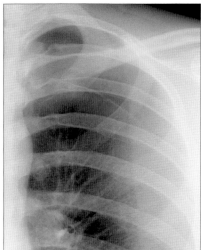

Figure 29.3 *Acute asthma. Pleuritic chest pain. Left pneumothorax.*

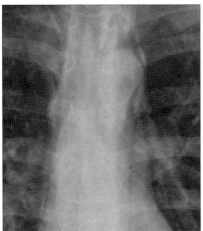

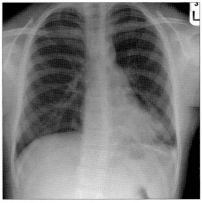

Figure 29.4 *Acute asthma. Pleuritic chest pain. Extensive mediastinal emphysema. The process causing the emphysema is explained on pp. 123–124.*

Figure 29.5 *Acute asthma. Unexpected clinical deterioration. Left-sided shadowing effaces the heart border. Pneumonia. The consolidation—pneumonia—is situated in a lingular segment of the left upper lobe.*

AN INTERESTING CONDITION—ABPA[4,7]

ABPA = allergic bronchopulmonary aspergillosis

Aetiology / pathology

A rare cause of asthma. Spores of the fungus *Aspergillus fumigatus* are inhaled. A hypersensitivity reaction is induced. The bronchi contain hyphae and the walls of the large bronchi become damaged resulting in proximal bronchiectasis; the upper lobes are especially affected.

Clinical features

Asthma unresponsive to conventional treatment. Blood eosinophilia. Immediate skin reaction to *Aspergillus*.

The CXR

Recognition of the classical CXR appearances resulting from ABPA may be the first signal that the patient does not have simple asthma. If the proximal bronchi become dilated and filled with mucus this causes a CXR appearance which is referred to as the *toothpaste shadow*, or a *finger-in-glove appearance* (Figs 29.6 and 29.7). Pulmonary densities, representing areas of acute eosinophilic infiltration of the alveoli[4] also occur. These shadows often come and go—they flit—sometimes spontaneously, sometimes in response to steroid treatment.

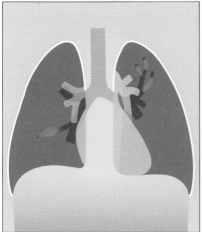

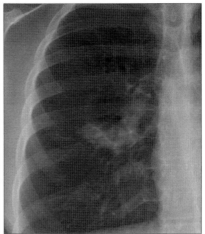

Figure 29.6 *ABPA. The dense plug of mucus and fungus within dilated proximal bronchi has given rise to the descriptions of "toothpaste" or "finger-in-glove" shadowing. The upper lobes are frequently affected.*

Figure 29.7 *Asthmatic patient with ABPA. The right mid zone shadow represents dilated proximal bronchi (i.e. bronchiectasis) containing a thick sticky mixture of mucus and Aspergillus fungus.*

REFERENCES

1. Findley LJ, Sahn SA. The value of chest roentgenograms in acute asthma in adults. Chest 1981; 80: 535–536.

2. Dawson KP, Capaldi N. The chest X-ray and childhood acute asthma. Aust Clin Rev 1993; 13: 153–156.

3. Tsai TW, Gallagher EJ, Lombardi G et al. Guidelines for the selective ordering of admission chest radiography in adult obstructive airway disease. Ann Emerg Med 1993; 22: 1854–1958.

4. Lynch DA. Imaging of asthma and allergic bronchopulmonary mycosis. Radiol Clin North Am 1998; 36: 129–142.

5. Mecoy RJ. When a wheeze is not asthma. Aust Fam Physician. 1993; 22: 941–945.

6. Scott PM, Glover GW. All that wheezes is not asthma. Br J Clin Pract 1995; 49: 43–44.

7. Patterson R, Greenberger PA, Radin RC et al. Allergic bronchopulmonary aspergillosis: staging as an aid to management. Ann Intern Med 1982; 96: 286–291.

30 HAEMOPTYSIS: WHAT TO LOOK FOR

Haemoptysis:	Coughing up blood or blood stained sputum.
Massive haemoptysis:	Definitions vary[1,2]. Typically—coughing up more than 200 ml blood in 24 hours (approximately one cup).
Mild haemoptysis:	Some blood in the sputum…often spotting or a few ml only.
Pseudohaemoptysis:	Spitting up blood that has not originated from the lower respiratory tract.

Some patients referred from primary care with suspected haemoptysis have had a pseudohaemoptysis. A patient will often have difficulty in distinguishing between blood resulting from epistaxis, gingivitis, gastrointestinal haemorrhage…and blood originating from the lower respiratory tract.

RELEVANT ARTERIAL ANATOMY[3–5]

An understanding of the dual blood supply to the lungs explains the differing origins of mild and massive haemoptysis (Table 30.1).

Table 30.1 Importance of the arterial supply to the lung.

Artery	Capillary contact	Clinical relevance
Pulmonary	■ Alveolar ❑ Main function: gas exchange ❑ Low pressure from the right ventricle	■ Haemoptysis occurs when the pathological process actually involves a pulmonary artery (e.g. pulmonary embolism). ■ Massive haemoptysis is rare.
Bronchial	■ An extensive plexus in intimate contact with the entire bronchial tree ❑ Main function: lung nutrition ❑ High pressure from the aorta	■ Haemoptysis can result from any disease which affects the bronchi or the bronchioles. ■ A massive haemoptysis usually arises from a disease process affecting the bronchial arteries (e.g. bronchiectasis).

The lung has two distinctive and separate blood supplies (Fig. 30.1):

■ Low pressure pulmonary arteries which end in a network of capillaries supplying the alveoli only.

■ High pressure bronchial arteries arising from the aorta. Their sites of origin can vary—usually from the proximal descending aorta. Typically, two bronchial arteries supply the left lung and a single bronchial artery supplies the right lung. These arteries feed the bronchial walls up to and including the terminal bronchioles. They also supply the connective tissue of the lung as well as the visceral pleural membrane.

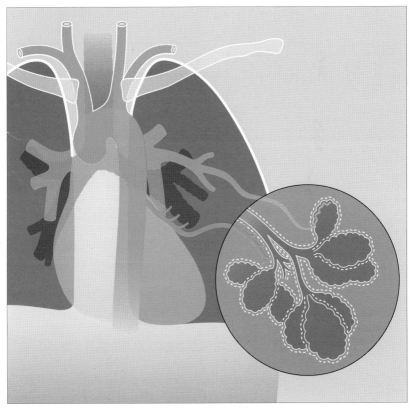

Figure 30.1 *The two separate blood supplies to the lungs. The bronchial arteries (high pressure) arise from the aorta. The pulmonary arteries (low pressure) arise from the right side of the heart.*

CAUSES OF HAEMOPTYSIS[1-3,5-11]

The patient who coughs up blood has one overwhelming fear—that he has cancer. Knowledge of the numerous causes of haemoptysis—and the frequency of their occurrence—is essential (Table 30.2).

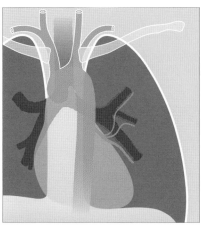

Figure 30.2 *Haemoptysis due to acute bronchitis. The bronchial arteries arise from the aorta and nourish the walls of the inflamed bronchi. Inflammation around and involving the bronchial arterial capillaries can cause a mild haemoptysis.*

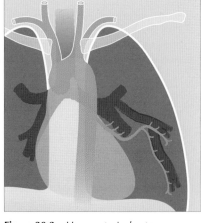

Figure 30.3 *Haemoptysis due to bronchiectasis. The chronic inflammation can cause localised proliferation of the bronchial arteries; these vessels may become friable and cause a mild haemoptysis. Sometimes the bronchial arteries are actually eroded by the inflammatory process and a massive haemoptysis results.*

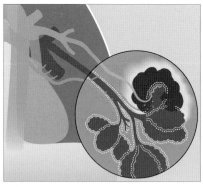

Figure 30.4 *Haemoptysis due to pulmonary tuberculosis. The high pressure bronchial arteries can be eroded by the tuberculous inflammation. In this example a cavity has involved a bronchial artery, and a potentially massive haemoptysis could result. Erosion of low pressure pulmonary arteries or capillaries may also occur in chronic tuberculosis.*

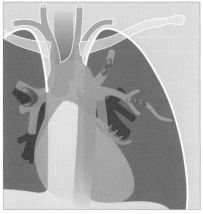

Figure 30.5 *Haemoptysis due to pulmonary thromboembolic disease. Emboli have lodged in the low pressure pulmonary arterial circulation. An embolus may cause a mild or moderate haemoptysis.*

Table 30.2   Causes of haemoptysis[1-3,5-11].

Cause	Notes
1. Infection	
❏ Acute bronchitis	Common in Europe and North America
❏ Pneumonia	Also common
❏ Lung abscess	Less common
❏ Tuberculosis	Less common
❏ ·Bronchiectasis	Less common
2. Neoplastic	
❏ Bronchial carcinoma	Haemoptysis is the presenting symptom in approximately 50% of primary carcinomas
❏ Other lung tumours	Metastatic carcinoma. Particularly: breast, kidney, colon, oesophagus, choriocarcinoma
3. Pulmonary embolism	
4. Cardiac	
❏ Mitral valve disease	The haemoptysis is usually mild and the expectorate is often described as pink and frothy
❏ Congestive heart failure	
5. Vascular	
❏ Vasculitis	
– Wegener's granulomatosis	
– Systemic lupus erythematosis	
❏ Idiopathic pulmonary haemosiderosis	Rare. Presents in childhood
❏ Arterio-venous malformation	
6. Trauma to the thorax	Lung contusion or penetrating injury
7. Drugs	
❏ Aspirin/warfarin/cocaine/ penicillamine	
8. Glomerular inflammation	Goodpasture's syndrome
9. Catamenial haemoptysis (menstrual-related)	Monthly. A very rare cause in young women
10. **UNEXPLAINED**	*Figures vary. As many as 20% of all patients presenting with haemoptysis[6]*

CLINICAL INVESTIGATION / MANAGEMENT

(1) MASSIVE HAEMOPTYSIS: RARE BUT AN EMERGENCY

Massive haemoptysis is arbitrarily defined as coughing up more than a cup of blood (200 ml) in 24 hours. This is a medical emergency and necessitates immediate hospital admission and in-patient investigation and treatment.

- The causes of massive haemoptysis are shown in Table 30.3. High pressure (i.e. aortic pressure) vessels are eroded. Severe haemorrhage results.

- Usually, the pathology involves the bronchial artery circulation. Asphyxiation by blood is a serious risk.

- Blood transfusion and embolisation of the affected artery may be necessary.

Table 30.3 Causes of massive haemoptysis[1].

Common	Uncommon
■ Bronchiectasis	■ Invasive aspergillosis
■ Cystic fibrosis	■ Mitral stenosis
■ Tuberculosis	■ Pulmonary arteriovenous malformation
■ Lung abscess	■ Arterial fistula with an airway
■ Aspergilloma	■ Bleeding diathesis
■ Pulmonary contusion/trauma	■ Inhaled foreign body

(2) MILD HAEMOPTYSIS: MUCH MORE COMMON

Mild haemoptysis is defined as some blood in the sputum...generally a little spotting or a few millilitres only.

■ Mild haemoptysis is relatively common.

■ The most frequent causes are acute bronchitis, pneumonia, bronchial carcinoma, bronchiectasis, and pulmonary embolism.

■ The prevalence of these diseases varies from country to country.

■ The patient can be investigated as an outpatient.

■ The CXR (frontal and lateral projections obtained as a pair) can have an important impact on the further management of the individual patient.

The vast majority of patients presenting with a mild haemoptysis and who have normal frontal—and lateral—CXRs have benign disease. A management algorithm can be constructed based on the CXR findings (Table 30.4).

Table 30.4 Investigation/management of mild haemoptysis.

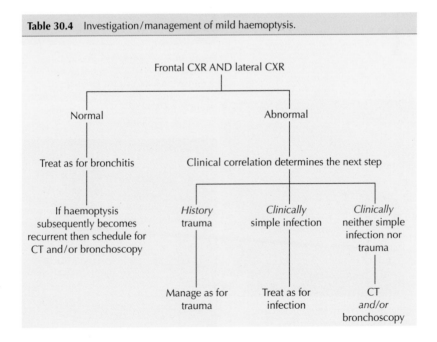

THE CXR: ABNORMAL AND NORMAL

CXR ABNORMAL (1) *PROBABLE* CAUSE SUGGESTED

Examples (Figs 30.6–30.9) include pneumonia, pulmonary oedema (heart failure), bronchial carcinoma, metastatic lung disease, bronchiectasis and traumatic pulmonary contusion.

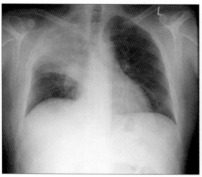

Figure 30.6 *Mild haemoptysis. Due to infection. Lobar pneumonia.*

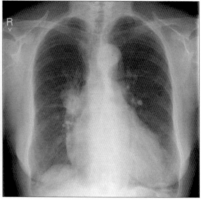

Figure 30.7 *Haemoptysis due to a bronchial carcinoma. A central tumour at the right hilum. In most instances of haemoptysis resulting from a lung carcinoma the bleeding is mild and caused by the tumour eroding small vessels.*

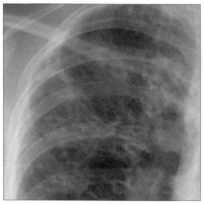

Figure 30.8 *Haemoptysis in a young patient with cystic fibrosis. The CXR shows extensive bronchiectasis: ring shadows (cystic dilatation of bronchi) and tramline shadows (bronchial wall thickening). The chronic inflammation erodes friable mucosal vessels and causes bleeding.*

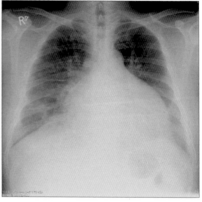

Figure 30.9 *Haemoptysis secondary to elevated pulmonary venous pressure. In this case due to mitral valve disease. The sputum was pink and frothy rather than red.*

CXR ABNORMAL (2) *POSSIBLE* CAUSE SUGGESTED

Examples (Figs 30.10–30.13):

■ Tuberculosis…from the distribution and features of the shadowing (p. 134).

■ Bronchiectasis (if minor/subtle CXR abnormality, p. 322)[9].

■ Solitary pulmonary nodule (SPN) suggests bronchial carcinoma, or metastasis, or a rarity such as Wegener's granulomatosis.

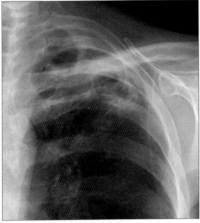

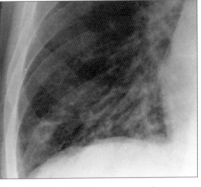

Figure 30.11 *Mild haemoptysis due to bronchiectasis. The crowding of vessels and the prominent tramlines (thickened bronchial walls) at the right base raised the suggestion of bronchiectasis. Bronchiectasis was subsequently confirmed on CT.*

Figure 30.10 *Haemoptysis due to post-primary tuberculosis at the left apex. The chronic inflammation has caused erosion of friable vessels. The bronchial arterial or the pulmonary arterial circulation may be affected.*

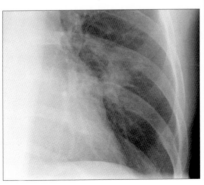

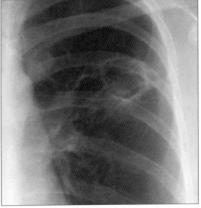

Figure 30.12 *Mild haemoptysis due to a SPN in the left lower zone. This SPN was a primary bronchial carcinoma.*

Figure 30.13 *Mild haemoptysis due to Wegener's granulomatosis. Necrotising lesions can erode blood vessels and cause bleeding. This left mid/upper zone lesion is cavitating.*

CXR NORMAL—IMPLICATIONS AND USEFULNESS

■ In most patients presenting with a mild haemoptysis and no other symptoms a normal CXR is good news. Remember that a lateral CXR should always be part of the haemoptysis CXR investigation protocol.

■ Many patients with a normal CXR will have either acute bronchitis or a pseudohaemoptysis.

■ If the haemoptysis recurs then CT and/or bronchoscopy will be indicated (see Table 30.4).

■ Any symptom or sign that could be attributable to a pulmonary embolus (PE) means that this must be the default diagnosis—even if the frontal and lateral CXRs appear normal (see Chapter 23).

FACTS AND FIGURES

■ A massive haemoptysis—200 ml or more in 24 hours—is most commonly due to an inflammatory condition eroding bronchial artery vessels.

■ Mortality from a massive haemoptysis can be as high as 50%[5]. Death results from asphyxiation because the airways are flooded with blood.

■ In the majority of cases of mild haemoptysis the underlying cause is benign and self-limiting[10].

■ Despite thorough investigation the cause of haemoptysis remains unexplained in a significant number of patients. Figures vary between different series, but may be as many as 20–30% of cases[6,11,12].

■ *Persistent* haemoptysis and a normal CXR. Approximately 5% of these patients will have a bronchial carcinoma[13].

■ The majority of patients with a PE have some abnormality on the CXR. Often minor—but an abnormality is present. Totally and unreservedly normal PA and lateral CXRs makes a PE unlikely[14] (see p. 293).

REFERENCES

1. Johnson JL. Manifestations of hemoptysis. How to manage minor, moderate and massive bleeding. Postgrad Med 2002; 112: 101–113.

2. Thompson AB, Teschler H, Rennard SI. Pathogenesis, evaluation, and therapy for massive haemoptysis. Clin Chest Med. 1992; 13: 69–82.

3. Fraser RG, Muller NL, Colman NC, Pare PD. Fraser and Pare's Diagnosis of Diseases of the Chest. 4th ed. Philadelphia, PA: WB Saunders, 1999.

4. Ryan S, McNicholas M, Eustace S. Anatomy for Diagnostic Imaging. 2nd ed. Philadelphia, PA: WB Saunders, 2004.

5. Marshall TJ, Flower CD, Jackson JE. The role of radiology in the investigation and management of patients with haemoptysis. Clin Radiol 1996; 51: 391–400.

6. Santiago S, Tobias J, Williams AJ. A reappraisal of the causes of hemoptysis. Arch Intern Med 1991; 151: 2449–2451.

7. Goldman JM. Hemoptysis: Emergency assessment and management. Emerg Med Clin North Am 1989; 7: 325–338.

8. Reisz G, Stevens D, Boutwell C et al. The causes of hemoptysis revisited: a review of the etiologies of hemoptysis between 1986 and 1995. Mo Med 1997; 94: 633–635.

9. Gudbjerg CE. Roentgenologic diagnosis of bronchiectasis. An analysis of 112 cases. Acta Radiol 1955; 43: 210–226.

10. Corder R. Hemoptysis. Emerg Med Clin North Am 2003; 21: 421–435.

11. Bidwell JL, Plachner RW. Hemoptysis: diagnosis and management. Am Fam Physician 2005; 72: 1253–1260.

12. Andersen PE. Imaging and interventional radiological treatment of hemoptysis. Acta Radiol 2006; 47: 780–792.

13. Lederle FA, Nichol KL, Perenti CM. Bronchoscopy to evaluate hemoptysis in older men with nonsuspicious chest roentgenograms. Chest 1989; 95: 1043–1047.

14. Worsley DF, Alavi A, Aronchick JM et al. Chest radiographic findings in patients with acute pulmonary embolism: observations from the PIOPED study. Radiology 1993; 189: 133–136.

31 SYSTEMIC HYPERTENSION: WHAT TO LOOK FOR

Causes of arterial hypertension:

1. Essential (95%)

2. Secondary (5%)

    ❑ renal: chronic renal failure, renal artery stenosis, acute glomerulonephritis, polycystic disease

    ❑ coarctation of the aorta[1-3]

    ❑ other: corticosteroids/oral contraception, Cushing's disease, Conn's syndrome—primary aldosteronism, phaeochromocytoma, acromegaly, toxaemia of pregnancy

Normal blood pressure and hypertension: Clinic measurements are often higher than those recorded at home or as 24-hour ambulatory values. There are no universally agreed absolute measurements…but general clinic values:

▪ Ideal normal: 120/80.

▪ Age 40+: < 140/90.

▪ High: > 140/90.

Coarctation of the aorta: A congenital narrowing of the aortic arch.

▪ *Infantile type:* a diffuse aortic narrowing between the left subclavian artery and the ductus arteriosus.

▪ *Adult type:* the narrowing is adjacent or slightly distal to the ductus. The obstruction develops gradually and presentation is commonly due to complications occurring between the ages of 15 and 30 years[1].

ESSENTIAL HYPERTENSION—WHAT WILL THE CXR SHOW?

In the vast majority of patients with essential or secondary hypertension the CXR features are unrelated to the underlying cause. The role of the CXR is very basic and simple: to show whether obvious cardiac changes resulting from the raised blood pressure are present. These are:

▪ cardiac enlargement

▪ features of elevated pulmonary venous pressure (p. 158)

COARCTATION OF THE AORTA

This is the one cause of systemic arterial hypertension in which evaluation of the CXR must include more than an assessment of cardiac complications. There are two circumstances:

- In a particular patient the physician may, on clinical examination, consider that coarctation is possible.

- The diagnosis may be completely unsuspected. The CXR findings may be the first intimation of coarctation. Most of the coarctations that present after the first year of life are usually post-ductal and these patients are often symptom free. Frequently aortic coarctation is discovered incidentally, not simply because of hypertension or a murmur but serendipitously because of an abnormal CXR.

EVALUATING THE CXR[3–5]

The narrowing of the aorta is shown in Fig. 31.1.

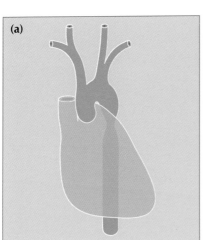
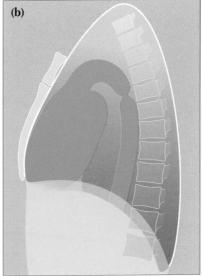

Figure 31.1   *Coarctation. To show the site of the aortic narrowing at, or close to, the isthmus of the aorta. (a) Frontal CXR. (b) Lateral CXR. The aortic isthmus is the anatomical site of the junction of the arch and descending aorta.*

Look for—rib notching[3,5]

- Resulting from the development of a collateral circulation involving the posterior intercostal arteries. The dilated arteries cause pressure erosion of the posterior and inferior aspects of the ribs. Only ribs 3–9 are affected.

- Usually bilateral; occasionally unilateral. The notching is often asymmetrical (Fig. 31.2). Notching is rarely evident below the age of five years.

- The roof of each notch shows some reactive sclerosis[5] (i.e. density), because the dilated posterior intercostal arteries exert a longstanding pressure effect on the ribs.

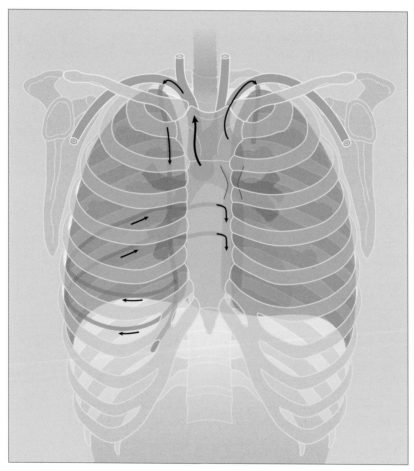

Figure 31.2 *Coarctation. The rib notching results from the anastomosis between the internal mammary arteries and the descending aorta—via the posterior intercostal arteries. The dilated posterior intercostal arteries cause the rib notching.*

Look for—an abnormal mediastinal shadow[3]

An abnormal aortic knuckle is usual in adults. It is often evident even in young children. There are a variety of configurations (Figs 31.3–31.6)[3].

1. Double knuckle:

   The "figure 3" configuration. The superior bulge is caused by an enlarged left subclavian artery and/or the aortic arch. The inferior bulge is due to post-stenotic dilatation of the aorta (Fig. 31.3).

2. High knuckle:

   Caused by an enlarged left subclavian artery and/or aortic arch...but there is no appreciable post-stenotic dilatation (Fig. 31.4).

3. Low knuckle:

   The post-stenotic dilatation is the dominant shadow (Fig. 31.5).

4. Flat knuckle:

   Due to an inconspicuous left subclavian artery, a small aortic arch, and no post-stenotic dilatation (Fig. 31.6).

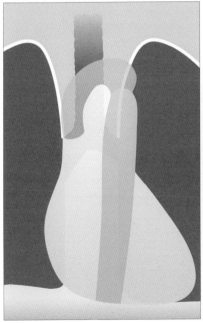 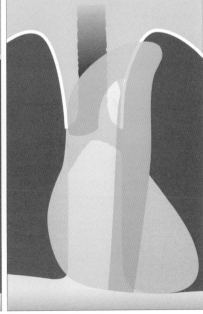

Figure 31.3 *Mediastinal shadow. Double knuckle or "figure 3" appearance.*

Figure 31.4 *Mediastinal shadow. High knuckle configuration.*

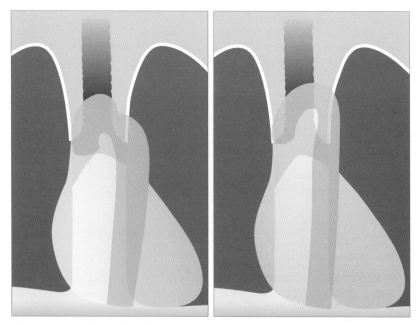

Figure 31.5 *Mediastinal shadow. Low knuckle configuration.*

Figure 31.6 *Mediastinal shadow. Flat knuckle configuration.*

Look for—cardiac enlargement

In children with coarctation an enlarged heart is common and is due to left ventricular hypertrophy[3]. Adults with coarctation usually have a normal cardiothoracic ratio unless there is accompanying aortic valve disease or heart failure.

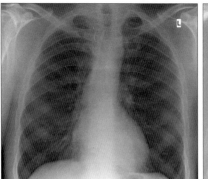
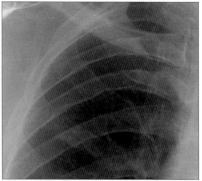

Figure 31.7 *Adult. Coarctation. The main finding is the posterior and inferior rib notching. The mediastinum demonstrates a (somewhat) high knuckle appearance.*

AN INTERESTING CONDITION — PSEUDOCOARCTATION (AKA KINKED AORTA)[6–8]

Aetiology / pathology

Closely related to coarctation but there is no pressure gradient across nor obstruction to the aortic lumen. An elongated and high aorta is kinked at the isthmus. There is no collateral circulation and so there is no rib notching.

Clinical features

No abnormal findings attributable to the kink. Often detected solely as an incidental left sided "mediastinal mass" on a CXR.

The CXR

A left-sided "mass" is projected above the aortic arch. A lateral CXR is very useful and will usually suggest that the mass is simply due to the high aortic arch. A CT examination with sagittal reconstruction will exclude a mass lesion or an aortic aneurysm and will confirm the diagnosis of pseudocoarctation.

REFERENCES

1. Swanton RH. Pocket Consultant: Cardiology. 5th ed. Oxford: Blackwell, 2003.

2. Rosenthal E. Coarctation of the aorta from fetus to adult: curable condition or life long disease process? Heart 2005; 91: 1495–1502.

3. Jefferson K, Rees S. Clinical Cardiac Radiology. London: Butterworth, 1980.

4. Cole TJ, Henry DA, Jolles H et al. Normal and abnormal vascular structures that simulate neoplasms on chest radiographs: clues to the diagnosis. Radiographics 1995; 15: 867–891.

5. Guttentag AR, Salwen JK. Keep your eyes on the ribs: the spectrum of normal variants and diseases that involve the ribs. Radiographics 1999; 19: 1125–1142.

6. Hoeffel JC, Henry M, Mentre B et al. Pseudocoarctation or congenital kinking of the aorta: radiologic considerations. Am Heart J 1975; 89: 428–436.

7. Cheng TO. Pseudocoarctation of the aorta. An important consideration in the differential diagnosis of superior mediastinal mass. Am J Med 1970; 49: 551–555.

8. Taneja K, Kawlra S, Sharma S et al. Pseudocoarctation of the aorta: complementary findings on plain film radiography, CT, DSA, and MRA. Cardiovasc Intervent Radiol 1998; 21: 439–441.

32 BLUNT TRAUMA: WHAT TO LOOK FOR

> Following an injury to the thorax, a CXR is usually the baseline radiographic examination.
>
> A normal CXR will often provide considerable clinical reassurance.
>
> Deciding that the CXR is normal depends on an informed and accurate assessment of the image.
>
> MVA: motor vehicle accident (USA)   RTA: road traffic accident (UK)

EIGHT QUESTIONS

A blunt injury. There are eight frequently asked questions:

- Fractures?
- Pneumothorax?
- Pneumomediastinum?
- Aortic rupture?
- Tracheo-bronchial injury?
- Lung contusion?
- Cardiac trauma?
- Ruptured diaphragm?

QUESTION 1—ARE THERE ANY FRACTURES?

MINOR THORACIC TRAUMA

There is no indication for a routine CXR in the majority of these patients. Demonstration of a simple rib fracture on a radiograph will not affect treatment. The only indication for a CXR is to exclude a pneumothorax in a patient in whom the pain or other symptoms raise this possibility. Oblique views of the ribs are not indicated.

MAJOR THORACIC TRAUMA[1-6]

Particular sites need special attention (Figs 32.1–32.3).

Double check ribs 1–3, the clavicles, and the scapulae[7,8]

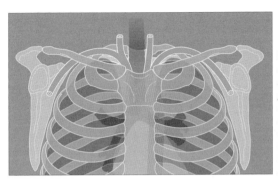

Figure 32.1 *There is a close relationship between the subclavian artery and the posterior aspect of the first rib and the clavicle. The first rib is very strong. If an injury causes a fracture of this rib then it should be assumed that a very powerful blow has been sustained.*

■ A fracture involving ribs 1–3 usually results from a very severe force. Important soft tissue and vascular injuries are potential complications. These include:

❑ Arterial or venous rupture; arising from the close relationship of the first rib to the subclavian vessels.

❑ Rupture of a bronchus.

❑ Brachial plexus injury.

■ A fracture of the clavicle or scapula may injure the subclavian artery.

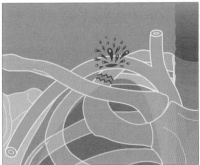

Figure 32.2 *Fracture of the first rib and a laceration of the adjacent subclavian artery.*

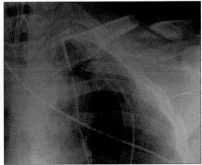

Figure 32.3 *RTA. Fractures of the left clavicle, third rib, and scapula. Clearly, a very violent force had occurred. The priority: clinical assessment to rule out a vascular injury.*

Double check ribs 11–12

A fracture of either of these floating ribs may cause a laceration to the liver, spleen, or kidney (Fig. 32.4). Look very carefully because this area of the radiograph is often underexposed.

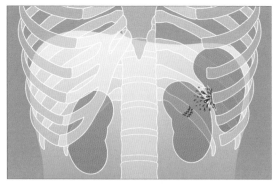

Figure 32.4 *The spleen, kidney and liver are at risk when a fracture of ribs 11 or 12 occurs.*

Look for a flail segment

■ A flail segment is clinically important because it may cause paradoxical movement of the adjacent lung, which can adversely affect gas exchange. This effect varies between patients. Mechanical ventilation may be required.

■ A flail segment is defined as two fractures in each of two or more adjacent ribs. It may also:

   ❑ Result from a fracture involving the sternum and/or a fracture extending across the midline to involve the opposite ribs.

   ❑ Involve the costal cartilages on each side of the midline. When this occurs the abnormal segment will not be recognised on a CXR because cartilaginous fractures are not visible on a radiograph (Fig. 32.6).

■ A flail segment is always associated with underlying pulmonary contusion.

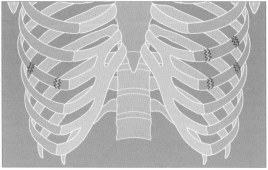

Figure 32.5 *The rib fractures on the right side do not indicate a flail segment. On the left side there are two fractures in each of two adjacent ribs: a flail segment is present.*

Assess the sternum carefully

Clinical suspicion of a possible fracture of the sternum must be relayed to the radiographer (technologist) because diagnosis normally requires an additional lateral (cross-table) radiograph.

Sternoclavicular dislocations rarely cause an important soft tissue injury, but a sternal fracture always raises the possibility of an injury to the myocardium.

CAUTION—INVISIBLE FRACTURES[9]

1. Through cartilage. A fracture through a rib cartilage or a costochondral junction (Fig. 32.6) will not be detectable on a CXR. Cartilage is not visible on a radiograph.

2. Undisplaced. Many rib fractures—through bone—are initially undisplaced and are often invisible. A fracture may only become evident on a subsequent CXR.

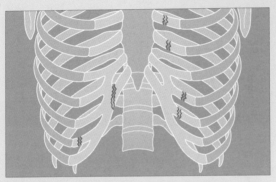

Figure 32.6 *Several fractures through costal cartilage. These will not be detectable on a CXR. Note that a radiographically invisible flail segment is also present because fractures are present on each side of the midline in two adjacent costal cartilages (i.e. in the ribs).*

QUESTION 2 — IS THERE A PNEUMOTHORAX?

Following violent trauma the CXR is obtained with the patient lying on a trolley or examination couch. A large pneumothorax will be obvious. Smaller pneumothoraces are more difficult to detect on a supine CXR. Recognising a small pneumothorax is important — particularly if the patient is to be treated with positive pressure ventilation.

The features indicating a pneumothorax on a supine CXR are described in Chapter 7, pp. 97–100.

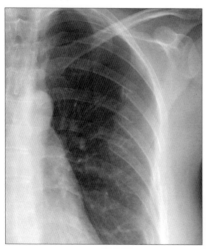

Figure 32.7 *Left-sided flail segment shown by two fractures in each of ribs 5, 6 and 7.*

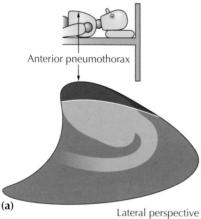

Anterior pneumothorax

(a) Lateral perspective

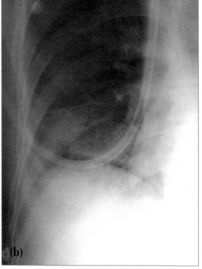

(b)

Figure 32.8 *Pneumothorax. When the injured patient is lying supine, air in the pleural space collects at the highest point — i.e. anteriorly (a). On the frontal CXR the visceral pleural line may not be evident. The diagnosis will need to be made by scrutinising the areas around the dome of the diaphragm and adjacent to the lateral border of the heart (b). The black line outlining the diaphragm indicates a pneumothorax: see p. 97 for a detailed description.*

QUESTION 3 — IS THERE A PNEUMOMEDIASTINUM?

- Pneumomediastinum following trauma may result from a:
  - ❑ tear of lung tissue
  - ❑ pneumothorax
  - ❑ rupture of the trachea or bronchus
  - ❑ rupture of the oesophagus
  - ❑ rupture of an intra-abdominal viscus

- The CXR appearances of a pneumomediastinum are described in Chapter 8, pp. 123–127. If serial CXRs show a persistent severe pneumomediastinum (+/− pneumothorax) then consider whether there is an unrecognised tracheobronchial rupture (p. 366) or an unrecognised oesophageal rupture.

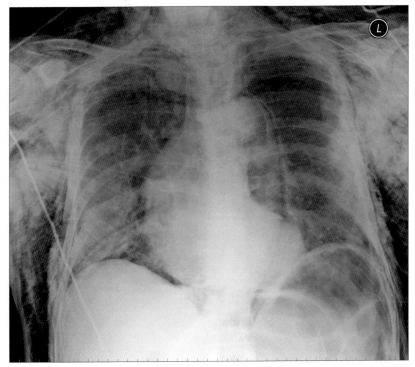

Figure 32.9 *Male. Age 56. Intoxicated and fell over. Supine CXR. Multiple rib fractures. Air outlines the descending aorta; it has also dissected outside the pleura and appears as a black line along the surface of the right dome of the diaphragm. This is an extensive pneumomediastinum. Several mechanisms could explain the presence of this mediastinal air — e.g. a traumatic pneumothorax or a tear through the trachea, bronchus or oesophagus. In this patient the air had arisen from a tear of the lung parenchyma with subsequent dissection through the interstitial tissues, thence to the hilum, and out into the mediastinum.*

QUESTION 4 — IS THERE AN AORTIC RUPTURE?

RUPTURE — STATISTICS

- 80–90% die immediately.

- 50% of early survivors die within 24 hours if untreated.

- 2–5% of untreated survivors will live. An aneurysm will eventually develop at the site of injury. It may rupture at any time during the following years.

CXR APPEARANCE

- In most cases of aortic rupture the mediastinum or aortic contour will appear widened. The following CXR features are very suggestive of an aortic injury[2,3,10,11]:

  - widened mediastinum

  - lobulated aortic outline

  - trachea displaced to the right

- A haemothorax should always raise the possibility of a large vessel injury (e.g. the aorta).

Major arterial injury

- If possible obtain an erect sitting-up CXR.

- A completely normal mediastinal contour on the sitting-up CXR will exclude the diagnosis of a major arterial injury[2].

- The following signs are of modest value in hinting at a definite arterial injury. Their importance lies in alerting the physician that a major abnormality might, just possibly, have occurred…but their positive predictive value is low[2].

  - An apical pleural cap. Haemorrhage dissecting external to the pleura and extending over the apex of a lung.

  - Mediastinal width greater than 8 cm at the level of the aortic arch on an AP radiograph.

  - Fractures of the first or second ribs.

Mediastinal widening

Mediastinal widening is not necessarily bad news. In approximately 80% of trauma patients with true mediastinal widening — this is not due to aortic rupture. The widening is due to bleeding from small arteries and small veins.

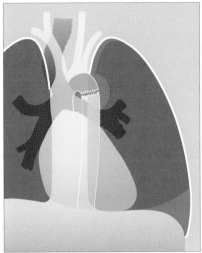

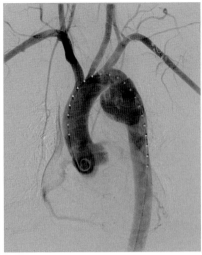

Figure 32.10 *Deceleration injury. Aortic rupture at the isthmus. The haematoma has widened the mediastinum, extended over the apex of the left lung, and it has also displaced the trachea to the right. Some blood has leaked into the left pleural space.*

Figure 32.11 *Male. Age 38. RTA. Aortogram following intravenous injection of contrast medium. Rupture of the aorta at its isthmus. Aortic isthmus: the junction of the aortic arch and the descending aorta.*

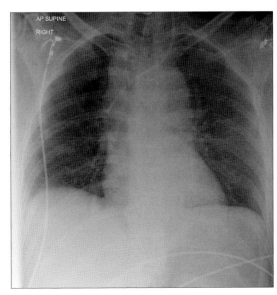

Figure 32.12 *Female Age 54. RTA. Widened mediastinum; trachea displaced to the right (i.e. by a large haematoma). Further investigation revealed a rupture of the aorta at the isthmus. The isthmus is a relatively fixed site and is thus vulnerable to a violent deceleration force.*

QUESTION 5 — IS THERE A TRACHEO-BRONCHIAL RUPTURE?

These injuries result from very violent trauma—usually a deceleration force applied to the anterior chest wall. An injury to the great vessels or an intracranial injury are recognised associations of tracheal or bronchial rupture.

■ CXR features[4,12] suggesting a tear of a main airway (transection or rupture):

❑ Pneumomediastinum.

❑ Lobar collapse. Either because the torn bronchus results in deflation, or because blood occludes the bronchial lumen. Whatever the cause, a lobar collapse may not occur for a few days.

❑ A pneumothorax that does not resolve following intercostal tube drainage[12].

❑ Pitfall: the significance of any one of these three important CXR features may not be appreciated…because their appearance can be delayed.

■ Consequences of a tear/rupture:

❑ High mortality.

❑ Broncho-pleural fistula.

❑ Eventual bronchostenosis (scarring with narrowing).

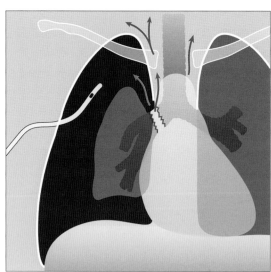

Figure 32.13 *Violent trauma. Rupture of a main bronchus. This can cause a pneumomediastinum (arrows), and/or a pneumothorax that fails to absorb following insertion of an intercostal drain, and/or persistent lung or lobar collapse (i.e. persistent lung deflation).*

QUESTION 6—IS THERE LUNG CONTUSION?

Contusion is very common following a violent injury. It appears as an area of consolidation, similar in appearance to lobar pneumonia.

■ The consolidation[2,3,5,13] may:

   ❏ Be present on the initial CXR. Usually, it will be evident within six hours of the injury.

   ❏ Cavitate.

   ❏ Take four to six weeks to clear. Clearing can be particularly slow if contusion has been accompanied by a laceration through the lung parenchyma.

■ NB: the differential diagnosis for an area of consolidation on the CXR:

   ❏ Lung contusion.

   ❏ Aspiration pneumonia.

   ❏ Adult respiratory distress syndrome.

   ❏ Fat embolism.

   ❏ A combination of any of the above.

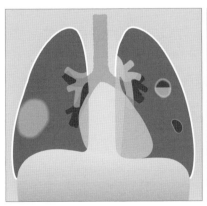

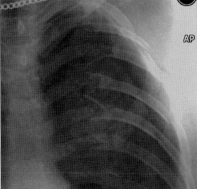

Figure 32.14   *Blunt trauma. Lung contusion. Various appearances may result: an area of consolidation (right lung); or cavitation; or a cystic area, i.e. a pneumatocoele (left lung).*

Figure 32.15   *Male. Age 23. RTA. Left-sided rib fractures (note that a flail segment is present). Pneumothorax. The consolidation in the left upper lobe is an area of lung contusion.*

QUESTION 7 — IS THERE AN INJURY TO THE HEART?

The sternum and thoracic spine protect the heart and pericardium from non-penetrating injuries. The demonstration of anterior rib fractures or a sternal fracture should always raise the possibility — not the probability — of a myocardial injury. The CXR is usually unhelpful in excluding the possibility of pericardial or myocardial damage. Echocardiography provides a much more sensitive evaluation.

QUESTION 8 — IS THE DIAPHRAGM NORMAL?[14–17]

Rupture of a dome of the diaphragm occurs in approximately 5% of cases of severe thoracic trauma[14,16]. A rupture is more common with blunt trauma than with a penetrating injury. The mechanism of injury is usually a sudden rise of intra-abdominal pressure from violent compression to the abdomen or lower thorax[1].

■ A rupture may affect either dome. The left dome is more commonly involved[14] — in the ratio of 4:1. A few cases are bilateral.

■ In 50% or more of cases herniation of abdominal viscera through the rupture is delayed[14]. Delay may be two or more years after the injury and results from a small tear subsequently increasing in size.

■ The following CXR features suggest a tear of the diaphragm[2,3,14–17]:

  ❏ Gas-containing viscus in the thorax (Figs 32.17 and 32.18).

  ❏ Abnormal contour of a dome (Fig. 32.18).

  ❏ A significant change to the shape of a dome compared with a previous normal CXR.

  ❏ Left dome: tip of a nasogastric tube situated unusually high.

  ❏ Right dome: small haemothorax with an unexpectedly high dome.

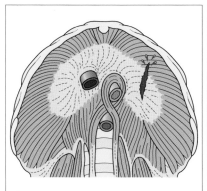

Figure 32.16 *The diaphragm viewed from below. Sagittal rupture through the central tendon and muscular part of the left dome from an antero-posterior compressive force. The tendon has a relatively poor blood supply and when ruptured it heals slowly and less effectively than the surrounding muscle.*

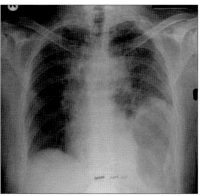

Figure 32.17 *Male. Age 35. RTA. Widened mediastinum (due to a haematoma from ruptured veins). Multiple rib fractures. Seemingly high left dome of the diaphragm with the stomach gas bubble also unusually high. Diaphragmatic rupture with herniation of part of the stomach into the thorax.*

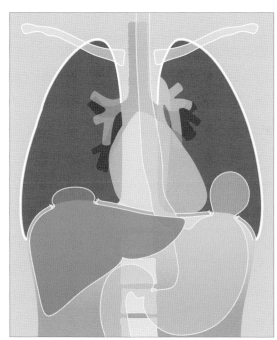

Figure 32.18 *Rupture of both the right and left domes of the diaphragm. The diaphragm is injured in approximately 5% of severe thoracic injuries[14,16] and 22% of all thoraco-abdominal injuries[3]. Some 33% of these injuries are diagnosed three years after the trauma… sometimes because the abnormal CXR features were previously overlooked[3]. The most common site of injury is at the apex of the left dome.*

FACTS AND FIGURES

- Following major trauma—20% of all deaths are due to a thoracic injury.

- Aortic rupture accounts for 16% of all RTA deaths[4].

- Pneumothorax occurs:

  - In approximately 40% of patients following major blunt chest trauma[4].

  - In 20% of patients following a penetrating injury to the thorax[4].

- Pulmonary contusion (lung bruising):

  - This is the most common cause of a pneumothorax resulting from blunt trauma[6].

  - The pulmonary haematoma around a tear of the lung may take weeks—sometimes months—to clear.

  - If the tear communicates with a bronchus then a lung cyst (pneumatocoele) may form.

- Post-traumatic pleural effusion[6] is usually due to bleeding from injury to one or more of:

  - Lung.

  - Chest wall.

  - Major mediastinal vessels.

- Intubated patients. On a supine CXR the endotracheal tube[18] should:

  - Not lie below the level of the aortic arch.

  - Lie a minimum of 3.5 cm (preferably 5–7 cm) above the carina.

REFERENCES

1. Schnyder P, Wintermark M. Radiology of Blunt Trauma of the Chest. Berlin: Springer-Verlag, 2000.

2. Mirvis SE, Templeton PA. Imaging in acute thoracic trauma. Semin Roentgenol 1992; 27: 184–210.

3. Besson A, Saegesser F. A colour atlas of chest trauma and associated injuries. London: Wolfe Medical Publications, 1982.

4. Collins J, Stern EJ. Chest Radiology: The Essentials. Philadelphia, PA: Lippincott, Williams and Wilkins, 1999.

5. Groskin SA. Selected topics in chest trauma. Radiology 1992; 183: 605–617.

6. Goodman LR, Putman CE. The SICU chest radiograph after massive blunt trauma. Radiol Clin North Am 1981; 19: 111–123.

7. Woodring JH, Fried AM, Hatfield DR et al. Fractures of first and second ribs. Predictive value for arterial and bronchial injury. AJR 1982; 138: 211–215.

8. Gupta A, Jamshidi M, Rubin JR. Traumatic first rib fracture: is angiography necessary? A review of 730 cases. Cardiovasc Surg 1997; 5: 48–53.

9. Ontell FK, Moore EH, Shepard JA et al. The costal cartilages in health and disease. Radiographics 1997; 17: 571–577.

10. Cowley RA, Turney SZ, Hankins JR et al. Rupture of thoracic aorta caused by blunt trauma: a fifteen year experience. J Thorac and Cardiovasc Surg 1990; 100: 652–660.

11. Mirvis SE, Bidwell JK, Buddemeyer EU et al. Value of chest radiography in excluding traumatic aortic rupture. Radiology 1987; 163: 487–493.

12. Kelly JP, Webb WR, Moulder PV et al. Management of airway trauma. (1) Tracheobronchial injuries. Ann Thorac Surg 1985; 40: 551–555.

13. Greene R. Lung alterations in thoracic trauma. J Thorac Imaging 1987; 2: 1–11.

14. Eren S, Kantarci M, Okur A. Imaging of diaphragmatic rupture after trauma. Clin Radiol 2006; 61: 467–477.

15. Iochum S, Ludig T, Walter F et al. Imaging of diaphragmatic injury: a diagnostic challenge? Radiographics 2002; 22: 103–116.

16. Nursal TZ, Ugurlu M, Kologlu M et al. Traumatic diaphragmatic hernias; a report of 26 cases. Hernia 2001; 5: 25–29.

17. Gelman R, Mirvis SE, Gens D. Diaphragm rupture due to blunt trauma: sensitivity of chest radiographs. AJR 1991; 156: 51–57.

18. Chan O, Wilson A, Walsh M. ABC of emergency radiology: major trauma. BMJ 2005; 330: 1136–1138.

INDEX